Mother's Journey

Sally's Story

Janet S. Gould

2018

Pin Curl Factory
Hot Springs, Arkansas

Library of Congress Control Number: 2018943320

ISBN – 13: 978-1-7323055-0-2, paperback

Cover production: Trevor Gould
Logo: Copyright © Pin Curl Factory

Published by
Pin Curl Factory
Hot Springs, Arkansas

This book is dedicated to my Mother.
This is Sally's story.

Introduction

My mother's journey with dementia began in 1999, when she was 73 years old. She had started to forget how to do certain tasks, such as how to make coffee and how to pay her bills. During that winter she experienced a drastic downturn. In February of 2000 my brother found her in her home lying on the floor unconscious with a broken hip. Over time her doctor determined that she had suffered a massive stroke brought on by a brain infection caused by burning moldy wood in the stove that heated her house. The smoke had been toxic.

After leaving the hospital she went into a nursing home for rehabilitation. Her hip healed and the brain infection healed. However, she was left with big gaps in her memory. After leaving the nursing home she lived with me for awhile. Then she lived with my brother for awhile.

My brother found a spot for her in an assisted-living facility. She lived there happily for quite awhile until her memory took another downward turn. One night the staff found her wandering around outside in the cold dark, not knowing how to get back inside. They moved her into the memory care unit. The prices for that unit became exorbitant and my brother took her out.

She next moved in with my niece and her growing family. She did very well for quite awhile until there was another downward turn. Needing 24 hour care, my niece was no longer able to care for her. My brother found her a spot in another nursing home, now permanently in the memory care unit.

I began this journal about my mother because memories of our life together kept flooding in. She was constantly on my mind. I want to remember everything and forget nothing. I want to remember all of those memories, the good ones and the not so good ones. And I want to remember all of my visits with her, every detail. The only way to preserve these memories is to write them down. I don't know what my future holds.

The journal also contains the research I did along the way about dementia and other health conditions. I discovered that with all of the studies done on dementia the information is sometimes conflicting, sometimes confusing, and sometimes just plain wrong.

The journal shows the struggles that go on in the family that has a loved one with dementia. Not only the struggle that the person with dementia goes through, but also the struggle the entire family goes through. I've included an abbreviated family tree so that relationships are clear. I've not listed any last names due to privacy.

This is my Mother's Journey.

Family Tree

Mother's name was Shirley, but she was always called Sally.

Mother's Sister: Laurie
　　　Daughter: Linda

Husbands: Bob(1), Ken, Bob(2)
　　　Bob (1): Father of all of her children
　　　　　　Mother: Ruth
　　　　　　Brother: Boyd, wife Jane, daughter Pam
　　　Ken's children: Judy and Mike

Son: David, wife Dorothy
　　　Children: Jason and Rebecca
　　　　　　Rebecca, husband Jamie
　　　　　　Children: Alexsis, Clyde, Steven, Vincent

Daughter: Nancy, husband Dave
　　　Children: Amy, Patrick, Caroline

Daughter: Janet, husband Tom
　　　Children: Tommy and Scott
　　　　　　Tommy, wife Trisha
　　　　　　　　Children: Kelley and Zakary
　　　　　　Scott, wife Ruth
　　　　　　　　Children: Trevor, Ben, TJ
　　　Friends: Kathy, Kippy, Delomia
　　　Past pets: iguanas Rex Anne, Ruffles, Buddy
　　　Pet tortoise: Chelsey

Daughter: Emily, husband Mark
　　　Children: Josiah, Annie, Holly

August 14, 2009

David and I went to see Mother today. I flew in a couple of days ago, but yesterday I was pretty sick with a really bad headache and wasn't able to go anywhere. I wasn't sure what to expect during this visit because I knew Mother's memory had gone downhill since the last time I had seen her. I'm ashamed to admit that it has been over a year since my last visit. I have no good excuse except that Tom and I had been having a really bad year financially. We came close to losing our business. Construction had come to a grinding halt. That, plus not getting paid for work we had done. We lost a lot of money. The economy was bottoming out and we were going along for the ride. It was awful, and it was scary. Still, I should have found a way to see Mother.

We parked in the small parking lot in front of the building. There were a lot of people sitting around outside the entrance, residents and visitors. The door opened into a large foyer area. There were doors here also, but they were standing open. I imagine that in winter they close all of these doors to keep the heat in. Passing through the foyer we entered a lobby containing several upholstered chairs and a couple of small couches. Against the right wall is a counter with a coffeemaker and condiments. Past the sitting area is another counter and small office. There was a woman, in her 60s, with short curly gray hair sitting behind the counter. We had to sign in before progressing any further. The woman was very friendly as David and I both signed in, noting the date and time and who we were there to visit. After signing in, we walked a short distant down the hall to the elevators. I noticed there were several hallways going in different directions. We got on an elevator and rode it to the second floor. It's a long walk to Mother's memory care unit.

We emerged in an area that was full of residents sitting at long tables playing bingo. We made a turn and began walking down a long hallway, what they call the bridge. There were numerous windows with potted plants sitting on the sills. There were padded benches here and there. It looked very cheerful. There were pictures along the walls and a glass case with some kind of memorabilia inside. There was also a collection of pictures on the wall that children had painted. About halfway down was a blood pressure machine. David said he sometimes tests his blood pressure on his way in to see Mother and then again after the visit. We stopped and tested ourselves. David was first and he put his arm in the machine. His blood pressure was 126/70. I said,"Wow, that's good." My turn – mine was 117/70. I was surprised because I was a little nervous. We continued on and there was a large bird habitat next to the wall. It was made out of wood and had glass on three sides. Inside was a row of different types of nests on the back wall and quite a few little birds flying around and chirping. I was surprised at how many birds were in there. I always feel sorry for birds like this, all cooped up in such a small place (like Mother).

We continued on. As we got near the end of the bridge there was a large rehabilitation room on the right. It had big windows and inside I could see exercise equipment, etc. The room was empty and the lights turned off. Leaving the bridge we turned right into another hallway. We walked past the kitchen, and finally arrived at Mother's unit. There is a button on the wall to open the door – making sure no residents are on the other side trying to make an escape I guess.

We entered into an area that had tables and chairs for visiting. There was a piano next to one wall. Next to this area is the dining room and then another area for sitting and visiting, lined with upholstered chairs. There are no walls between the areas. Residents were scattered throughout the entire place. As we passed through the dining room we could see an elderly lady sitting in a wheelchair. She was saying, "Help me, Help me," over and over, like she was chanting. David told me later that she does this constantly; sometimes she gets a rhythm going like she's singing the words help me, help me, over and over. David finally spotted Mother heading for an outside door that was on the far side of the waiting area. I could see that she was slightly stooped over because of her osteoporosis.

When we caught up to her she was pushing on the door trying to get out. It was locked of course. I was shocked at her appearance. She had aged so much since my last visit. And her hair was cut shockingly short. Her beautiful white curls were gone. She looked so much like her mother at that age. In a joking way I said, "What are you doing?" That was obviously the wrong thing to say because she instantly became defensive and said, "Nothing." She had a small glass of milk in her hand. I noticed it wasn't a pure white like milk should be and wondered if it even was milk. She was also holding a kitchen towel. No telling where she picked that up. David tried taking the glass out of her hand so it wouldn't get spilled, but she held on to it with all her might. He finally won, jerking it out of her hand, and set it on a nearby table. Mother glared at us. I said, "Don't you recognize me?" She said, "No." I said, "I'm your daughter, Janet." Pointing at David I said, "You recognize him, don't you?" "No." She started to look outside and I said, "What are you looking at?" Pointing with her head she said, "That." I said, "That plant?" and she said, "Yes. It's pretty." I really didn't know what to do at this point but David is used to this. He said, "Would you like to sit down and talk with us?" She said, "No." "Would you like to go for a walk?" "No." "Would you like to go get ice cream?" "No." She had gotten angry and turned to David and said, "What are you doing?" He said, "We're here to visit you." She started to soften at that and said, "Really?" I had brought along a small beanie baby teddy bear. It was a soft, white bear and said 'With Love Mom' on it. I pulled it out of my purse and handed it to her saying, "I brought this for you." She took the bear from me, and David was able to get the towel out of her hand.

The expression on her face as she looked at the bear was so sweet. Mother used to have a huge teddy bear collection. She started it when she was a young girl and continued it all of her life. Her collection was wide, stretching from tiny bears to huge Danbury bears wearing tuxedos and what not. The collection is now scattered between us siblings. When Mother finally retired she started making teddy bears. Her favorite were little mini bears. She used all different types of fabric and colors. She even had an assembly line set up on her dining room table. One spot had a basket of bear arms, the next spot had a basket of legs, the next spot had bodies, and one spot had heads. She would move from chair to chair putting the little bears together, stitching on ears and embroidering the faces, granny glasses perched on the bridge of her nose. When the bears were finished she'd sell them in a craft shop in town – and share with her family, I have many that I absolutely treasure.

Mother finally agreed to sit with us. We moved away from the doors and entered the sitting area. There were two chairs with a table in between and David steered her in that direction, motioning to the chair on the left. She tried sitting on the table first but David took her arm and sat her in the chair. I pulled up another chair and placed it facing them. Mother was wearing a long-sleeved red plaid blouse over a dark T-shirt along with beige slacks. She had on black socks but no shoes. She was also wearing a red, plastic beaded necklace; the beads were different sizes and kind of a square shape. She looked so pale. She had always had a deep tan, living on the lake like she did. She loved spending time outside. She loved living in Crosslake, it was her dream finally achieved.

We talked about many things. David has always loved teasing her about her lack of memory, asking her what she had for breakfast, if she had any visitors, things like that. Mother has always responded with humor and just says, "I don't know. I can't remember," and then laughs. David and I talked about other things, just catching up with our lives, and sometimes Mother would make a response; it would usually only be about two words like, oh really, or, how awful. We'd stop and listen to what she was saying and then realize she was about two topics behind. But we always listened and encouraged her to say more, although she never would. She seemed very comfortable with us and our conversation flowing around her. We'd talk for awhile and then turn our focus back on Mother.

David asked her who had cut her hair and she said she didn't know. I asked if she knew her hair had been cut really short. She got a puzzled look on her face and reached her fingers up to feel the back of it. I knew she was disappointed. She has never had her hair that short. David said he didn't know who had arranged for it to be cut because that's something he always does. David takes care of every part of Mother's life. He makes the arrangement to get her hair done and to arrange the payment. He was at a loss about this haircut.

Mother recently had all of her bottom teeth pulled out. It was actually done right there in the nursing home. The dentist has a space there so that the residents don't have to travel into town. Mother went for the procedure during the afternoon and an anesthetic came in and put her under; that way she would just go to sleep afterwards for the night. But she didn't sleep all night. The nurse called David and said Mother had awakened during the night and got out of bed. She was walking down the hallway and fell, but it was just on her butt. The nurse asked why she was out of bed and Mother said she was hungry. A sandwich was prepared; she ate, and then went back to bed. I can't imagine eating a sandwich right after having all of my teeth pulled out. The pain would have been unbearable I would think.

Mother's teeth had rotted. Her own mother's teeth were the same way when she and Grandpa moved back to Minnesota from Florida so that Mother could take care of them. I was so shocked at the time, seeing Grandma's rotten teeth. But Mother took care of that right away. When Mother's teeth became rotted and her gums were bleeding a lot they needed to come out. Her top teeth were pulled out many years ago. I remember that being on a fixed income she couldn't afford to have all the work done so she had to "borrow" the money from husband Bob(2). He was a jerk. But they weren't living together any more by that time.

Bobs are a joke in our family with Mother. She married (and buried) two Bobs. When she moved into the assisted living place she took up with another Bob. That was so cute. She wrote me a lot of letters about him. I was able to meet him and he was very nice. He was in a wheelchair; he had lost one of his legs due to diabetes. The day I met him Mother sat on his lap and they shared a sandwich. But he had serious medical problems and after awhile he was transferred to the VA hospital. Mother was very upset and her letters showed that, she missed him so much. But he called her on the phone often. In the end they had to take off his other leg and he didn't survive. Mother was heart-broken. He was buried in a cemetery very close to the nursing home and I asked her if she visited him often and she said no, she never goes. I asked why not and she said that he was buried next to his wife. "He's with her now," she said, "that's where he belongs." When David was making the arrangements for Mother to move into this nursing home David, with his sense of humor, asked if they had any Bobs living there. Alas, there wasn't.

David asked Mother how her mouth was and she said fine. "It doesn't hurt where they pulled out your teeth?" he asked. She just looked puzzled, and David told her that her teeth had been pulled out. He said, "Run your tongue over your gums and you'll feel it." She did that and then she stuck her tongue out, like a little kid. We laughed and finally got a smile out of her. She used to smile all of the time. I was always amazed that she could smile so much. It reminded me of a woman who sometimes attends my aqua exercise class. The woman is in her 80s and has a very active life. She sings in a choir and participates in a small theatrical group. And when she's in the pool she is always smiling. I mentioned this to her one day, about her always having a smile on her face, and she said, "I'm happy to be alive." I wonder if Mother would say the same thing – I'm happy to be alive. They didn't make any dentures for

Mother, there was no reason to. After arriving here she stopped wearing the top ones. She just doesn't care. She looks so different without any teeth. Her voice hasn't changed though.

I said, "That's a nice necklace. Where did you get it?" She just had a blank look on her face. I said, "Touch it." She just sat there. I went over to her and took her hand and placed her fingertips on the necklace. But she just couldn't understand what I was talking about. I noticed that she was wearing red fingernail polish that was all chipped on the ends. Her long, tapered slender fingers were so white, and her skin looked so thin. The red polish made me think about how she had always worn bright red lipstick. She always looked good. I could never wear red lipstick. It always looked ghastly on me. When she had lived with me she would always run into her room when she heard Tom pull into the driveway and put on her lipstick. I always thought that was funny; that she wanted to look good for Tom when he got home from work. The last time I remember her wearing lipstick was for Rebecca's wedding. She was in assisted living then. Emily and I took her shopping for a pretty outfit to wear. It was funny all of us in the dressing room at the store getting Mother to try on clothes. Emily got her ready for the wedding and even put her own red lipstick on Mother.

As we talked a woman resident came over and sat on the table facing me. She was also wearing chipped red nail polish. She started gesturing to me with her hands to come over to her. I didn't of course. Then she sighed and dropped her hands onto her thighs. Then she gestured again. We had stopped all talking at this point and Mother just stared down at her hands. The woman reached over and started rubbing her hand up and down Mother's arm. Mother looked so angry but she wouldn't look up (she's had some fights in this place with the other residents). The woman gestured to me again, and I shook my head no. A nurse finally came and took the woman by the arm and led her away. David said she does things like that often. I had to feel sorry for her, obviously she needs to have visitors also.

I noticed that all of the nurses were wearing purple scrubs. Good idea, there in the memory care unit, for the residents to have that little sign of recognition, of being able to identify the nursing staff.

Mother was just sitting there looking at me. I asked, "Do you remember me now?" She said, "I remember having a daughter Janet." "That's me!" I thought well, at least that's something. I wonder if she thinks I'm too old to be her daughter, after all I'm getting up there in years myself; I'm 57. Last time I was here there was a large photograph on her nightstand of me and the boys. I was only in my 20s at that point. Is that how she thinks of her daughter Janet, not the older me?

A nurse came over and said they were getting ready to show a movie. David asked Mother if she wanted to go watch the movie and she said yes. We went down the hall to Mother's room so that we could sign David's calendar. He set the calendar up when she first moved in so that he could see who visited since Mother can never remember. When we got to the room Mother's roommate was in her bed, she was quietly saying 'help me' over and over. I wonder how many residents recite this mantra. I took the teddy bear from Mother and put it right under the covers in her bed. I said this way you'll have it tonight when you go to bed. We signed the calendar and I noticed that my photograph was gone. So was the photograph Emily had set up on her last visit of her and her family. But there was a snapshot of Mother with David and Emily. I wonder where my photograph went, maybe that woman who was gesturing to me had it, maybe she thinks I'm her daughter.

Things have a way of disappearing in this place. Residents wander in and out of rooms, if they get tired they lay down in the first bed they see (David actually found Mother napping in someone else's bed one day). If they see something they want they take it. Vases of flowers disappear; even the small live Christmas tree Emily sent last year didn't stick around long. I suppose it's like that in every nursing home, especially in the memory care unit. As we left Mother's room David said the little teddy bear probably wouldn't last long; I didn't write her name on it or anything. I said that's why I put it under the covers, and he said, doesn't matter. Then I felt guilty for taking it from her but figured she wouldn't remember it anyway.

When we got back to the visiting area the movie was getting ready to start. Mother was very excited and started to make a beeline for it. We had to grab onto her so that we could say good-bye. I said, "I love you," and she repeated it back. The nurse saw her coming and set a chair in place for her but Mother didn't see that. She saw an empty chair at a table and went to it and tried to pull it out but the nurse intercepted her and sat her in the first chair. She had already forgotten about us. David said she loves movies, sometimes he watches with her and she seems to follow the storyline and laughs in all the right places.

We left the unit and made our way back to the front doors. We signed out. The woman behind the counter was very friendly once again.

Later David told me that he doesn't know what to expect whenever he visits. Sometimes she's in a good mood. Sometimes he takes her downstairs for ice cream. Sometimes she's in such a foul mood that he only stays for 10 minutes. Sometimes she's trying to get out the door and says, "I have to get out of here!" And he'll say, you can't get out this door, should we try another? He'll lead her to different doors (he knows which ones are locked) until he gets her to the front door and then they'll go sit outside. By then she's perfectly calm. What makes her like that anyway? Why is she sweet one day but foul the next? What puts her in a bad mood? I'd love to know what goes on in her mind. It can't be completely blank, can it? There must be something going on in there.

August 17, 2009

David and I went back to visit Mother today. We got up to her unit and walked throughout the entire area but didn't see her. We walked down to her room. The door was closed. We weren't sure if we should go in, we didn't want to interrupt anything that might be going on. A nurse came walking down the hall so we asked her if she thought it would be okay for us to go in. She said she would check for us and she disappeared into the room. She came out a moment later and said that Mother was in the bathroom with a nurse; she was getting ready to put Mother down for a nap. When she told them that Mother's family was here to visit the nurse with Mother said she would bring her out. A minute later they walked out. The nurse had her arm around Mother's shoulder. Mother was wearing a light green short-sleeved shirt that said Crosslake on it, cream colored slacks, and tennis shoes. She was pulling on the bottom of her shirt like she was self-conscious about her looks. And she was crying. I asked, "Why are you crying?" She said, "I'm happy." I put my arm around her and she wrapped both of her arms around my waist. She's so small, always was, 98 pounds soaking wet. We walked down the hall that way and I thought what a difference from the other day.

David asked her if she'd like to go downstairs and get some ice cream and she said yes. We stopped at the nurse's station to sign her out, her arms still around my waist. The nurse said, "Are you crying because you are happy or because you are sad?" And she said, "Because I'm happy." I was so moved at her tears and in a broken voice I told the nurse that I was sure she didn't know who I was. I wondered if she did know who we were or if she just was happy that her 'family' had come to visit, whoever they were. Was it the word family or did she on some level know who we were. I asked David later if she cries like that often when he visits and he said she's never cried like that. Did she remember my visit from the other day; was she afraid I wasn't coming back?

We walked to the door of the unit and when we got close David told me to stand back with Mother otherwise her bracelet would set off the alarm. As he punched in the code to open the door I noticed the bracelet for the first time. The last time she was wearing long sleeves so I didn't see it. The bracelet was a plastic wrist band (similar to what you wear in the hospital) with a square plastic box on it. I took her hand so I could see it better. Her wrist was so tiny. There was a large bruise on it under the box. Had she been trying to get the bracelet off, or had it just been rubbing on her skin? I ran my fingers over her skin. It was smooth – soft and silky, and looked paper thin. Her hand was cold.

We walked back down the long hallway, across the bridge and back to the elevator. We rode down with a girl who was about 14 years old and a white haired elderly lady in a wheelchair. The lady asked if we were going out and David said, "No, we're going for ice cream." The lady asked, "Where do you get that?" David told her that you can get it in the store. The lady seemed surprised by that information. When the elevator door opened she went one way and we went the other. Downstairs we had to walk down another hallway. I held Mother's hand the entire way. At the end of this hallway was a small store and an area with a couple of tables and chairs and a row of vending machines. We sat Mother down at a table and David handed her a VCR movie he was going to donate to the nursing home, asking her if she'd like to have it. She said, oh yes. It was an old Fred Astaire and Ginger Roger movie. The picture on the front showed Ginger wearing a pretty white dress. We told her we'd be right back with her ice cream and David and I went into the little store. David started picking out ice cream and I wandered around a bit to see what was there. There were a lot of snacks, toiletries, greeting cards, and gifts, etc. I guess we were in there a little too long because the young girl who was in the elevator with us suddenly came in and said, "Your Mother just took off down the hall." I rushed out and saw Mother boogeying down a different hallway, carrying the movie. I ran after her, caught her arm and said, "Where are you going?" I brought her back to the table and sat her down, and then sat down myself.

David came out with Klondike bars; unwrapped Mother's and put it down on the table in front of her. Mother started digging in with her fingers. She has always loved ice cream. I got a handful of paper towels for the mess that was about to occur. David also had a Klondike bar but I just got a cup of coffee out of the vending machine. We talked about different things. Mother didn't say much, too focused on her ice cream, but at one point she called David by name. Later he told me that she hasn't done that in a very long time. It looks like she is having flashes of memory. After awhile Mother's nose started dripping from the cold ice cream. I handed her a paper towel, telling her that her nose was dripping. She took the paper towel but just started wiping her fingers instead of her nose. I got another paper towel, put it to her nose and said, "blow." She did, just like a child. Funny how she forgets the simplest things. After a while she started just picking at the ice cream with her fingers. David said, "You're done," and wrapped it all up and threw it away.

By then her fingers were covered with ice cream. There was a restroom down the hall so I took her by the elbow and off we went. She was holding her hands slightly out in front of her as we walked. Her nose started dripping again, of course. We got inside the restroom and I turned on the hot water faucet. She put her hands in right away before it had even warmed up. My fingers were also in the water regulating the temperature so it wouldn't get too hot. She started saying, hot, hot. I kept turning it down until the water was like cold, but she kept saying hot. I said it's not hot. By then her fingers were freezing. I finally realized she meant to say cold, not hot. I turned off the water then saw that there were no paper towels. I dried her hands the best I could with toilet paper until we could get back to the table and paper towels. We left the restroom and I said, turn left, and she did. We got to the hallway and I said, turn left, and she did again.

David asked if she wanted to go outside for awhile and she said yes. We walked back down the hallway and went outside. At first we sat on a bench right outside the door. I wondered how long it had been since she'd been outside. She has always loved being outside. It was a beautiful, warm, sunny day but we were sitting in the shade. I suggested we find a bench in the sun. We were directly in front of the building and there were a lot of residents sitting out there. We crossed to the other side and Mother actually waved at someone as though she recognized her. Maybe she did, but I doubt it, those people were all out there on their own (meaning from a different unit). We sat down on another bench. There was a group of women sitting nearby, in the smoking area, including the lady who had been in the elevator with us. They were having a lively conversation with each other. I wished Mother could participate like that.

We sat side by side, holding hands. We didn't even bother to talk, just enjoyed the sun and watched the other people. I could feel a slight shaking in Mother's fingers. They were still cold. I noticed a small flaky spot on her face. Over the years she has had many spots removed from her face. When she was with me that year the doctor froze several spots. One was on her nose and she was not pleased when he blasted that one, claiming that it really hurt. While she was living at the assisted living place she developed a cyst right in the fold under her eye. It had to be surgically removed. David asked Emily and me to come up for the surgery. Afterwards Emily and I took turns spending the night with her, sleeping on the hide-a-bed.

The evening I spent with her we had dinner in the dining room with the other residents. One of them was her new beau, Bob. After dinner he asked Mother if she wanted to go to his apartment for ice cream. She said sure. We went back to her apartment briefly to give him time to get settled in. Bob's apartment was elaborately furnished. He had a large screen television and a cabinet full of glassware. It was a beautiful place. Bob was in a wheelchair, a very big wheelchair; it was fully padded with a high back and built-in headrest. He was severely disabled and had a hydraulic lift next to his bed to help get him in and out. Mother fixed us the dishes of ice cream. Bob had the same taste in movies that Mother does (westerns and the old classics) and she spent many evenings with him watching them. After finishing the ice cream I could see that Mother was settling in to watch the movie. I was feeling like a fifth wheel so I excused myself and went back to Mother's apartment. Mother had a little tiny television, very old. The knobs were broken off and I had to use a pair of pliers to turn the channel and maneuver a small antenna to get a clear picture. I was glad Mother had this nice relationship with Bob. I didn't want her to be lonely; like she is now.

The next morning Mother got totally frustrated while getting dressed and finally asked me for help. She said she couldn't find her bra. But before I even got into her bedroom she had found it. I had noticed that little things like that were off track with her. We went down to the dining room for breakfast. Bob joined us again. After we finished eating Bob asked Mother if she'd like to go play bingo. She said oh, yes, then turned to me and asked, "You don't mind do you?" Actually, I had thought I would play also. After all, I was without a vehicle. I was planning on sticking by her side. I said no, I didn't mind, then I wondered what I was going to do, but just then Dorothy popped in and asked if I was ready to go. That was in 2003.

Sitting outside in the sun today we stayed for quite awhile. At one point David went back inside the building briefly, only 5 to 10 minutes. I watched Mother as he came back out so I could see her reaction when she saw him coming. She sat straight up and said, "Oh, don't we know him?" I said, "Yes, we do." He came and sat down again beside us and she didn't say anything else. She was so calm. I'm sure she didn't know who we were but felt comfortable with us. We were family. I was thinking that she really needs a companion.

A nurse came out looking for our elevator smoking lady. She said, with a smile, "I knew you'd be out here." She said it was time for her to take her medications and she pushed her back into the building. One by one the other women finished their smoking and went inside until only one was left. She turned to us and said, "You have to be careful with these ashtrays because sometimes they catch on fire. I saw one on fire once." The ashtray was one of those vase shaped iron jobs with the narrow neck and a hole near the top where you drop the cigarette in. I always wondered about that because the cigarette is lit when you drop it in. I said, "Really? That's good to know." She dropped her butt in and left.

After awhile Mother started to doze, but when I said something to David she said, "I'm not asleep." Something she had said quite often when we tried to get her out of her chair in front of the TV every night, even though her head would be snapping back and forth. We took her back inside, into the elevator, and the long walk back over the bridge. As we came to the bird habitat David asked her if she had fed the birds today. She said no. I remembered that there had been a similar habitat in each nursing home she had been in and David always asked Mother the same question – did you feed the birds? They look so comfortable together. He has always taken care of her. He became very protective after Daddy died.

Once we got back to her unit David went to sign her back in and I took her to her room. I let her lead as we were going down the hallway and she went right to her room announcing, "This is my room." Her roommate was still lying in her bed but she was quiet, no help me chanting. As I took off Mother's shoes I noticed a card sitting on her nightstand that I had recently sent her. I send her a card in the mail every week. She can't read so I always just pick out a children's card, knowing she's just going to look at the picture on the front. However, she can see my name signed inside, so she has to think of me whenever she looks at it. Right? Hopefully. I handed her the card and said, "Oh you got a card." She looked at it like she was reading, she was really studying it. Was she trying to read it? She didn't have any reading glasses on, of course, so how could she read it. Maybe her blurry vision was causing her to be even more frustrated. I noticed there was no white beanie baby bear in sight. She finally handed the card back. I put my arms around her and told her that I loved her and that I would see her again soon. Then I laid her down on the bed for a nap.

David and I left the unit and made the long walk back to the elevator. We were very quiet, lost in our own thoughts. We got in the elevator, David pushed the button, but nothing happened. He pushed the button again but still nothing happened. We thought maybe something was wrong with the elevator so we got out. We were getting ready to try the other one but just then a woman staffer walked up and entered that elevator. David said he couldn't get that one to work. We followed her back in and she pushed the button and down we went. David was amazed and said, "I kept pushing the 2 button but nothing was happening." I said, "David, we were on 2 already." We laughed and he said, "You don't have to make me look stupid." The woman said, "We do that all by ourselves."

David had to stop on the way home and run an errand. I waited in his truck and when I was alone I couldn't stop my tears from coming again. This is all so sad. Back at the house we talked about Mother. How her memory has taken a downturn recently. David said, "I hate her being there!" I agreed with him but pointed out that we don't have any other choice. I said we could always move her to a different home but she needs 24 hour nursing care and none of us can provide that. It's just so frustrating. But as long as this place is taking good care of her there's no reason to move her.

August 23, 2009

I've been home almost a week now, but I can't stop thinking about Mother. I can't go to sleep at night. I can't focus on anything but her. She broke my heart. I feel such a loss of time. I just have to spend more time with her. I need to be with her as often as possible. I know this will cost me a fortune but I have to find a way to do it. I really don't know how much time I have left with her. I know that she is on the downside of the proverbial hill. I'm afraid it's not going to be very long. I hope I'm wrong, but I just have this feeling. I'm going to have to talk with Tom about this.

August 24, 2009

I talked with Tom today about Mother. I told him about my emotional state and that I had decided that I need to see her every couple of months, if possible. I said that I had slept on it a few nights and nothing had changed, I need to spend time with her. I said it's hard to explain, but I just have to do this. Tom actually volunteered to start driving me up there. I was so surprised. I thought he would be upset about the frequent plane trips. I'd much rather drive than fly. I said, once you see her you will understand. We have set up the first trip for the last weekend in September.

August 27, 2009

An amazing thing happened this morning. I was getting ready to make my bed when I saw a small piece of paper lying on the floor. I picked it up and saw that it was a tiny envelope, only about 2 inches square, and it had my name on it. I opened the envelope and inside was a message from Mother. She was telling me that the necklace she had just given me was made from the diamonds from her wedding ring from Ken. She had started out the note by saying I love you. I don't remember the note but I remember when she gave me the necklace about 20 years ago. It's a thin gold heart with four diamonds embedded in a design. It's really beautiful. I don't know where this note has been for the last twenty years or how it came to be on my bedroom floor this morning, but I know that spirit works in mysterious ways.

September 3, 2009

This evening I was out walking among the pine trees. The smell of pine always makes me think of Mother. She would love this place. She did see it while she was here. We had just bought the land and we brought her out to see it. She didn't seem very impressed. But that's because it looked like a cow pasture, which it had been before the owner split it into lots and sold it all. We got the last two lots, no one wanted them because they are odd shapes, but we fell in love with them. Although it was a pasture the back of the land is a wooded area bordering on a railroad track. There is a row of shade trees on one side and two huge trees on the other side. There is a variety of trees: oak, maple, persimmon, pine, cedar, and in one area there is a large hickory tree. Tom wanted a Christmas tree farm but out of the 400 trees we planted over the course of two years less than 20 have survived. A couple of years ago I was walking near the two huge trees and discovered an entire stand of tiny pine trees that had seeded themselves. It was spring and I hadn't walked in a while. I was so surprised. I stopped counting at 100. Now those trees are big enough to put out that heavenly scent of pine. I always think of Mother when I walk through there because that's how it always smelled at her place.

Mother loved to walk through her woods. The last time I was there visiting her was when she had just started her serious decline although we didn't know it. It was 1999. I had gone to spend Thanksgiving with her. She seemed fine except for her chronic coughing. During that trip we went out exploring and I took photographs of whatever caught my fancy. There was no snow yet so I took a lot of forest pictures. One evening after dinner we went up on the road for a walk, along with the dog of course. The clear, crisp night air was so refreshing. Funny, when Mother was in the house she coughed almost constantly but outside in the fresh air she didn't cough at all (I suppose that should have been a sign of something going on). The night was beautiful. The stars seemed really close and there was a full moon that illuminated our way. There's not many street lights out in the north woods. We probably walked two miles that evening.

September 8, 2009

I was out walking this evening and came upon a small turtle. We have a lot of wildlife around here. Like our trees, we have a variety of different turtles, some that I can't even find in the identification books. Whenever we find a turtle near the house we run and grab some fruit to feed it. Today I brought out some strawberries and sliced them up in front of the turtle's face. I sometimes had pet turtles when I was a kid. One year I had a tiny one; about the size of a half dollar (didn't everyone have one of those). One day I had taken the turtle out of its bowl and was playing with it, however I wasn't watching it very closely and all of a sudden it was gone. I was heartbroken and we searched everywhere but couldn't find it. That winter Mother was going through the front closet and she found the tiny turtle, dead of course. She gave it to me and I cried and cried. Then I remembered learning that you could put a turtle in milk and it would soften the shell. I begged Mother to let me try it. She said it wouldn't work, the turtle was dead. But I pleaded, please, please. So she got out a glass of milk and I plopped the turtle in. And waited. And waited.

September 14, 2009

I was driving home from town this afternoon when I passed a horse ranch. They had just mowed it and there were big, round hay bales scattered all over. It reminded me of the time when I was a child and we were driving up to Crosslake. We passed by a field and it was covered with the round hay bales. I asked Mother what they were and she said, "They're fairy houses." I was amazed and I spent a lot of time trying to picture those fairies and what the inside of their houses looked like. I don't know how long it took me to figure out it wasn't true. I mean, you believe everything your Mother tells you, don't you?

September 17, 2009

I went to the pool this afternoon and actually found myself alone, which was nice. Since I first started going there I had wanted to try out those aqua moves Mother had taught Emily and me when we were kids. Mother grew up near Lake Calhoun. Every year on May 1, or maybe it was June 1 (probably June 1, considering it was Minnesota), she and her sister would go jump in the lake and have their first swim of the year. Mother had been part of a group of women who performed water ballet. I don't know whether Aunt Laurie did it also. One year Mother took us all down to watch a performance. It was so neat. It was evening and there were lights in the bottom of the pool. The performance was like watching an Ester Williams show. After the performance we walked around the marina. We looked at the sailboats and then Mother bought us homemade ice cream from a little stand. I loved it all and wanted Mother to teach me everything about water ballet. That summer she taught us some of the simple moves. Now that I am spending so much time at the pool I wondered if I could remember any of those moves. I thought this would be a good time to try. I was in the deep end and tried floating on my side and raising my leg straight up. After nearly drowning myself I moved to the shallow end. After about thirty minutes I was finally able to do it. Wow. I need to do that more often.

September 19, 2009

Last night I had a dream about Mother. In the dream I was in some kind of shop or flea market. Mother had a space where she was selling things. There was a pile of VCR movies. I was looking through them and was holding one that I wanted to buy. It had a picture on the front of a woman wearing a long, white dress. There was something white bulging out from the tape case, like a part of the dress in the picture. Mother had left the area and when she returned I told her that I wanted to buy the movie. She said that I couldn't buy it but I could rent it. She pointed at a tape player and said that I could rent that also. I said okay. That was the dream. I believe that the movie was representing Mother and that I could have her for awhile (rent her) but would not be able to have her forever (couldn't buy her) like I wanted. Meaning, I would have a limited time with her. However, the white dress bulging out of the case was showing me that my time with her would be a full, rich time. Interesting, the picture on the tape case looked like the one on the movie David had just given to Mother, well, had donated to the nursing home.

September 22, 2009

Last night when I went to bed I could hear all kinds of night sounds outside that made me think of Mother. The pond right behind the house is back because of all the recent heavy rains. As I was going to sleep I could hear the insects singing and a loud chorus of frogs chirping. Just like at Mother's! The way it used to be anyway.

September 24, 2009

We are on our way to Minnesota, spending the night in Chillicothe, Missouri. David called me earlier on my cell phone. He told me about when he had stopped to see Mother last Friday. He had found her in front of a big TV screen watching a movie, well not actually watching the movie because she was asleep. He woke her up and she stayed awake for about ten minutes then went back to sleep, so he left.

We are at the Super 8 Motel. It is so bad in here. All of the white towels are dingy and stained. There's actually a used, dirty bath towel hanging on the hook on the back of the bathroom door; like the housekeeper hadn't seen it. There is another towel sitting on the rack all folded like it's clean but it's dirty; there are rust stains on it but it also looks like someone had wiped their dirty hands on it. That leaves one semi-clean towel for Tom and me to share. It's hard enough for a woman to bathe with only one towel, we really need two, one for the hair and one for the body, but then to have to share the one towel makes it extremely unpleasant. I can't get Tom to go back to the office and get more towels because he's already asleep and I'm not waking him up. Besides, it started out bad with the night clerk. Tom had paid in cash and when he got back in the truck he looked at the receipt and it said that there was a balance due in the same amount he had already paid. He got mad and went back inside and made the man write on it that it was already paid. We didn't want any surprises when we check out in the morning. The clerk was not pleased at Tom's attitude, and Tom was not pleased by the clerk's attitude.

The bathtub didn't drain properly so while I was taking a shower I was standing in dirty water. The temperature of the water was inconsistent so I was always fiddling with the knobs. The pillows are so flat that they barely make a bump on the bed. The pillow cases and sheets are also dingy and stained. The comforter has a big slit with the filling coming out. The bottom sheet popped off as soon as we got in the bed. There's no mattress cover of course; Tom is already lying on the bare mattress. We'll never stay here again.

September 25, 2009

I had this dream during the night: I was walking around a department store. There was some kind of sweepstake going on. There was a big grand prize and then a secondary prize. As I was walking through the store I heard that there was a problem with the cards. The cards, which were like credit cards, was how you won a prize. There was a woman and her teenage daughter nearby, in front of a counter. The woman asked the salesclerk, "What do you want us to do with the cards, just set them on the counter?" The salesclerk said yes. The woman had her card on her key ring and she took it off and put it on the counter. I wasn't sure what I'd do with my card. I knew the sweepstake wasn't over yet, although there was some kind of problem. The daughter said to her mother, "Well, you already won the treasure chest." The mother agreed. I knew that the treasure chest was the secondary prize. Then the dream ended.

I wonder if this dream was representing Mother and me in some way, maybe in a reversed way. In the dream the mother was hoping for the grand prize but knew she would only get the secondary prize. The daughter was saying she should be happy with that. Me, in the dream, was reluctant to give up the card, to give up the hope of winning. Was the dream telling me that I already have the prize? Not the grand prize – that would be Mother with a full memory – but the second prize, which is a treasure. And I shouldn't expect anything else. Mother is a treasure, no matter how I find her. And I will treasure whatever time I have left to spend with her. The woman having her card on her key ring could also signify this dream is about Mother and me because we are in route to her now. Or, the key to her heart!

Back on the road and I'm wondering if I am overreacting. Is it worth it, will it be worth it? About eight hours into the trip yesterday my back started hurting really bad from the traveling. And it didn't take long today for it to start hurting again. Can Tom handle making this trip every couple of months? 850 miles is a lot of driving. And that's 850 miles twice in a four day period. Take this trip alone, we left home early afternoon on Thursday. We'll arrive late afternoon on Friday. Then we'll leave out again Saturday afternoon and get home Sunday evening. However we work it Tom will have to take two days off work, then we have gas, motels, and food; plus, the 1700 driving miles in four days. Can I handle making this trip every couple of months? Maybe that's what the dream actually means – that Mother is worth the pain and hard traveling to get to her and spend time with her.

It was 5:00 when we got to the nursing home. We spent about an hour in rush hour traffic driving through Minneapolis. It was raining lightly and the sky was dark and cloudy. I hoped that I could find my way back to Mother's unit; it was the first time by myself. Tom wanted to stay in the truck since we knew I wouldn't be in there long, at that hour they would be setting up for dinner, but I made him go with me. As we walked towards the entrance we could see a couple of people sitting outside smoking. I shivered and hoped they wouldn't get sick being out in this weather. We could smell the coffee as soon as we walked in – not the good smell of fresh coffee but the strong, bitter, bottom of the pot smell. We approached the desk to sign in and a woman with shoulder length blonde hair, about 50, was sitting there. She was very friendly and I asked her for directions to the little store and she pointed out the proper hallway. I hadn't been able to remember where it was. I had just followed behind David. We walked down to the store so Tom could see it, went to the restroom, and then back to the elevator.

We found our way okay and then walked through the areas and finally found her near the outside doors again. Tom didn't even recognize her with that short hair. He actually thought that she was the woman standing next to her because they had identical haircuts. I had decided that I would just walk up to her and give her a hug.

I went over and said, "Hello Mother," and started to put my arms around her. She stiffened up immediately and in a slow, deep, angry sounding voice said, "DON'T YOU TOUCH ME." I said, "It's me, Janet, we're here to visit you." She said, "I know who you are," and then she stomped off. The look on my face must have alarmed Tom. He said, "You know that she doesn't know who you are." I nodded. She crossed through the room and sat in a chair. I was at a loss of what to do next. Tom told me to go sit next to her. She was slumped forward, kind of curled up on herself, looking at the floor. I went over and sat in the chair next to her. She was wearing dark blue slacks and a navy blue pullover sweater. I noticed that she now had maroon nail polish. Although the polish was again chipped at the edges her nails looked perfectly manicured and I couldn't help but wonder if they were fake. My nails never look that good. I can't imagine though that they would actually put fake nails on her. She was holding a small plastic cup, like maybe she had just taken some medication. She kept twisting it around in her fingers. After a minute, with just a brief glance at me she said, "Are you going to try to talk to me too?" I didn't really say anything to that but asked her, "Why are you so mad?" She did look at me then and said, "I'm mad because...," then her face kind of went blank when she realized she couldn't remember, and then said, "I'm not mad." She got up and stomped across the room again to another chair. They were getting ready to serve dinner so we decided to give it another try in the morning. I'll try a different tact, and I'll leave Tom outside; that was a little embarrassing.

After leaving we went over to David and Dorothy's house to have dinner with them. The grandkids were spending the night. Alexsis is ten, the twins (Clyde and Steven) are three, about to turn four next week, and Vincent is now three. What a group! David said that when he had visited Mother earlier this afternoon she was in a good mood. She was watching a movie again (I guess they show one every Friday afternoon, perhaps every day?). He was sitting with her, also watching the movie, and he noticed tears running down her face. He asked, "Why are you crying?" She said she was just tired. But I wonder – maybe she knew that she knew him but didn't know who he was. That would be very frustrating. He's there so often that she must find him familiar even if she doesn't know who he is. David continued, saying that while he was still there they brought around the afternoon snack, today it was ice cream with chocolate syrup, and she gobbled it right up. So what happened between David's visit and mine that put her in such a foul mood?

We talked about how researchers have been saying that the amount of people who have dementia, for whatever reason, has risen dramatically and is expected to keep rising, although they don't know why. Grandma developed dementia when she was in her 70s. At that time they didn't call it dementia, but senility, people were senile. When she died at the age of 82 Mother was by her side although Grandma didn't know who she was. Is this stuff supposed to be hereditary? I think so. But I hope not.

I think there is supposed to be ways to prevent dementia. Things like exercising the mind – doing puzzles and games, etc. I need to do some research on this. I'm at a good age to start with some prevention. I don't want to end up like Mother and Grandma!

September 26, 2009

We spent the night in a motel in Anoka. There sure aren't many motels around here. None near Mother's nursing home. I had a dream that seemed to last all night. In the dream I was sitting in front of my computer playing a game on Pogo. The game was all laid out and I could see several different moves. I was trying to plot it out, thinking that if I make this move, this will happen, if I do this that will happen. I kept going over it but wasn't making a move. I never sleep well in a motel and I wake up several times during the night. Each time I woke and then went back to sleep the game was laid out exactly in the same way and I went through the same routine never making a move.

I think the dream was my mind trying to come up with some different ways of approaching Mother without her reacting in such a hostile way. Especially if she's trying to get out of the building or just looking out the window. Both times I tried that it didn't work; first when I was with David and then last night.

I usually play games on Pogo before going to bed, so I dream of it pretty often. Usually in my dreams I play and play and drive myself nuts trying to make it stop. But this was the first time that I didn't make any of the moves. Playing Pogo games is a really good way for me to exercise my mind. At least that's my story, and I'm sticking to it.

I had another dream during the night. I was with a group of people inside some kind of settlement. We had gathered together because something bad was getting ready to happen. Not the apocalypse or doomsday or anything like that but something temporary. Each family had their own small space. The power had just gone out, meaning that whatever was going to happen had begun. The people who were not in the settlement when the power went out were stuck wherever they were. The rest of us, in the settlement, were frantically looking for supplies, including me. At the end of the dream I had come back to my space and said, "I found some potatoes. They should last us six months."

Is this dream representing Mother? You could say that Mother is in a settlement (nursing home), everyone has their own small space (bed, nightstand, closet), and every-one is there temporarily – which is kind of a bad way of saying it, but the truth. Basically, they'll be there until they die. And my time to have Mother is temporary. Gathering supplies could be my way of getting some response from Mother, some recognition. Or it could mean Mother, and the other residents (I almost said inmates), trying to get, or find, some kind of strength, energy, or manna (potatoes) from their visitors. Remember the power has gone out. Have they lost their own personal power? They are after all in the memory care unit.

There is also the symbolism of potatoes I have to consider. Potatoes provide energy, so perhaps my visits with Mother will provide her with energy. In numerology the number 6 represents love. I hope the 'six months' wasn't a warning.

September 27, 2009

By the time we checked out of the motel and got to the nursing home it was already going on 11:00. The weather was beautiful, sunny and in the 70s. I went up to the unit alone. Tom stayed outside with his seemingly endless supply of paperback westerns. My approach this time was going to be not approaching her at all. I knew they would be setting up for lunch so I wouldn't be there for very long. And I knew I'd have all afternoon after lunch. So if I wasn't able to talk to her right then it would be okay. Really I just wanted to see what would happen if she saw me but wasn't approached by me.

I found her near the outside doors again. But there was now inside doors that were closed. I guess those outside doors are in a vestibule and I didn't realize it. Mother was sitting in a chair near the inside doors, next to a window. She was asleep. I sat down in another chair near her with a small table between us. I sat and waited, watched her, and looked out the window. There are a lot of squirrels around there.

She finally woke up and started looking out the window. She was holding a small plastic glass in her hand, twirling it around gently in her fingers. She would look out at the room then back out the window. I knew that she knew I was sitting in the chair, at least she knew that someone was sitting in the chair, although she never looked directly at me. I made sure that I was sitting in such a position with my legs crossed so that she would have to see at least my foot. After a few minutes she dropped the cup. She tried to pick it up but it had rolled under her chair and she couldn't reach it. I said, "Do you need some help?" but she ignored me. She continued looking out at the room and the window. I did the same, being very patient.

She was wearing light green slacks and a short sleeved cream colored knit top with some type of picture on it. I wondered if she missed wearing her old blue jeans or having a dog around. She always had a dog. I was looking at her nail polish and remembered when she was in the first nursing home in Pine River. Tom and I went up and got her and we drove down to Nancy's for Caroline's high school graduation party. Along the way she said, "Look what they did to my nails," and held out her hands for me to see. All of her fingernails were cut straight across. I couldn't believe it, why would they do that? Mother was very angry. Unfortunately I didn't have a manicure set with me or I would have fixed them immediately. It's nice that she's receiving a little bit of pampering here.

A man approached us; another resident. While I had been sitting there I had seen him walking up and down the hall. He walked right up in front of me and stood there. I didn't say anything, rude I know, but I didn't want Mother to think that I was there to visit him. Mother really perked up though and said, "Hi." He looked at her but didn't say anything then looked back at me. Mother curled forward, rejected. The man started rubbing his face really hard, like in frustration. He looked back at Mother and she perked up again and said, "Hi, how are you?" Her voice sounded so young. Again he looked away and again she curled forward in rejection. Mother always liked the men, but this was sad. The man then turned around and walked away. As he crossed the room I heard a nurse call him Ray.

Poor Mother. She just wants someone to talk to, someone to acknowledge her, her existence, to pay attention to her. I am a person! I have thoughts and feelings just like everyone else. Don't ignore me, I am right here. I am real, not just a part of this chair. I am not my Social Security number, but real flesh and blood. Mother continued looking out into the room and out the window. I was so tempted to say something, she looked so lonely, but I was sticking to my plan for now. I really wanted to observe her in her environment.

I wondered if the man thought he knew me. Did I look familiar in some way? He may be going through the same thing as Mother. After all, he is in the memory care unit also. Was he upset because I didn't acknowledge him? Do unto others. I need to change that in myself. I need to treat the residents the same way I want everyone to treat Mother. That means acknowledging anyone who approaches me, even by just saying hello. I'm still a little new at this dementia stuff.

A male orderly approached Mother. He was Jamaican and dressed all in white. Mother perked up again and said, "Hello." They were already bringing the residents to the lunch tables so I think he was coming to get her. He started to say something to her then noticed me sitting there and said, "Are you here to visit her?" I said, "Yes, but she doesn't know it." He said, "Are you her daughter?" "Yes." And he said, "You look just like her." He must have seen a strange look on my face – come on, no one wants to hear that you look just like an 83 year-old, and he said, "You have similar features." Okay, that's better. He turned to Mother and said, "Did you know that your daughter is here to see you?" She finally looked right at me, got all excited and said, "I know that!" I had a brown and white teddy bear for her and I tried to give it to her but she didn't seem interested so I set it on the table. The man said, "Get up and give her a hug." We both jumped up and she threw her arms around my waist, holding on tightly. Wow. I told him that I would just be there for a few minutes because they were getting ready to have lunch. He asked if I wanted to have a space set up for the two of us but I said no that I would come back after lunch. I am determined not to interrupt any of her normal routines; she needs to keep them consistent.

The man left and as Mother and I began holding hands she said, "Let's go." I asked where and she just waved her hand and I said, "For a walk?" And she nodded. I grabbed the teddy bear off the table. We walked through the sitting areas and then I asked if she would like to go to her room for awhile and she said yes. We began walking down her hallway, holding hands still. We got to her room and I said, "Here's your room." As we entered it was as if she had never been there before. That was really strange. I said, here's your bed and she said, really? She was looking at the blanket which was white with pictures of teddy bears all over it. She rubbed her hand over it gently and said this is so cute. I agreed and remembered when Emily and I were there for her 81st birthday. Rebecca had given her the blanket. Mother was living with Rebecca and her family at the time. She has changed <u>so much</u> since then.

I put the teddy bear on top of the nightstand and noticed several items sitting there. There were some ceramic figurines and there was that white beanie baby that I brought during my visit with David! Now where had that been? Mother sat down on the edge of the bed and I took David's calendar off the wall so I could sign my name on it. I opened the drawer looking for a pen, Mother watching me. The drawer was full of the cards I had sent her and numerous small framed photographs. I started taking some of the cards out and set them up on the top. Then I started taking the photos out one by one. They were of some of her great grandchildren. I showed each one to her, telling her who they were and then set them up. But there was one of a baby who I didn't even know. I gave it to her and she said, "Now this one looks familiar." I thought how she must be reaching for <u>anything</u> that looked familiar. How frustrating it must be not to recognize anything or anyone. In the back corner was a photo of her mother, probably in her 20s. I pulled it out and handed it to her saying you must know who this is. She said no and didn't even take it from me. I said it's your mother and then put it back in the drawer; we don't want that to disappear. The snapshot of her with David and Emily was still on the wall and I pointed it out and said, "And of course this is you with David." She said, "And you." And I said, "No, that's Emily." Of course she hadn't even gotten up from the bed to look at it.

I told her that there had been a photo of me and the boys and another one of Emily and her family but I didn't know where they were. I suggested we look in her closet and she agreed. We opened her closet and saw all of her clothes hanging there. There was a long sleeved white shirt folded up in the front. It had little pictures of birds all over it. She gently stroked it saying how pretty it is and asked me, "Did you do this?" I said, "No, it's yours." I picked it up so she could see it and then turned to the label inside with her name on it and said, "See, here's your name." She didn't say anything. I wonder if she knows who she is. I started looking around saying let's see what else we can find. I found the large photograph of Emily but I couldn't find mine. When I turned back around she was sitting on the edge of her roommate's bed. Luckily the roommate wasn't there, she was probably already at lunch. That would have been very awkward if she had been in the room when we first got there and Mother couldn't remember ever being there. But maybe she goes through that all the time. The staff here must have the patience of Job. I asked her if she was ready to go eat lunch and she said yes, she was always ready to eat lunch.

We walked back out to the dining area. We were walking between the tables, they were all pretty full, and I saw one resident taking food off the plate of the woman next to her. One of the nurses was stopping her. I asked her where Mother's place was and she, and another nurse, both rushed forward and found an empty spot and brought up a chair. She said, "She can sit here." I thought they had assigned seating, thought that would be part of the routine, but then maybe no one can remember an assigned seat. I put Mother in the chair and someone went to get her food. I bent down to kiss her and she looked so distraught that I was leaving. I assured her that I would be back after she ate.

I was so surprised at Mother's reaction to her room. It was like she was getting the grand tour for the first time. It was totally opposite from my visit with David. It was like she had no sense of identity. I felt so sorry for her. I can't imagine living like that. She must be confused all of the time. Again, she must reach out for anything familiar.

Tom and I drove into Crystal for lunch. We hadn't eaten anything yet and were starving and desperately in need of coffee. Ah, Crystal, my old stomping grounds. It should have brought back a lot of memories but it didn't. Everything was totally different. I wouldn't have even been able to point out where Tom and I first met. Of course we hadn't been in Crystal for decades. We drove around a bit at first trying to get the layout of the streets that we could remember and get our bearings somewhat. We found a small café, like a small neighborhood place where everyone knows your name. We sat down in a booth and ordered then I just started watching the people around us. I was feeling kind of rum drum, a little light-headed. A woman came in and saw someone she knew; they started talking and she said, "We lost Mother this year." I had to stop listening; it almost brought me to tears.

Back at the nursing home Tom waited outside again. I told him that I was just going to run up there, get Mother, then bring her back down. I left my purse in the truck because I was just running up and running back down. I said we are going to sit on this bench and when I'm ready for you to come over I will wave at you. Okay, no problem. I rushed up to Mother's unit and found her sitting on a chair, right on the edge of it, hands folded between her legs. I sat down next to her and she looked right at me. I said, "Are you waiting for me?" She said. "Yes, I knew you'd be back." I thought wow, she remembers me! I asked if she would like to go outside and she said yes. I said she'd have to put her shoes on first and she said, "They're already on." I said, let me check. I reached down and touched her black stocking and then said, nope, no shoes just socks. I stood up and said come on let's get your shoes. We walked down to her room and I started to put her tennis shoes on. This turned out to be very difficult because she didn't help at all. She was just like a little child. I kept saying, push, push your foot. She'd just sit there looking at me like she couldn't figure out what my problem was. Finally I said, "Can you stand up?" She did and the shoe finally went on. Same with the other foot. "Okay," I said, "let's go."

We walked out of her room, hand in hand, and went to the nurse's desk and signed her out of the unit. I didn't have the door code and that caused a problem. No one wanted to open the door for me or give me the code. They basically told me to wait until someone came in from the other side. We finally got out and began walking down the hall. I asked her if it had been a long time since she'd been outside. She said she had gone to the zoo yesterday. I said, "Really, they took you to the zoo?" "Yes." I knew David had visited Mother yesterday and that today he was taking his grandchildren to the zoo so I figured he had told her about his plans and the zoo part had stuck in her mind. We got to the end of the hallway and found ourselves in an area that was not familiar to me at all. It was full of tables with residents sitting at them. I wondered what happened. I said, "This isn't right. We must have made a wrong turn; we'll have to turn around." We went back up the hall part way then turned and went back and ended up in that area again. I couldn't figure it out. We went in a straight line so how could we have made a wrong turn. Later I realized that I had missed the turn altogether. It was just a little opening in the hallway going back over the bridge.

Well, we'll just go a different way. How hard can that be? A couple of women nurses were moving amongst the residents sitting at the tables and I tried asking them how to get to the front door but they just ignored me. So we just kept walking until I found an exit sign leading to an outside door. The door was standing open and we sailed right out, setting off the alarm with Mother's bracelet. A nurse had been sitting at a nearby desk so I was sure she had seen us. I told Mother we'd have to walk a bit and get to the front of the building. She said okay. I wasn't sure which way to go. I started one way but it led in between the buildings. I wasn't even aware there were different buildings. I guess that's where the bridge comes in. I didn't want to start wandering in there so we turned back in the other direction. We went out onto the sidewalk which skirted a parking lot on our right and the city street on our left. Mother did very well this first stretch, probably because I told her we just had to go around the corner. However, when we got to the corner I realized I didn't know where we were. Tom and I had driven around the front part of the building before parking and this wasn't it. Nothing was familiar. I told her we'd have to walk to the next corner. We walked at a steady pace. I told Mother that Tom was waiting for us around the corner. She said, "Tommy's here?" We haven't called him Tommy in about twenty years of course, not since it had become too difficult having two Tommys in the house. So, father became Tom and son became Tommy. So who was she remembering, father or son? Tommy and the kids had been with me during a previous visit.

We got to the next corner and as we turned my heart sank. Ahead of us was another unfamiliar stretch. By now I was wishing I had my phone with me so Tom could come and get us. I said, "We just have to go around that corner." She was looking a little tired by now and I asked if she was okay. She said she was but all of a sudden she started walking faster. I said, slow down a little. She did at first then started going even faster. She's bent over slightly so it was like her head was leading and then it was like she just wasn't able to stop. She was going faster and faster, her head leading the way. I was afraid she was going to fall. I thought, oh my god, if she goes down my ass will be in big trouble. I could just see her lying on the sidewalk with a broken hip. I'd have to flag down a passing car to go get Tom because I don't have my cell! I will never leave my phone in the truck again. I said, "You've got to slow down. I'm afraid you're going to fall on your face." I still had a hold of her hand, pulling on it, trying to get her to slow down. Finally I just stopped, which caused her to stop also. But then she started swaying from side to side and she was making little noises, like oh, oh, oh. I didn't want to know what that was about. She was breathing hard. I looked around, no benches anywhere, just another parking lot. I pointed at the curb and said let's sit down and rest. She nodded and I led her over. I sat down and was trying to lead her down next to me but she wouldn't bend her knees. I was finally able to pull her down on the curb. Then she started squirming around. I said it wouldn't be so uncomfortable if you didn't have such a bony butt. She started taking deep breaths and sighing. I knew she would sit there all day if I let her. So I gave her about two minutes then said let's go.

I knew there couldn't be too many corners left. I couldn't believe we'd been around as many as we had. This place must be set up really weird to have this many corners. I suppose if I had turned the other way in the beginning we would have been right in the front. We walked to the next corner and as we turned I could finally see a familiar area. We had driven through it earlier, it wasn't the front but if we cut through this parking lot we would get to the front, which we did. What a relief. I could see Tom sitting on the tailgate with a puzzled look on his face as we came walking up the sidewalk instead of out the front door. But he knows me very well; he really isn't surprised by anything I do.

We made our way up the long sidewalk and over to the bench we had sat on before with David. Mother sat down with obvious relief. After we got settled in I turned and waved to Tom to come over. When he reached us I told him about getting lost as we were coming out. He thought it was funny of course. I have the worst sense of direction; I can get lost in my own backyard. He greeted Mother and she acted like she knew who he was. He said, "Can I have a hug?" What a surprise, I don't remember him ever hugging her before. She said, "Sure," and they both leaned forward and hugged. I asked her if she minded if Tom took some pictures and she said okay. He got the camera and took a few shots then said she had stuck her tongue out. I said "Really?" She said she had a hair on her mouth, but then she turned to me and said, "I just couldn't resist," and she was smiling. Just like a kid.

I asked her if she wanted to see my pet tortoise and she said, "You have it here?" When I said yes she said she really wanted to see it. Tom pulled Chelsey out of her tote bag and held her up. Chelsey has been on a lot of road trips with us. We discovered that if we just carry her around in a tote bag no one knows she's even there. And she's a good traveler. We just put her in a small bed with baby blankets in the back seat and she pretty much sleeps all the time. Or I hold her and she'll look out the window for awhile then snuggles under her blanket and goes back to sleep. Simple. I asked Mother if she would like to hold her and she reached her hands out. Tom put Chelsey in her hands but it was like Mother didn't know how to hold her. I suppose it could be confusing on where to put your hands on a tortoise. Soon Chelsey was looking straight down at the sidewalk and I said, "You're holding her with her head down." She said, "Oh," and then looked confused. Tom reached over and helped her in the proper way of holding a tortoise. She didn't bring Chelsey close to her, like she was a bit wary – kind of like 3 year-old Vincent last night. But they looked at each other, eye to eye for a moment. Tom took Chelsey back and they returned to the truck, to the paperback western, and the pet bed.

I said, "You know I've always liked unusual pets," and she said, "Yes, I have," and looking me right in the face she said, "haven't I?" I nodded in agreement thinking, all I remember you having were dogs. She always had a dog. I, on the other hand, always had something not a dog. It's not that I don't like dogs, I do like them, I'm just allergic. Then she said, "This has been going on for a long time…this…" She was holding her hands slightly outstretched, palms up and I said, "Journey?" She nodded and said again, "This has been going on a long time." I said, "Yes, it has." I was really surprised because she rarely speaks on her own. And I was surprised because her mind now seemed clear, at least clearer. She seemed to know who she is or some sense of it anyway. She was noting the passage of time instead of being in a fog. She was right; it has been going on for a very long time. And she seems really, really tired.

She relaxed back on the bench and I wondered if she was in any pain because of her osteoporosis. We sat in silence for awhile then I asked her if she'd been having a lot of visitors and she said yes. I asked if David had been to visit her and she said, "Oh yes, he was here yesterday. He visits me every day." And Nancy? "Oh yes, she was here yesterday. She visits me every day." And Emily? "Oh yes, she was here yesterday." "So everyone was here yesterday except me?" "Yes." "Well you know I live a long ways away. It's hard for me to get here very often." She nodded.

There was an elderly man sitting in a wheelchair at a nearby table. He said, "You two look just alike." Again someone telling me I look just like her. Funny, I've never thought I looked anything like her. I'm going to have to take another look in the mirror. I said, "Did you hear what he said? He said we look just alike." "Of course, you're a lot older," I continued with a smile. "But I'm getting up there myself." And she said, yes, like she knew I was getting older. I said, "But all of us are, even Emily is getting older." She said, "I know."

We sat in silence awhile. The sun was feeling good. It's hard to know what to say to her. It's pretty much a one-way conversation with her just agreeing to everything I say, even when I realize that she usually doesn't know what or who I'm talking about. I said, "It's good that you have been able to see all of your grandchildren." She nodded, saying yes. "And you've been able to see all of your great-grandchildren. Scott brought all of his kids to see you. Tommy brought his kids to see you. You were able to see Emily's grandchildren when you were out there." She kept nodding, saying yes.

I am so glad that all of my grandchildren have seen Mother since this journey has begun. She was able to spend a lot of time with Kelley, Zakary, and Trevor when she was with us that winter. Ben and TJ weren't born yet so they missed out on that. At that time I was picking Trevor up from daycare every afternoon and bringing him back to the house until Ruth got off work. Each afternoon Mother would be waiting for him and when he ran in the door she gave him a big hug and they both got down on the floor and started playing with whatever caught their interest that day. We had celebrated Mother's 75th birthday at Tommy's house that year and Kelley and Zakary were able to get Mother to wear a party hat. It was a lot of fun. Since that time Kelley has been to Minnesota once and Zakary twice. I thought about the trip Scott and his family made with me that one year, Mother still in assisted living. It was right before Christmas and there was a lot of snow. All of them were absolutely thrilled; we don't see much snow in Arkansas. Ben was only 3 at the time and TJ was 5 months. They may not remember and Mother I'm sure doesn't remember, but that's okay.

While we sat there a woman wheeled herself out, parked her chair on the sidewalk full in the sun, stretched her body out, head leaning back, and went to sleep. Basking in the sun. The man who had been sitting nearby in his wheelchair had gone back inside then came back out, this time with some visiting family. They were a young family, including two boys - grade school, maybe middle school. The boys ran around a bit, not that there was much landscape. The man parked his wheelchair back at the table. The couple stood up the entire time, even though there were chairs around the table where they could have sat with the man. It was like they were thinking, how long do we have to stay, when can we leave? There's something about people who visit but won't sit down, it's like they're just fulfilling a duty and want to hurry up and get it over with. It's Sunday, nursing home day. The family was there for about 10 minutes then left. Nice visit; nice tiny visit.

I was running out of conversation so I just asked the normal questions, "Are they treating you good here? Is the food good? Is your bed comfortable?" She kept nodding, saying yes. "Well, that's all that matters then, isn't it?" She nodded yes. We sat in silence again until I noticed she was falling asleep then told her it was time to go.

I helped her up from the bench and we walked back into the building and into the elevator. Going up to the second floor I asked her if she was tired and she said yes. She even seemed a little weak and was leaning against the wall. I said that when we got back I was going to lay her down for a nap and she said, "No." Just at that moment the elevator door opened and she refused to get out. I said, okay, I won't lay you down. She got out and we began the long walk back to her unit. As we passed the first area we could see residents sitting at long tables playing bingo. I said, "Look, they're playing bingo." Mother said, "Yuk." I said, "You don't like bingo?" She shook her head no. I thought, that's funny, she sure did like it with Bob in the assisted living place. We went back over the bridge and down her hallway. We entered the unit and began walking across the area and I asked her where she wanted to go. She didn't answer at first so I said, "Do you want to go lay down for a nap?" "Oh yes." We went down the hallway to her room. I sat her down on the bed and took off her shoes. At least they came off easily. I helped her lie back on the bed and then lifted her legs on; making sure the pillow was under her head. I leaned over and kissed her on the forehead, telling her how much I love her, and that I would be back very soon. It was so hard to leave her. I wiped away tears as I left her room.

I made the long walk back to the elevator. There were three people waiting there already. There was a woman in a wheelchair about my age and a younger woman, her daughter I'm guessing, and an elderly man. The way the two women were talking I believe the woman was only there temporarily; an accident or illness maybe. I wasn't paying much attention to them at first until they started wondering why the elevator was taking so long. Then I realized they hadn't read the little sign over the button. I said, "You have to punch in the year and then this button." They laughed saying they hadn't even noticed the sign. I said I had done the same thing the first time. Just another security measure. Once inside the elevator the woman noticed that the back wall also had sliding doors. She asked me where those doors opened up to. I said I didn't know. She asked if I thought they led outside and I said they probably open to another part of the building. She said to her daughter, "If you got a call saying I was lost, would you think I was lost outside or inside?" The daughter said, "I would think you were lost somewhere inside." The mother said, "Really?" like she was surprised by the answer. As I left the building I passed by the group of smoking women and there was my elevator lady. She saw me, got a big smile on her face, and said hi. I smiled and said hi back.

Back on the road heading home. I am always so drained of energy after visiting Mother. I hope she is more energized as a result. I was telling Tom how hard it is to make conversation with her and he suggested I try talking about the past. Good idea, maybe it will even jog her memory a bit. As I relaxed I thought about how all of the staff, except for one nurse, were Jamaicans. David had told me that Minnesota was the number one state now for immigrants. They have immigrants from pretty much every country and culture. I wondered if it was because it was a weekend that today they were all Jamaicans. It seemed like some of them were receiving training. The men were dressed all in white and the women wore the purple scrubs. All of the men were very nice to me but not all of the nurses were. As I drifted off to sleep I thought that as long as Mother was treated well it didn't matter where the staff was from.

September 28, 2009

I was walking this evening and could smell something burning. It smelled just like a campfire. That smell always brings back memories of growing up camping in Crosslake. We had the piece of land right next to Grandma and Grandpa's. They weren't there very often. We had a big six person tent and sleeping bags, no cots for us. I didn't really like camping out, too many bad things for my child's mind; like mosquitoes, biting flies, wood ticks, too hot, too cold, hard ground, no television, too much work, no bathroom. I'm sure Mother wasn't too thrilled with all of the hard work. She had to cook on a small propane cook stove, or over the fire. Food was kept in a big cooler. Daddy had dug and put in a pump which had to be primed whenever we used it and then we had to haul buckets and buckets of water. I'm sure Mother didn't enjoy washing dishes in a metal tub – wait, did she wash the dishes or did us kids wash the dishes? Teeth brushing was done with just a glass of water, no running water.

And the bees. One summer some friends left their pontoon boat with us since they were going to make frequent visits. One day we had been out fishing and when we got back to shore I jumped off right into a swarm of bees. I took off running and when I looked back I could see that one stubborn bee was still in pursuit. I panicked, you can't outrun a bee. The only place to hide was the tent so I dived in there. I was the first one off the boat so I guess no one had seen what had happened with me. I was afraid to come out and I watched as all of the kids took off into the woods to play and the adults gathered around the picnic table. I've always hated having attention put on me, I've always been extremely shy, and so I didn't want to come out of the tent into the middle of the adults. Besides, no one was supposed to be in the tent. I thought surely they would walk off somewhere and I could sneak out, but they never did, of course. It was hot in the tent and I soon fell asleep. When I finally awoke it was late afternoon and the kids had come back. I heard Mother say, "Has anyone seen Janet?" I thought that sure took a long time for anyone to miss me. At that point I had to come out of the tent and when she saw me she said, "What were you doing in there?" I said I had been taking a nap. She didn't look very happy, but really, can you get mad when your child takes a nap?

We didn't even have an outhouse. All we had were some pieces of lumber and plywood thrown together. There was a wall on the back of it but no sides or front. A make-believe toilet was made out of more plywood that just had a hole cut out in the top. Underneath was just a deep hole in the ground. It had a slightly raised floor so that at least we weren't directly on the ground. It was a scary place, right out in the woods. There was absolutely no privacy and always a fear of wild animals. If we had to use it after dark we went with a flashlight. I remember one time someone came running back screaming "skunk!"

David was having his own memories of this place and he shared them with me last month. He said he remembered me coming back from the 'facility' and when I got back he said, "Did you flush?" I got all flustered and went back and looked all over the place but couldn't find a way to flush it. He thought it was hilarious of course. Such a loving brother. Oh, the stories I could tell about him, like when he got me to put my hand on a hot stove burner, or when he caused me to receive a powerful electric shock, or when he talked me into putting my tongue on an icy steel fence post, or the time we were standing in front of a barrel fire and a strong wind came along and burned off my eyebrows. Oh yes, I could tell some stories about him. But I won't. I wonder if all of us are having a lot of childhood memories right now.

Of course there were some good parts to the camping, not just bad. The fact that we could swim all day, the lake was just a few steps away. Fishing was always fun. Turtle hunting. There were other lakes nearby. One time David and I were out walking and exploring. We came to a shoreline and started messing around. Suddenly I spotted a small lizard in the water. It was really something with a pretty blue tail. I reached out and grabbed it and the tail came off in my hand. I was horrified, thinking I had injured the lizard, but it took off running. David thought it was funny of course. One autumn we all found turtles, they were all a pretty good size. They were probably gathering in preparation of hibernation. We were curious as to whether the same turtles would be there the next spring so we all put our initial on our turtle's back in nail polish. The next spring we began turtle hunting but could only find one with an initial. I can't remember whose it was. Down the road there was a huge, high hill covered entirely with sand. We loved to run and tumble down that hill, finally ending up in the lake. Yes, we did have fun.

September 30, 2009
We've had a lot of rain this year. This evening I was out walking and in the soft mud I saw deer tracks. We get a lot of deer here but we don't get to actually see them very often. Around our walking paths we can see where the foliage is all bent down in a circular manner where they spend the night. I really need some night vision binoculars. Mother loved her deer. Every activity would stop when a

deer was spotted. She took numerous photographs of the deer down by the lake edge. Most of the time they came at dusk or early in the morning. She had a big feeder fixed up right outside her kitchen window. It was actually a wooden planter but she used it as a trough. She filled it with various foodstuffs that deer like, such as dried corn. She could sit quietly at her kitchen table and watch them eat. She also loved the ducks. She would watch them from the gosling stage, swimming behind their mother, to full grown. She got so excited whenever she saw them. In the evening she would take a huge amount of dried corn down to the lake and start throwing it out. It was fascinating to watch because ducks would come from everywhere; even the loons would come flying in for their evening meal. Mother loved living there. I was so worried when she first went into the nursing home that she would miss it so much. But, as it happened the infection destroyed only certain brain cell memories. She didn't remember living in Crosslake, she didn't remember her dog, and she didn't remember her husbands. I don't know whether that was actually a good thing or not.

October 2, 2009

I was sitting outside today with Chelsey and watching the hummingbirds. I've always been fascinated with the tiny birds. I've been hanging up feeders for years. Last year I started setting up my lawn chair quite close to the feeder and I was able to start watching their behavior. I don't remember seeing very many hummingbirds when I was a child but I remember Mother telling me about them. She said they never stopped moving except at night when they nested. That really intrigued me. I was sitting in front of her picture window in Crosslake one day when I saw one of the tiny birds land on a branch right in front of me. I said, "Mother, that hummingbird is sitting on the branch." She didn't seem very impressed and I said, "Don't you remember telling me they never stop moving?" Funny how you can remember certain things said to you as a child; and we always believe what our mothers tell us, don't we? Of course I know now that it's not true; they sit quite often, on a branch or on the feeder as they drink.

I've also discovered hummingbirds are quite territorial, often running other hummingbirds off. Last year we had one that was quite aggressive so I started hanging up more feeders to give everyone a chance. One feeder was in the farthest tree. Tom said I was mean, but I said the hummingbird shouldn't be so greedy. Our little guy got quite a workout as he tried to defend every feeder. I wondered if the same bird would show up this year. I don't know whether they return to the same area each year but in the spring if I don't get the feeders out in time they actually buzz my windows. It's really fun having a hummingbird looking in the window at me and it always brings a laugh; but this year we have different birds. Although they are hard to tell apart the coloring is often different.

October 5, 2009

Today I got the photographs developed from our trip to see Mother. Looking at the photos, holding them up to the mirror, I wondered, do we look alike? I do look like her (up close), same chin, same mouth, same blue eyes, but not the same hair. Our hair was never the same; mine was always red, hers was always black. I asked her one time, as a child, why my hair was red when hers was black and Daddy's was brown, she said Daddy had red whiskers. As I was looking at the photos I noticed that Mother's hair was even shorter than it had been during my visit with David. I got upset all over again. I can't believe someone would just cut her hair off; her beautiful white curls. Now it looks gray and a dingy white, no curls, just scraggly looking old hair.

Being so obsessed with Mother's hair got me thinking about my own hair problems as a child. At the beginning of every summer Mother would sit Emily and me down and cut off our hair. She would cut our bangs super short so that we would be 'set for the summer.' We hated it. I swear we looked like the Campbell Soup kids; like someone put a bowl over our heads and cut around it. There were other hair fiascos over the years. My hair was always completely straight and when I wanted some curl Mother would get out the bobby pins and make little pin curls. One night she had me all set up with the bobby pins because I was having school pictures done the next day. I went to bed and in my sleep I took some of the pins out, they must have been too tight. I woke up and realizing what I had done I called out to Mother. But Mother refused to put the bobby pins back in. I cried and cried. I knew it would look really bad. Sure enough, the next morning one side of my hair was curly, the other side straight. I looked awful and the school picture was awful. I have always taken bad photographs anyway; I needed all the help I could get. One year as a young adult I destroyed all of the school photos of me that I could find. But I didn't find all of them because they have been turning up over the years. I guess I'm glad now that some have survived.

One year Mother decided to give me a home permanent. Grandma Ruth was taking us kids to a veteran's Christmas party. I can't remember where it was, at the American Legion maybe, or the VFW. Oh, what a mistake that permanent had been. My hair was a complete frizz ball. I was horrified and tried to stay home but Mother made me go. I was so embarrassed. At least I didn't know anyone there. I was afraid Grandma would be embarrassed to be seen with me but she wasn't.

Once I gained control over my hair I let it grow long. I loved long hair. When I was 15 I was mad at Mother about something and decided to get it all cut off. I'd show her! I told Mother that I wanted to get a haircut and she took me to a beauty school (cheap cuts). She waited in her truck while I went inside. The place was really full, with students all lined up doing various things to people's hair. The young woman who got me asked how much I wanted cut off. She held her fingers about an inch from the bottom of my hair (it was very long) and I said "shorter," she started moving her fingers up and I kept saying shorter, shorter. I told her exactly the way I wanted it styled. She became a little wary and finally said, are you sure? I said yes. I understood her concern, it was a drastic change. When she started cutting off my long, beautiful red hair she began giving the long locks to the other students, for experimentation I guess. When it was finally completed one side was very short, above my ear, and the other side was longer, curving along my chin. I liked it. The look on Mother's face when I went outside was well worth it. It was a sign of my rebellion, of course, so I had probably sashayed out with an attitude. She was angry but didn't say a word.

Shortly after receiving my new do Grandma Ruth took me with her on a trip to Norfolk, Virginia. We had a great time going to cousin Pam's wedding, having lunch on Uncle Boyd's ship, and hanging around the naval base. We then went up to New York State and stayed with some relatives I had never met before. We had to share a bedroom and one morning while getting ready to go out Grandma said, "For God's sake, can't you put a part in your hair?" She then grabbed my comb and with all her force carved a part in my hair. I couldn't understand it – short hair on one side, longer hair on the other, why did I need a part? And to this day there are times when I make sure there is no part in my hair, just to make a point (to myself I guess since Grandma is long gone).

Grandma bought me my first mini dress on that trip. It was so cute; it was a light gray sailor dress with white pin stripes, a collar, and a tie. I loved it and wore it home on the plane. Mother picked us up from the airport and boy was she mad when she saw the dress. It had been an argument we had been having, about me having a mini dress. But she didn't say anything, although she wouldn't let me wear the dress afterward.

Grandma also bought me my first pair of pierced earrings on that trip although I couldn't wear then for quite a while. That was another argument Mother and I were having. She wouldn't let me get my ears pierced. I had tried to go against her wishes by having a friend pierce my ears one day after school. It was easy really, we just used an ice cube pressed against the ear until it was numb and then my friend poked the needle through. I couldn't feel a thing. My reasoning was that if my ears were already pierced what could Mother do about it. The only problem was that I didn't have any earrings to put in my new holes so I had to borrow some from my needle wheedling friend. However, the only earrings she would let me borrow were some ugly gaudy looking things. But then maybe Mother would hate them so much that she'd let me buy some new ones. But I was wrong. When Mother saw me she threw a fit and made me take the earrings out. I cried and cried, and begged, but she wouldn't budge. She finally promised that when I turned 16 she would take me to the doctor and have them professionally pierced.

Nancy had her ears pierced by this time. Mother had taken her to the 'earring doctor.' I'll never forget it. She came home with little brown threads hanging out of the holes. She had to turn the threads several times a day to keep the holes open. She also had to put alcohol on the holes to keep them from getting infected. I don't remember how long she had to wear those threads. Once the holes healed she was able to put the earrings in. After she got the earrings in she became a little paranoid about it and kept pushing the earring backs in, afraid they would fall off. Eventually she pushed one in so far that she couldn't get it out. I don't remember if the hole got infected or not, but she did have to make a trip to the doctor to have the earring removed. The entire thing was hilarious, although Nancy didn't think so; there had been a lot of crying and panic.

Mother was true to her word and when I turned 16 she took me to the earring doctor. The process had evolved by then and they had an earring gun that just kind of implanted the earrings (fake gold studs) right into my ear lobes. It hurt like hell, but it was done. I just had to turn the earrings to keep the holes open and use the alcohol, but it was a lot better than having threads hanging from my ears.

October 6, 2009
The weather turned pretty cool today so I went in search of a long sleeved shirt to wear. I pulled out a pretty, light green knit top. It has a scalloped neckline and tiny brown leaves printed all over it. It is lightly lined and very warm. I

realized that this is the last Christmas present Mother had given me before she started this journey.

October 7, 2009
Early this morning after Tom left for work I was in a deep sleep and was abruptly awakened by some very loud music. I couldn't imagine what it could be, it sounded like music box music. I jumped out of bed and in the dark I followed the sound. It was coming from the living room. I turned on the light and it was coming from a music box sitting on a shelf in the entertainment center. I thought, "What the hell…that thing hasn't worked in years." I picked it up and tried to turn it off but there is no way. The music was very loud. I finally took it to my office (the furthest reaches of the house), set it down and went back to bed. Way too early for me to be up. As I was going back to sleep, still hearing the music faintly, I thought about Aunt Laurie. She loved music boxes. Not only did she collect them, but she even made her own in a ceramic class. When Mother and I went to her funeral Linda took us to Aunt Laurie's apartment and gave us some of her things. I received one of the music boxes that she had made. It is so special to me. Right now it is still packed up in a box from when we moved out here. I really need to get it out of storage and find a place for it. I don't know what made that music box come on this morning but it eventually stopped while I was sleeping. The only explanation I can come up with is that one of the kids had been trying to play with it and had turned the knob and it wouldn't come on. And then over time the vibrations of the house just loosened it up until it was free and the music started. We'd been having trouble with it for quite a while, which is why it hadn't been played. Another one of life's mysteries.

October 9, 2009
This afternoon we went to the Mountain Pine Homecoming ceremony. Kelley was an 8th grade maid. She looked so beautiful wearing a floor length sleeveless aqua colored dress. Ever wonder what kind of shoes they wear under those dresses? Kelley was wearing flip flops! At least she never stumbled. I wish Mother could have seen her. At

thirteen Kelley is already taller than me. She is tall and slender with beautiful long, red hair. I remember when Emily and I reached Mother's size. We were in high school and one day we realized that we could now wear Mother's clothes, if we wanted to. So we decided to raid her closet. She had some nice cashmere sweaters. It didn't end too well though. We took one of the sweaters to the dry cleaners and when we went to get it we were told that they couldn't find it. It was a couple of teenage girls working and we knew they had stolen it, but we didn't know what to do, so we did nothing, didn't even tell Mother. She never mentioned it. We felt horrible.

I was taking photographs of Kelley and the ceremony and I thought about recently going through one of Mother's journals. She was writing about my last visit with her in Crosslake before she went down. It was November but there was very little snow. We had gone out in the woods and I was taking photographs of trees and stuff. Mother had written that I was beautiful and how proud she was that I was a photographer. I was surprised at what she had written and thought how nice that would have been if she had told me what she was thinking. She never was one to share her feelings. I made sure I didn't inherit that trait from her. I always shared my feelings with the boys as children, and now. And the boys don't have any problem sharing their emotions. The word love comes out of their mouths quite often. Still, this reminds me that I need to express my emotions even more.

As we were leaving the ceremony we walked out with Trisha's brother. He started talking to Tom about his car racing last weekend. Since I was already thinking about Mother it brought up memories of the time she had gone to the races with us. She had flown down to spend two weeks with us. At the time Tommy was racing a pure stock car. That weekend he wanted to race in Murphysboro, so we made the 80 mile drive. Tommy was packing the track and asked Mother is she would like to ride with him. She said sure. The doors are welded shut, of course, so she couldn't figure out how to get in. Tommy just picked her up (little as

she is) and slid her in, feet first. It was so funny. Afterwards he pretty much got her out the same way. It was a
late night and she was sound asleep by the time we got
back home.

October 10, 2009

I am having so much trouble with my washing machine.
It's thumping and grinding and vibrating all over the
laundry room. A couple of times it has stopped working
altogether. Tom has got the mechanism zip-tied in place. I
do not want to have to buy a new one until it is absolutely
necessary. At least I don't have to go to the laundromat.
Mother always seemed to like doing the laundry. She
always had a wringer washer. For a while, when I was a
child, she took in laundry for extra money. She picked up
and delivered to the neighbors. There were always rows of
laundry baskets and stacks of hangers in the basement. I
always hung out where Mother was, so I watched
everything she did. I remember a big press she had where
she would iron people's sheets. I asked her one day if I
could help her and she said that I could do the ironing. She
taught me how to iron men's shirts and pants, etc. I think
she paid me ten cents for each piece I ironed. As I went
along I realized how calming it was to iron. I wondered if
she felt that way about the washing.

When Mother married Ken and we moved into his house
she brought that washing machine with her. But she never
taught us how to use it. After Ken's mother died he came
home with his truck full of household items. She'd had a
wringer washer also, so then Mother had two. She was like
in heaven – she'd have both of them going at the same
time. It looked like so much work to me. The clothes would
first go in a big iron sink of water then into the washer, as
they came through the wringer they'd go into another sink
of water then into the other washer and through that
wringer…When I was in high school I got a job at IHOP
and had to wear a uniform. I didn't really think about
washing it. I would have just kept wearing it every day
until it was able to stand up by itself. Although I never

asked Mother to wash it, that uniform was clean and ironed for me every day. I was so thankful for that.

Mother also sewed Barbie doll clothes. She'd make complete wardrobes and sell them. I asked to learn how to sew and she taught me a few simple things. I was able to make dresses for my baby doll although there were no hems or sleeves. There was a large standing blackboard down there also that we fiddled around on. One day I came across a magazine ad that was titled "How well do you draw?" On the ad was a simple drawing of a dog with long, floppy ears. The ad was for some art school and they wanted us to draw the picture and then send it to them for evaluation. I started drawing that dog over and over again with the chalk. I finally got where it looked pretty good then drew it on paper and mailed it in. I never heard a word from the place. Years later, I was already in high school, I think, Emily came across the same magazine ad. She sat down, drew the picture, and mailed it in. Pretty soon a man showed up at our front door! They wanted her in their art school. But Mother said no, we didn't have the money for art school.

October 11, 2009
I had a dream last night that I was walking through the kitchen and saw a small plastic bag of potatoes sitting on the floor leaning against the chair leg. I picked it up and saw that several of the potatoes in the bottom had big chunks missing. It looked like something had gotten in the bag and was eating them. It had to be big, though, because the missing parts were pretty big – like a rat had gotten in. I wonder if this dream is referring back to my earlier potato dream in September. In that dream the potatoes would last for six months, if so then it looks like a chunk of that six months has passed. Time is moving by.

October 14, 2009
Today I was buying Halloween cards for the grandkids and Mother. Mother used to always send cards to the boys and later the grandkids. She loved to send cards, she sent them for every holiday and occasion. She even sent me a

sympathy card once when my pet died. She never missed a birthday or anniversary. When we were packing up her things after her house sold I found a handful of Halloween cards that she never sent. They were for grandchildren and great-grandchildren. I brought them home and will use them myself someday. It's sad that we won't receive any more from her. It was always nice to know that she was thinking about us.

October 17, 2009

Tonight I made meatloaf for dinner and it made me think of when I first learned how to make it. I was in grade school still and Nancy called me into the kitchen. She said, "Mom said I have to teach you how to make meatloaf." Nancy looked pretty mad that she had to teach me, and I sure wasn't crazy about learning it from her. I felt a little betrayed that Mother wasn't going to teach me herself. I knew Mother was extremely busy, she almost always had a full-time job, it's hard to support a family of six. Nancy went on to teach me quite a bit about cooking and then I was taught more when I was in high school; we learned all about setting up and running a household. I wonder if they teach that nowadays, family planning classes. We also had classes on manners and etiquette. Mother didn't know how to cook when she married Daddy. She didn't have to so no one taught her. Once married she had to learn fast. Daddy probably taught her a lot himself. He cooked occasionally for us. He had special dishes he liked to make.

October 19, 2009

I was watching TV today and a doctor was talking about depression. He made this statement: "Memory loss is caused by depression." I thought, are you kidding? Memory loss caused by depression? Is that why my Mother has memory loss? Wouldn't it be the other way around – memory loss causes depression? I know that when I am depressed my memory is excellent. I can remember every bad thing that has <u>ever</u> happened to me. I can remember them in precise detail and will dwell on them until the depression passes.

October 20, 2009

I found a small box of stuff out in the storage building that had been packed away since we moved. I brought it in and started going through it. Funny, when we moved we just started throwing stuff in any box we could find figuring we'd straighten everything out later. Some of the boxes are a collection of all different kinds of items and they're fun to go through. This box had some interesting items. Among them were some iron soldiers Mother had given Tom. The family has always had a hard time deciding what to give him as gifts. Mother saw these soldiers in a flea market and thought he'd like them. He loves them; he loves all antique toys. She followed it up with a few more that she found. Mother loved shopping flea markets and I think she was happy to have this little mission of something to look for. I know Tom felt touched that she would do that for him.

October 22, 2009

We have just received 17 hours of rain. Our pond is overflowing and we have a fast moving stream going through the entire property. As I was standing at the door watching it made me think of one summer when I was young. It was a beautiful warm, sunny day and David and I were getting ready to play in the sprinkler. We were wearing our swimming suits. All of a sudden a storm blew in. Mother had laundry hanging outside on the clothesline and she yelled for us to help her take it in quickly. We were pulling that stuff off the line and running it into the house. The wind was blowing so hard that on one trip the back door slammed shut violently on my back. Glass went flying everywhere, a large piece slicing open the back of my leg. I started howling with pain. Mother took me in the bathroom and started cleaning me up but said I'd have to get stitches. I'd never had stitches before and the thought scared me even more. Even though I was holding a towel to the bleeding wound Mother laid out a large sheet of plastic on the back seat of her car. I could understand that she didn't want blood on the seat, but it still hurt my feelings a little that she was even thinking about that. It was my first time in an emergency room. They were a lot different back then, back then you got immediate attention. As we were being led to a room, still holding the towel to my leg, I noticed a man staring at me. I looked down at myself; I was wearing a raincoat, but it was standing wide open, with just my swimming suit underneath. I pulled the coat closed, holding it closed until I was out of the man's sight. That really creeped me out. I still have the scar from the stitches behind my knee. And the memory of being creeped out.

October 23, 2009

I was at the pool today and there were two new women in the exercise class. One was an elderly woman and the other, younger, was her caregiver. They were actually there at the last class, but they weren't anywhere near me, so I didn't pay much attention. Today, however, I was still in the locker room when they arrived. The elderly woman is in her 80s and her name is Barbara; the younger woman, about my age, is Judy. When they entered the locker room Judy told Barbara to take off her clothes (they already had their swimming suits on underneath) and Barbara said no, she didn't want to take her clothes off. I left the locker room at that point and a few minutes later they entered the pool area. Barbara was still fully dressed but Judy was in her suit. Judy sat Barbara on the bench next to the door, nestled in amongst our towels and bags, telling her to sit right there. Judy entered the pool and took a spot near me. I was surprised that Judy was still going to attend the class; I would have turned around and left when Barbara refused to participate, but I guess she had her own reasons. After a few minutes Barbara got up from the bench. Judy said, "Barbara, sit back down." Judy had an accent so it sounded like, "Ba bra, sit back down." Barbara sat down. A few minutes later it happened again, "Ba bra, you must sit back down, the floor is wet and I don't want you to slip and fall." Barbara sat back down. After awhile people started leaving, one at a time, and Barbara would stand up again. I realized that every time someone left Barbara thought the class was over and she would stand up to leave. "Ba bra, you must sit down." Barbara always replied that she was ready to leave, one time very loudly, shouting it really and Judy would say it wasn't time, class wasn't over yet. She really was in the way by then as people would have to reach around her to get their belongings. I suggested to Judy that maybe she would like the other bench better. Judy agreed and moved her to the empty bench on the other side of the door. Barbara still kept standing up to leave and they'd have the same conversation.

During the class Judy and I talked quite a bit. Barbara reminded me of Mother, of course. Judy said that when Barbara started having memory problems she moved in with her daughter, who lives in a condo. Judy goes in during the day, while the daughter works, to take care of Barbara. What a nice set-up that is; they're lucky they can do that. I discussed Mother a little. Judy said Barbara is usually sweet but some days she's in a horrible mood. I asked if she has Alzheimer's and Judy said the daughter won't answer that question. At one point Barbara actually called Judy by her daughter's name. Judy asked me what the difference is between dementia and Alzheimer's. That kind of caught me off guard. What is the difference exactly? I said, "Well, in dementia the gray cells in the brain die, leading to memory loss. And with Alzheimer's it's chemical. They basically have the same symptoms, but different causes." I really need to do some research on this.

At the end of class I left the pool before the two women. I had just finished with my shower when they came in. Judy was getting ready to get in the shower and she was giving directions to Barbara to sit right there in that chair and not move until she was finished. Barbara said, "I'm not going to get up." I told Judy I'd wait with her while she took her shower; which I did. I wonder if they'll be back. Barbara is so lucky to have a full time companion; that's exactly what Mother needs.

October 30, 2009

Tom and I went into town today and received our flu shots. Tom gets one every year now, ever since he got the flu really bad several years ago. We now get the free shots that the government gives out. It made me think about when Mother got the flu a couple of years ago. I didn't get to see her but David called and told me about it when she was getting steadily worse. It scared the hell out of all of us. He said he had just gone to see her and the nursing home people had her dressed and propped up in a wheelchair, sitting at the dining table with dinner in front of her. David said she was nearly unconscious and he took her back to her room and put her to bed. That is so crazy; she should not have left her bed until she was over it. I asked David if he was going to take her to the doctor and he said they had one there that had looked at her. She probably should have been in the hospital where she could get the care she needed. Especially since at the onset she had vomited up a blood clot. But the doctor said he believed the blood clot was caused by her osteoporosis medication. So he just took her off the medicine, so now she isn't being treated for that. They now have all kinds of warnings about osteoporosis medications so it's probably good that she's not taking it. Still, osteoporosis is serious and can even cause jaw bone loss. I wonder if that's why she lost all of her bottom teeth, but David said her gums were healthy, just not her teeth.

When Mother was living with me my doctor had her tested for osteoporosis. She was put onto a huge scanning machine. I was able to sit with the nurse and watch the results roll out of the computer. The scan showed that there were actual holes eaten out of her bones. It was severe. The doctor put her on the medication immediately, she also needed exercise. I had trouble getting her to do that. When she complained that her shoulders (or whatever) were hurting I'd tell her it was because she didn't exercise. She would say, "But there's nothing to do." Yeah, right, nothing to do; however, I'd tell her to walk. "But there's no where to walk." And I'd say, just walk around the yard. And she did, she started walking around and around the yard, even getting friendly with my neighbor next door who was often working in his garden. Once she returned to Minnesota her new doctor took her off the medication for some reason, even though her medical records had been forwarded on to him. I'm not sure when she was put back on it, one of the nursing homes. I'd like to see a new scan and see what her bones look like now. She can't stand up straight and she can't or won't turn her head.

I remember having the flu one time when I was a child. It was extreme. I was pretty much unconscious the entire time. I knew Mother was really worried about me one night when she woke me up and had placed stuffed animals all over my bed. She said, "You have company. Look who came to see you." I looked at my bed and the animals and I felt such love coming from her and I fell back to sleep.

November 2, 2009

I went in this morning and received my allergy shots. I'm allergic to so many things; a lot of food: chocolate, peanuts, onions, cucumbers, and walnuts; along with cats and dogs and almost everything outside; the usual allergens. I had a lot of allergies as a child also, but this time around it affects my breathing. As a child my allergies affected my skin. I had eczema extremely bad. The itch was unbearable. It was the worst in the winter and cleared up in the summer.

Mother tried everything to control my eczema. I remember the two of us riding the bus downtown to see a doctor. I received shots in the butt while we were there and then received a sucker that would have a little plastic kitchen appliance on the end of the stick – like a tiny vacuum cleaner or iron.

Mother set up big bright lights that I had to lay under. I had to wear small plastic things to cover my eyes. There were pills and salves. Nothing worked. I couldn't eat chocolate or peanuts or fried foods or whole milk. The alternatives were pretty bad, such as skim milk or strawberry flavored instant milk. I couldn't wear wool or use a wool blanket. Being around cats and dogs would make me wheeze. Poor Mother. Grandma Ruth used to give me the white Easter bunnies and the white Santa Claus. They were probably white chocolate and we didn't know the difference; the taste was a lot different however.

One year Grandma Ruth brought me an Aloe Vera plant and said that the liquid inside was supposed to be healing. Mother cut it open and put it on the rash but it didn't work.

The only thing that would ease it was Aquaphor, but even that didn't stop the itch. I was in grade school and didn't have enough self-control not to scratch. It drove Mother and Daddy crazy of course. I was miserable. The eczema finally went away by itself when I got to high school. I was able to eat chocolate and peanuts and anything I wanted to; at least until some years ago when the allergies started back up. I read that that is quite common – allergies as a child presents as eczema and allergies in an adult (same person) presents as asthma. At least I'm normal!

November 3, 2009

Today I was out on the back deck shaking out a rug when I backed up and fell through a hole. My entire right leg went all of the way through up to my thigh. I thought my leg was broken at first the pain was so incredible. I visualized lying there all day until Tom got home from work. I couldn't let that happen. I had to get up. I was still for a minute and then carefully pulled my leg out. I was able to stand so I hobbled on into the house and went into the bedroom. I pulled off my jeans and saw that my leg, especially my thigh, was in bad shape. The pain was so bad and as I lay there my temperature started spiking and my immune system started screaming. I knew the bruising would be horrific. It made me think about the time when I was a child and I was playing in the park. It was early evening and I was the only one there. I climbed up the ladder to the top of the slide and since I was alone I thought I would try a fancy move and go down the slide backwards. However, I fell from the top of the ladder and landed on my right arm. I just knew that it was broken and I ran home crying, cradling my arm. I ran in the back door and Mother was preparing dinner. I cried, "I broke my arm!" She just looked at me and said, "It's alright," I was shocked and hurt, how could she know that by just looking at me? She was right, of course. I was fine.

November 4, 2009

Today I was reading James Hillman's book *The Soul's Code*. In the book he was talking about what he called depersonalization reincarnation. He said that moral theology from the East considers the suffering of isolation to be the task imposed on this life by past karmic actions in another incarnation or as a preparation for the next. This is an interesting concept. One time when Mother and I were talking about my writing aspirations she said, "I remember when you sent me that strange story." Strange story? I said, "Do you mean the one about reincarnation?" We talked about reincarnation and whether she believed in it. She said she wasn't sure whether she believed in it or not, but she did believe there was something beyond this existence after death.

Hillman went on to say moral theologies whether Eastern or Western subtly transform the sense of loneliness, exacerbating its unhappiness. Another interesting concept. I wonder if dementia has a purpose. Does it prepare the soul for reincarnation? Are there some souls that need to completely empty their memories for an easier transition? But along the way the soul suffers from the isolation and loneliness that it creates. Because when you have no memories there can be no new friendships; no meaningful conversations, there is just isolation from the world. And that causes unhappiness.

November 5, 2009

Zakary and I were watching TV this evening and there was a big fish tank on the program. I said, "Wouldn't it be fun to have a fish tank like that? I had one when I was growing up." We had a huge tank right in the living room. I loved it and could sit for an hour watching the fish. We each got to pick out the fish we wanted for ourselves. I picked out little tiny ones that has a red and silver stripe down their sides. When the light hit them just right the stripes would flash. Mother, of course, had the job of occasionally cleaning the tank. She'd have to transport the fish in buckets to the bathtub. Then she'd have to scoop out all of the water and clean the glass sides. Everything would have to be done quickly so as to get the fish back in the tank with the air bubble tubes. One day Mother brought home some big, pretty angelfish. Unfortunately, the angelfish ate all of the other fish and that was the end of that.

November 6, 2009

This afternoon Trisha, Kelley, and Zakary came over. Zakary is spending the night with us and Trisha and Kelley were headed for a football game where Kelley's boyfriend is playing. Kelley is now fourteen. I remember my first date, at least I thought it was a date, turned out it wasn't. I was also fourteen, and I got invited to a dance by a guy I barely knew. I was surprised when Mother said I could go. I don't remember his name, however he said it was a dance with a battle of the bands, and he was in one of the bands. Mother and I were very excited and we went shopping and she bought me a frilly pink party dress and shiny, white patent leather shoes. Since we were only fourteen the boy's brother was driving and they picked me up at the house. There was another couple with us so I sat in the front seat with the brother and off we went to the dance. When we entered I was shocked to see that I was the only girl wearing a dress, and a pink frilly thing at that! I was so embarrassed that I spent most of the evening trying to keep hidden as best as I could. I never saw the boy again afterwards; thankfully we didn't attend the same school.

My real first date happened about a year later. Again I was surprised Mother said I could go. My "special" guy was a few years older than me. Mother was dating Ken at the time. When the big night arrived I was surprised when Ken showed up. He never hung out at our house. I said, "What are you doing here?" I was nervous enough without him being there. He said he was waiting to meet my guy. As I got ready for my date I put on a little more makeup than usual – primping. When I was ready and went into the living room to wait Ken took one look at my blue eye shadow and told me to go wash it off. I said, "You can't tell me what to do!" He insisted I wash it off and I finally called Mother, who was in the other room, and she came in. When I explained what was going on she told me to go wash it off. I was mad, but did what I was told, thinking this was going to be a long, difficult teenage stage to go through with those two. Luckily, my date was wise enough to come up to the door to get me. I remember when Nancy was dating her "special" guy and one night he just pulled up and started honking his horn for Nancy to come out. Daddy hit the roof!

November 9, 2009

I was watching a health program on TV today. The program was about osteoporosis. They had a celebrity on that was talking about her own experience with the condition. She was touting a certain medication, of course, but at the end she said, "It doesn't matter what you do, if God wants you to have osteoporosis, then you'll have osteoporosis." The hosts of the show didn't comment on what she said, just continued on about how you can prevent osteoporosis. That was funny. They claim osteoporosis can be hereditary so I paid special attention to the prevention information.

November 10, 2009

I got an email from David today. He said that last Tuesday Mother had a bad fall. He said she was walking down the hallway and got to moving too fast. One of the nurses tried to get to her and slow her down but she got there too late. Mother fell on her right shoulder and the side of her head smacked into the floor. The nurse said Mother never even tried to break her fall as she went down. The nurse helped her up and thought she was okay, but then her face started turning black and blue and her eye swelled closed. They checked her vitals and her blood pressure was over 200. They took her to the emergency room and X-rays showed that some of the bones around her eye were broken. The doctor said she should see a specialist.

David was working out of town all week so the nurse was talking to him by phone. They made an appointment with the specialist, David wanting to make it next week when he'd be working in town, but the specialist wanted to see her right away. So, David got up at 3:30 am and drove from Detroit Lakes to the city. The specialist looked at the X-rays and decided not to do any surgery, that the breaks would heal on their own and the black and blue would be gone in about a week. David said Mother wouldn't take any pain medication, but finally agreed to take some Tylenol.

Poor Mother! She fell on the same day I did, exactly one week ago today. And on the same side of the body. Freaky. I'm glad Mother didn't have to have surgery. My bruising is so bad that I can't go to exercise class at the pool. My entire thigh is black with a big muscle sticking out. I even have to wear loose clothing. Ouch!

I sent an email to David telling him that we'd be coming up in a couple of weeks. We are waiting for Tom to finish up the job he is working on.

November 12, 2009
I looked out my office window and my roses are blooming! Amazing, it's the middle of November and my roses are in full bloom and very beautiful. Gardening has never been a talent of mine. I have the blackest of thumbs. The only reason these roses have survived is because I don't have to do anything, they take care of themselves.

Mother, on the other hand, had the greenest of thumbs. She could grow anything. When I was growing up she always had big gardens. One year I got a garden of my own. It was small and round. I planted colorful flowers in it and took care of it for a while. One day Daddy said he wanted to plant a tree right in the middle of it. I was upset; a tree in my garden? I pretty much lost interest after that.

Mother always had amazing things growing. She had a big strawberry patch set in risers. One year she had some huge sunflowers. I remember picking the ripe seeds. She popped them in the oven and we enjoyed them roasted. Peas picked right from the plant were delicious. One year she tried her hand at grapes. She constructed a wire fence and trellis. The plants were growing but I think the winter killed them off. Ken built her a small greenhouse in the backyard after they got married. She was always cutting and pruning something. Even after Mother retired to Crosslake she had a garden. She also grew her own herbs and we'd find them hanging around in the process of drying. I wish I had inherited that trait.

When Tom got home from work this afternoon he said there's a chance we could be leaving for Minnesota tomorrow. He may have an unexpected couple of days off.

November 13, 2009
Tom called about 9:30 and said the trip is on. We left about noon. The old Mountain Pine School burned down a few nights ago. All of the sirens woke me and looking out the window I could see the glow from the flames though the trees, amazing because we're a few miles away. I wanted to stop there on our way out of town and take some photographs to go with the ones I had taken inside the school a few months ago. I suppose it could have waited until we got back but I didn't want to take the chance that something else would happen – a berserk bulldozer or something. They were getting ready to demolish the old school but the fire got to it first.

Pulling up to the site we could see the total devastation. The structure of the school was now only scorched cement blocks; the entire outline of the school. And right in the middle was a still-standing brick chimney. I pulled out my camera and had the first shot posed; I pushed the button and the shutter closed, but it didn't reopen. My camera was completely dead! Crap, I didn't check the batteries before leaving. I got out a disposable camera I had in my bag and took a few shots. We got back in the truck, preparing to leave, and I looked at the camera again trying to see what was wrong and suddenly it was working fine. I got back out and took some more pictures.

Finally out on the road headed for Minnesota. In the afternoon I called David and said there had been a slight change in plans and we were on our way now. I knew that he was on his way to the deer woods but I wanted to let him know we'd be in town over the weekend. He was telling me that deer hunting was really bad this year. Since there was no snow the deer just laid down in the middle of the corn fields and nobody could see them. As we were talking my cell phone went dead. I thought we must be in a dead zone, but when I flipped it shut and then back open it was just fine again and I was able to call him right back. Welcome to freaky Friday the 13th.

Tonight we are at a motel outside of Des Moines. I can't get David and his deer hunting off my mind. I love the story about the first time he went hunting with Daddy and some of the neighbor men. He was probably 14. They went up to the North woods and there was a lot of snow. David went off by himself and got lost. Ha Ha Ha. He finally made his way out of the woods and started walking down a road until someone found him. I have photographs somewhere. They all wore bright red, wool jackets in those days. And there is one photo of David proudly posing with his first deer kill. I don't like that picture.

November 14, 2009

We had an uneventful drive today and got to the nursing home a little before 4:00. Once I got up to Mother's unit I found her right away sitting at a table in the dining area. I sat down in the chair nearest to her, smiled, and said hello. She smiled back. I was a little surprised by that. I said, "I'm here to visit you," and she said, "I know that." I said, "Really, do you know who I am?" "Yes, I do." "Who am I?" That got a puzzled look from her, like she was thinking. I said, "I'm Janet," and she said, "I know that." I said, "I look familiar, you know that you know me, but don't know who I am?" She just kept smiling with a puzzled look on her face.

There was a woman in a wheelchair on the other side of Mother. She was holding a brown teddy bear and was kissing it all over. After greeting Mother I said hello to the woman, but just briefly. The woman tried starting a conversation with me and at one point I said, "really," to something she said, although I couldn't hear what she was saying. But I was keeping all of my attention on Mother. I wanted her to understand that I was there to visit her. The woman then wheeled herself over and wedged herself in between Mother and me. She couldn't get too close because of the table so she didn't block my field of vision and I just kept talking with Mother. When the woman couldn't get my full attention she went to the other side of me. She started pulling up her pant leg to show me something but when she still couldn't get my attention she left. I don't want to be rude to anyone, but I have precious little time with Mother.

The orderlies (are they orderlies, or male nurses, or CNAs, I don't know) were bringing residents into the dining area in preparation for dinner. I asked Mother if she wanted to show me her room but she said no. Okay. I just stayed there, no problem, and it gave me the chance to watch her in her environment. I said, "David is in the deer woods this weekend." She said, "Really, I was hoping he'd be coming to see me." Interesting, was she remembering David, the real David? I said, "Sorry, you get me instead." She was looking off into the room then said, "There's..." I looked and saw Ray walk into the area and I said, "Ray?" She said yes. I asked if she likes Ray and she said, "Oh yes." I wasn't talking really because I could see that she was watching everything going on around her. Then she said, "Oh look, there's David." I looked around, but it was a male nurse pushing a man in a wheelchair into the area. I said, "That's not David." "It's not?" She kept saying 'there's David' and I finally caught on that every time a man was brought in she said it. That happened four times.

There were tables placed throughout the area all the way into the first visiting area. They were bringing in people in wheelchairs and placing them at various tables. They wheeled one woman up to the table nearest to Mother's; I noticed that it was the same woman who was always loudly saying 'help me, help me.' They had moved her from another table and she was not happy about it. One of the nurses said, "Come on, you can take your coloring with you. Your husband, Carlton, will be here in a few minutes." I saw that there was a metal plate built into the right arm of her chair which could hold a page from a coloring book. She started coloring it with a purple crayon. She colored continuously. They placed another woman in a wheelchair at the same table across from her. The first woman started chanting, "help me, help me, help me..." The second woman said, "Shut up!" The first woman looked at her and then continued her chanting, help me, help me, help me, only faster. The second woman started up, "Shut Up, Shut Up, Shut Up..." Then she started pushing the table into the first woman, her chair anyway, who kept up her help me chanting faster and faster. They chanted back and forth for about ten minutes. The help me woman looked really normal; her hair was well done, she was dressed nicely – still, she's in the memory care unit. Two black male nurses (dressed all in white) came over and said they wanted to take her to the bathroom. She said she didn't need to and they said they wanted to take her now, before she needed to and off they went.

Everyone was put in the main dining area at first then they started spacing them out. There was another woman nearby. She was dressed in purple and she had pure white hair. She had a very high-pitched voice and she was yelling, "Where's my son? He's supposed to be here!" Then she'd say, "I want to go home!" They took her and wheeled her all the way to the other end of the room and put at a table. That pissed her off even more and she started yelling even louder, "What are you doing? I don't want to be down here! Where's my son? He's supposed to be here. I want to go home!" Mother and I smiled and I said, "She's already home." Suddenly two nurses ran down to the woman and I saw that she had scooted herself forward and was about to fall out of her wheelchair. They lifted her back in. The woman continued to yell out off and on.

A man was wheeled up and put near Mother and me, but not at a table. Suddenly he just bent himself forward, like he was looking at his feet. I thought how that would kill my back if I did that. I couldn't figure out what he was doing, he looked like he was going to fall out of his chair. Someone finally noticed and came over and sat him back up and then moved him over to a table.

In the meantime Mother and I were talking. I stroked her face and her nose, looking at the bruises left from her fall. I asked her if the bruises still hurt and she shook her head no.

I said it must have hurt when she fell. She sat up straight, eyes wide open and said, "I don't know what happened." I explained that she had been walking down the hall and got going too fast, that the nurse tried to get to her in time, but she fell on her shoulder with her face smashing into the floor. I stroked her hair; it's not quite as short as on my last visit, having grown out a little. She was wearing dark blue slacks and a white top with a small flag design on it. She also had on a very soft, light blue jacket that had a zipper. I have one like it. I ran my hand down the softness on her arm and told her how pretty her jacket was. She didn't have any trouble with my touching her.

I wanted to try out my idea (Tom's idea really) of talking about the past. I started to ask if she remembered jumping in the lake every spring with Aunt Laurie and I got as far as, "Do you remember when you and Aunt Laurie…" And she said, "Oh yes," very loudly. I laughed and said I didn't even finish my sentence. I asked if she remembered them jumping in the lake every spring and she said yes. Since it had just been Veteran's Day I asked her if she remembered how she had celebrated the holiday. She said, "Well, ah, um, I had fun." I asked her what her daddy did during the war. She said, "My daddy?" When I said yes she said she didn't know. I said, "Well, he was in WWI and we know that he was wounded, that he had a big scar down his arm from a sword, I think." She listened to me but didn't remember anything. I continued, saying that during WWII she worked in an airplane factory and asked if she remembered and she said, "Oh yes." I asked her what my daddy did during the war but she didn't know.

I asked if David had visited lately and she said, "No, I haven't seen him." I asked if Nancy had visited lately and she said, "No, I haven't seen her." Conversation wasn't going so well so I just went back to what we had been doing, which was watching what was going on around us. I've never seen her as part of the group before; she had always been off by herself.

A nurse turned on some music and Mother got excited and was really listening to it. I asked if she knew who was singing but she didn't know. It was Big Band music. I said why don't you dance but she said no. I said why don't you sing along but she said no. She was watching everything and everyone. One of the nurses started dancing around the area. The room was now completely full of residents and staff. A lot of them were gathered around one table in particular and Mother was watching them closely. The dancing nurse was now sitting at that table and she was swaying to the music. Mother leaned towards me and said, "You're dancing." I didn't quite get that, but let it go. She seemed to be fully in the moment and enjoying herself.

A man came into the area and was very friendly to everyone, everyone seemed to know him. A woman in a wheelchair was sitting behind one of the tables and the man went over and greeted her and started talking to her. Mother leaned forward, looked directly at me and said, "He must think you're really cute." I was puzzled. Then the man left the unit.

A man in a wheelchair got wheeled in and was put at the table with the woman. He was wearing headphones. He started complaining really loud about something. Mother leaned toward me, looked directly at me and said, "What did you do?" I finally got it. She wants to be talking to them and was using me as a surrogate. Strange. And sad. After awhile they moved the man to a different area, near the nurse's desk, and I could see that he only has one leg. He was wearing underwear on the bottom but was fully dressed on the top. His left leg is only a stub.

The nurse stopped dancing and left the area. Mother started having a conversation with me, but I couldn't hear her words clearly, she was talking very quietly. She seemed to be talking about the music and she said, "Oh, that's..." She never seems to finish her sentences (out loud anyway). I said, "That's what? You didn't finish your sentence." But she just gave me a puzzled look, like yes, I did. This happened many times and each time I tried to get her to finish the sentence but just got that look on her face. She started tapping her nails on the table in time to the music. She was wearing red polish that is all chipped. I'm so surprised by her animation with the music and the people.

There seems to be three conversations going on, the one I'm having with her that she doesn't understand; the one that she's having with me that I don't understand; and the one we're having together which we do understand. Four really, the one she's having with herself. It's like she understands the concept (or thought) but not the words. She knows what she wants to convey, she just can't think of the right word, so she doesn't finish the sentence. It's frustrating. I do it myself occasionally and I'll catch myself not finishing my sentence because I know what I meant.

The chanting woman was brought back in and placed at the table. She saw that the other woman was still there and looking at her very sternly she started in, "help me, help me, help me..." The other woman started right up, "shut up shut up, shut up..." The help me's husband arrived and she immediately stopped chanting and started talking with him. They seemed so normal, yet she's in the memory care unit, and she chants.

The entire time I was there, about an hour and a half, Mother never put down a little plastic cup she was holding. She would play with it, turning it or tapping on it, or something, but never put it down. I asked what had been in the cup – milk, medicine, pills? But she doesn't know. I asked how many pills she takes. Ten? "No, probably two." "What are they for?" "I don't know."

She really confused me today because everything she said yes to last time I saw her she now said no to. Are you hungry? No. Did you eat lunch? No. Breakfast? No, I never eat, I never get hungry. When I questioned that she looked at me like I was nuts. I don't know when her no's mean no or yes. It was very frustrating for both of us. It was difficult for us to communicate.

During this time Ray was walking, walking, walking. He'd walk up to someone and look them right in the face, not like he wanted to say something, but like he was looking for someone familiar. He did that to me the first time I saw him. It's really quite disconcerting because he doesn't say anything. He would walk between people. Sometimes have to squeeze through tight spots and walk between objects. Suddenly he came up right behind Mother. He wasn't looking at her and she didn't see him, but he was walking at a fast pace. All of a sudden a nurse said, "He's going to fall," and two nurses came running up, each grabbing an arm to stop him. One nurse grabbed a chair, put it behind him, and they sat him down. He let out a little squeal then put his head down and went to sleep. I realized he was going so fast that he was about to collide with Mother. She would have been seriously hurt. He's a big man. Occasionally he let out a jerk while he was sleeping. Mother also jerked off and on the entire time. What are those jerks? I understand why Ray would be jerking, he was asleep; but why did Mother jerk? Was there a short circuit somewhere or something?

A woman came over and stood right between us. She was fumbling with the buttons on her sweater. I asked her if she needed help. I buttoned her up and said, "There you go." She said, "Am I ready to go?" I said yes. I then realized it was that obnoxious woman from my visit with David. I noticed that Mother looked very angry suddenly. The woman reached out and patted Mother's left arm. Mother reacted very strongly, she jumped and yelled, "Stop that!" I became on alert. The woman just stood there and didn't say anything. Neither Mother nor I looked at her. I placed my hand on the table, ready for action. She reached towards Mother again and I brought my arm up and said, "Don't touch." She was just able to touch Mother's shoulder briefly. Mother was very angry. I placed my arm on Mother's chair, waiting. We made no eye contact with her. A nurse finally came and led her away. I asked Mother if she was okay. I said, "You don't like her, do you?" She said no. She was really steaming. I touched Mother's arm and she jumped in anger. I see how she can get in such a foul mood.

I waited a few minutes and then told Mother that I was going to leave. I asked if she wanted me to come back tomorrow and she said, oh yes. I had asked her earlier if she wanted me to come back tonight and she said no. I said, "Really, you don't want me to come back?" No. I said, "Why not?" And she said, "Because I don't like it." Did she mean no or yes? I think she meant yes. I said, "So, I'm leaving." "Okay." I got up, kissed her on the forehead and said I love you. She said, "I love you too." "I'll see you tomorrow." "Okay." As I stood up to leave she started to stand up also. I thought she didn't want me to leave so I sat back down. She said, "What are you doing?" And I said, "I can stay a few more minutes," and she said, "Go on." I said okay, but that I needed to go to her room for a minute. She said okay. I got up, went to her room, signed the calendar and then went back; she was gone. I didn't look for her, just left.

November 15, 2009

Tom and I had breakfast with Dorothy and then headed for the nursing home, arriving shortly after lunch. Upon entering I went to sign in. Behind the counter was a woman with short dark hair. 50ish. She was knitting and didn't even look up. I wonder if these women are volunteers. I went up to the second level and crossed the bridge with the purple, blue, and beige patterned furniture and carpet. It's the same furniture as in the front lobby and in Mother's unit. There was a display case containing items from the Minnesota Historic Masonic Society and Museum. There were photos of people in the other unit, flower water colors, and metal flower wall sculptures. Near the end of the bridge a man and woman were walking with therapists. They were wearing straps like the ones they had used with Mother when she was in the Pine River Nursing Home, recovering from her broken hip, at the beginning of this journey.

Arriving in Mother's unit it was pretty empty of people. I found her in the dining area. She was sitting at the end of a table, sound asleep. Across the table from her was an elderly white haired lady in a wheelchair and next to her was a young, pretty, dark haired nurse. I pulled up a chair close to Mother and quietly said, "Mother." The nurse said she had just gone to sleep. I said, "I hate to wake her up." I did, but I didn't just drive 850 miles to watch her sleep. I started saying Mother, Mother, while tapping her arm and stroking it. I went to her other side and said, "Mother," thinking maybe that would work better. It didn't. I knew it would be a risk waking her up like this, who knew what her mood would be getting jerked out of sleep. She finally opened her eyes and looked at me. I smiled and said, "Hello." She smiled back and said, "Hello." Whew, that's good I thought. I asked her if she'd like to walk down to her room and she said yes.

I took her arm and we walked down to her room, holding hands. I had to steer her into the room. I sat her down on the edge of her bed and she started crying. I said, "What's wrong?" She didn't say anything. I sat down next to her and put my arms around her. I asked, "Are you okay? Is there something wrong?" She shook her head no. I asked, "Are you just happy to see me?" She nodded her head yes. Her nose started dripping of course. I said, "Your nose is dripping," and she said, "Oh, mine does that too." I got up and looked for a tissue but couldn't find any anywhere. I finally had to get a paper towel out of the bathroom. Her tears stopped and she pointed towards the wall and said, "Give me that." I looked and saw a red, plastic Christmas ball hanging in front of her calendar. I took it down and said, "This?" She nodded and took it from me. I said, "It's very pretty." She said, "Yes." She held the ball, turning it around and around in her hands.

I sat down on the floor in front of her so that she could easily look at me. I started talking to her although she didn't really say anything. She pretty much kept her eyes on the red plastic ball. Sitting where she was she could see into the hallway and I noticed that every time someone walked by her head would jerk up with a look of hope on her face. After several minutes a Jamaican female nurse was walking by, saw Mother looking, and came in. She had short black curly hair and was very robust. She sat down next to Mother and put her arms around her. "How are you doing today, Shirley?" Mother started crying again. "Now Shirley, I'm not going to come and play with you if you're going to act like this," she said in a very friendly way. I said, "She always cries when she's happy." All this time she had her left arm around Mother's shoulders very tightly and squeezing. Then she said, "I'll be back later to play with you, okay?" And Mother said, "Okay." Mother stopped crying immediately when the nurse left. She definitely needs personal attention like that. I'm sure it's very lonely not being able to remember anyone.

Today Mother was wearing olive green corduroy slacks and a light green sweatshirt that has designs on it; there was a moose, a bear, a canoe, a pine tree, and a couple of other things – almost like symbols of Crosslake. It was interesting because I was wearing a sweatshirt with pictures of bears, wolves, fish, eagles, and pine trees – symbols of Arkansas. Mother's hands were very dry, like mine right now. She focused on the images on my sweatshirt and said it was pretty. She seemed to be in a world all her own; sweet – like my friend Fran said recently; describing the Alzheimer's patients she used to work with.

When we first got in her room I noticed that the entire right side of Mother's face was an ugly yellow, the remnants of the bruising from her fall. I hadn't noticed it at all yesterday. I guess because the other side of her was facing me. I got my camera out and took some pictures. Her eyes were all bloodshot and her nose was red. I reached in my tote bag and pulled Chelsey out. I said, "Look Mother, Chelsey has come to visit you. You remember Chelsey, don't you?" Mother looked at Chelsey but didn't say anything. I said, "Would you like to hold her?" Mother said no. I said, "Okay, but I'm going to let her sit next to you a minute." I put Chelsey on the bed right up against Mother's thigh. Chelsey sat there for a minute then took off across the bed. I took her blanket out, put it on the bed, and she went underneath and hunkered down, not moving again until it was time to leave.

Meanwhile Mother was still watching the hallway. I happened to glance out there when a man walked past and Mother said, "There goes David." I said, "Where is he going?" She just shrugged her shoulders, "Just going." I had brought her a pretty, short sleeve blue and white top and I pulled it out and showed her, asking if she liked it. I didn't have a name label so I had just written her name on the tag with a magic marker. I put it in the closet for her. She was still holding on tightly to the red ball. I asked if she would hold my hand for a moment and she said, "Oh yes." I took the ball and she grasped my hands tightly. It was like she had to hold on to something. There was almost like a sense of urgency to it. I took off the long crucifix I was wearing and asked if she would like to hold it. She held it for the rest of my visit.

I noticed that Mother's attention was really wandering; and sometimes she acted like she was listening to something. At one point she said, more to herself really, "What are they talking about? Oh, they're talking about…" I said, "Do you hear people talking?" She said yes. I couldn't hear anyone talking. Her roommate was in her bed sleeping, sleeping very loudly. We heard her stir and Mother leaned towards me and said, "Are you still tired?" I said, "Yes, I'm tired, are you?" She said no. The roommate's sleeping returned to normal and Mother lost interest.

She started to focus on something in the room across from her. There was nothing there, of course, so I started watching her. She was so intent and the expression on her face would change with whatever she was looking at. After a brief time her eyes got really wide and she said, "Oh, that's pictures of you." Her eyes would jump to different spots in that area like she was watching something. I said, "Is there someone in the room with us?" She said no, without taking her eyes off of whatever she was seeing. Then she said, "You were such a cute kid." The entire thing was very strange. It really looked like she was seeing a series of photographs of me. She continued like that for quite a while and seemed to be enjoying herself. Was that her memory trying to kick start?

She had started to doze so I decided to leave. I had been there for a couple of hours. I said, "Are you ready for a nap?" She said yes. I took my crucifix from her and put it back on. I would have left it with her if I didn't think it would disappear as soon as I left. I put Chelsey back in her bag. I hugged Mother and told her that I loved her then helped her lay back on the bed, making sure the pillow was under her head. I kissed her on the forehead and told her again that I loved her and that I would be back soon. She said, "I love you too." It's always so hard to leave her. There are times when she looks so desolate, so tragic – that word keeps coming to my mind. As I walked back through the unit I could see a group of residents sitting in front of a small television watching a movie. There are rarely any visitors in this unit but today is Sunday so there were a few coming in and out and I was able to slip out the door easily.

As I reached the elevator an elderly woman got in with me. She was bundled up in a coat and a scarf around her neck. I recognized her from the group of smoking women who hang together outside. I said in a smiling, joking way, "I guess it's okay for you to go outside," acting like maybe she was trying to escape. She said, "Oh yes, I go out twenty times a day." We rode down together and at ground level the smell of bad coffee was overpowering. Tom was once again waiting for me in the lobby, sitting and reading. Yesterday he had moved around from sitting outside, to sitting in the truck, to sitting inside, all the while with Chelsey at his feet. Today he had moved around by himself. He must be so bored; what a patient man he is.

As we began our long drive home I thought about Mother's strange behavior. I wondered if her fall had caused it. Had her blood pressure spiking to 200 have something to do with it? Did she have another stroke? Or was this just a part of dementia I wasn't aware of?

Driving through Iowa we passed an apple orchard, funny, I had never noticed that before. It made me think of the apple trees we had in the backyard when I was growing up. There were only two trees and they were still small and we didn't have many apples. When the first red apple was ready to be picked Mother would cut it into six pieces so that we would all have some. It was like a little ritual. After all of the apples were ripe there were enough so that we would all get one. We didn't get a whole lot of food out of the gardens so we really savored those apples.

While we were driving through Missouri we stopped at a convenience store for gas. It actually had a bakery. A lot of the convenience stores sell doughnuts, but this place had a working bakery and boy did it smell good. The scent led me to the back and placed me in front of the shelves of beautiful pastries. I was surprised to see sugar coated jelly doughnuts! I haven't seen those since I was a kid. Grandma Ruth always had them for us when we visited. I had to buy one of course. As I wandered through the store I was surprised again to see an entire rack of fresh fruit and a section with hot food. We hadn't eaten dinner yet and I was hungry. Looking at the pots of hot food I was surprised once again to see goulash! It smelled so good and I reached for a Styrofoam bowl. I told Tom to find something for his dinner because I had mine – goulash and a jelly doughnut. I know, I know, all that sugar, but I only ate one. We'll probably never be able to find that place again.

Tonight we are in Springfield and will get home tomorrow evening sometime. I can't wait to get in my own bed. I'm always feeling sad on these trips home, Mother on my mind continually. She looked so sad. I hated leaving her.

November 16, 2009

We're finally home. We stopped for gas at a place right on the Missouri/Arkansas line. It had a big flea market next to it. I wish we had more time to really examine the place but we took about half an hour to browse through it. They had some Amish dolls just like the ones Mother used to make.

It was strange because they looked just like hers. They had the black bonnets with no faces. There was also a rabbit with big, floppy ears, also just like Mother used to make. I don't know how her items could have gotten all the way to southern Missouri so I'm guessing someone used the same patterns Mother did.

November 19, 2009

There's been a commercial on TV that has a family eating mounds of butter. The family looks like they are from the 1950s. The scene is in black and white, but the mounds of butter are bright yellow. The commercial is pretty funny and of course the message is not to eat butter. It brought back a memory of when I was very young. Butter was being rationed at the time. We would receive a plastic package that contained oleo; it had a small, yellow dye tab in it. You had to squeeze and squeeze the package until the oleo looked like yellow butter. It was fun actually. I don't remember the taste but I'm sure it probably wasn't very good. I remember going to visit Aunt Laurie during that time in Illinois and we brought her some. I don't know why we brought her some, I just remember riding in the car late into the night and when we got to the house Aunt Laurie gave us cupcakes. Funny how little things like that can stick in your mind for 50 years.

November 22, 2009

There was an article in the newspaper today about the warning signs of Alzheimer's. It was pretty interesting. The list includes things like changes in memory, and difficulty performing familiar tasks. But there were also a couple of things that were interesting in regard to Mother. One is losing track of time or place. The person may lose track of time or forget what season it is. Many times the person only understands things that are happening immediately. That fits Mother.

The other thing is difficulty with conversation. Sometimes the person has trouble maintaining or joining a conversation. Some people struggle with vocabulary, such as calling things by the wrong name, while others might stop in the middle of a conversation and not be able to continue. Most typical is when the person cannot find the right word to express a given idea. Exactly like Mother. Mother doesn't have Alzheimer's, however. But that shows how Alzheimer's and other dementias have the same symptoms.

November 24, 2009

Kelley and Zakary didn't have school today so we asked them if they wanted to spend the day with us. Tom wanted to take them to Cedar Glades Park for some hiking. The park is really nice with a big RC track. The sun was out and I thought it would be warm enough to hike comfortably but once we got out on the trail it was really cold. I even made Tom go back and get my jacket out of the truck. I was watching Zakary hike up a small hill and it reminded me of when we were hiking with him at Minnehaha Falls that year. Tom and I had been planning a trip to Minnesota to help Mother and David pack up the house in Crosslake. She had written me a letter asking us to come and help. Tommy and Zakary decided to go with us.

Packing up the house was a major job. Mother had so much stuff. When she retired she took her money and had the little log cabin made into a big log house. There was already electricity but no indoor plumbing. She also built onto the cabin making it a lot bigger and even had the house jacked up and put in a full basement. Ken had already built a big two vehicle garage that had a full loft on the top. When all the construction was finished the house had two bedrooms upstairs, two bedrooms downstairs, a bathroom on each floor, and a lot of space for chairs, tables, and her sewing and craft supplies. She also had a nice fireplace in the living room. It was a beautiful home sitting on top of a big hill overlooking the lake.

Mother had every inch of that place full. When we got there the two of them had already sorted through a lot of the items and either given the stuff away or had them packed up. We spent two days with them, sorting and packing. The roof on the garage was damaged and she had never had the money to repair it, so by this time it was starting to fall in, which made a major mess up there. Plus, the outside staircase leading to the loft had fallen down. The only way to get up there was climbing a big metal ladder. We had to either carry everything down or lower it with a rope. Mother wanted to go up there, but we wouldn't let her climb that ladder. We didn't get it all done by a long shot. David had to finish it by himself. We stayed in a local motel and David and Mother stayed in the house – for the last time. It was very sad. We hated giving up the house. Mother was living in the assisted living place at that time and the bills were rolling in, the house had to be sold.

It was Zakary's first trip to Minnesota and Tom wanted to take him to Fort Snelling. We asked Mother if she would like to go along and she said yes, so we went and picked her up. It was October and extremely cold. Fort Snelling still had their program running; it was the last day until the next spring. There were actually quite a few people there. We toured all of the buildings, listened to all of the talks, watched the soldiers with their muskets, and took pictures of all of the cannons. We had fun even though we shivered through the entire thing.

Then Tom said we should go over to Minnehaha Falls since it was right down the road. I said, oh no, it's too cold. No, it's not, come on let's go, it'll be fun. He finally convinced us. There is no doubt the place is beautiful no matter what time of year it is. The Falls weren't quite frozen yet; they look spectacular when fully frozen. But Tom wanted to hike. We headed into the woods and the wind was blowing; and dam it was cold. Mother was wearing her dark green corduroy winter jacket. She was wearing the same jacket the year before when she came and stayed with me and not once, that entire winter, was I able to get her to button up that jacket. Mother didn't want to hike so we found a bench for her near the hiking trails. I said, "Mother, Please button your jacket." And she did, it was that cold. We still had fun.

There is a tunnel on Interstate 35 that leads into and out of Minneapolis. The tunnel goes under the Mississippi River.

Every time we've been through this tunnel we always open the windows and start yelling like crazy. It is so cool with all of our voices bouncing off the tunnel walls. So of course when we took Zakary through we just quietly opened the windows and let loose. Zakary was so surprised. It was fun.

November 28, 2009

I had a dream early this morning that I was playing a game on Pogo. I was playing Mahjong Safari and I kept seeing a box-like form and a matching pair of animals that kept popping out of it and moving around the board. It started getting chaotic with a couple of boxes and animals moving rapidly around, always in a straight line like in the actual game. I said, "Let it be clear so that I can understand." The activity slowed down and I watched as two polar bears came out of the box, moved around the board, and then went back in. I was instantly wide awake. I thought, "That's just like Mother. She lives in a box (the nursing home), leaves it occasionally, then she has to go back in." But what did the dream mean? If I put myself in that position it would be utter boredom. Is Mother bored? She seemed to be during my previous visits, but not during the last visit. During the last visit it was more like her mind was in a box. A box of dementia, and sometimes she comes out of it; sometimes her mind is clear. Why I had the dream I don't know. Maybe just so I'd know that sometimes she's lucid. Maybe when things got chaotic on the board it represented Mother's mind at times; chaotic, trying desperately to find something familiar. Maybe it was showing her frustration.

November 29, 2009

I had another dream early this morning. I couldn't really see anything during the dream, instead I was sensing it. There was a party going on and there was a young woman who was very excited to be there. I said, "This is a wrap party. If you're here it means it's all over." I meant that it was a wrap party like after finishing a movie or some kind of production. It doesn't sound too good. I wonder what it was referring to. Was it about Mother? Is she so far into dementia that she'll never come out? But we already know that. Plus, I just had that box dream. Has she changed any further since I last saw her? There's no way to find out without seeing her.

Maybe it's not about her at all. The only other thing going on is that Tom is out of work. The dream could fit this situation also. That's a wrap! The work is over for this year. And we're in the same spot we were in this time last year. No work and very little money, with people owing us a lot of money who's not paying. Will that money come in or will we be screwed again? We don't have enough money to last even a month. Is it the end of our business? Is it all over? However, in the dream it was a young woman who was at the party. A naïve woman who didn't realize that the party meant that it was all over. So, it makes me think of Mother. I feel that something has changed. Something has ended with her. It scares me a bit.

November 30, 2009

Today I was looking at the photos I took of Mother during my last visit. There was no eye contact. Even when I said, "Look at me," and she did, as the button on the camera was pushed she averted her eyes. She looks so incredibly tired. She also looks guarded and a little wary, like she doesn't know what I want. Sometimes the expression on her face looks tortured; she looks so sad. The photo of her bruised face also shows blood-shot eyes and even a look of fear in them. She looks like she's going to cry, and that makes me want to cry. I wish there was something I could do to make her life easier, more enjoyable in some way, worth living. She breaks my heart.

December 1, 2009

The squirrels are real active right now. We love watching them. We keep them (and the birds) supplied with bird seed and nuts. The squirrels go through the seed and pick out the good stuff and leave the rest for the birds. One summer Mother came down to visit for two weeks. At the time we had our first iguana, Rex Anne. Rex Anne started out as Rex until we found out she was a female and then she became Rex Anne. One day we were sitting outside and put

Rex Anne in a little swimming pool. I had a new video camera I was trying out. Mother was on a roll and talked nonstop; she didn't realize it would be on the video. Later, after she had gone back home I was watching it and it was so funny because it shows Rex Anne swimming back and forth, back and forth, in the pool. But in the background you can hear Mother talking about her crusade against the squirrels; her efforts about finding the perfect squirrel-proof bird feeder. Her talking was what kept me taping; you can only watch an iguana swim back and forth in a pool for so long. I never showed her the video; I think she would have been somewhat embarrassed about her nonstop talking. I loved it.

Mother was funny about Rex Anne altogether. When Scott first brought Rex Anne home he had built a huge habitat for her. It had a big log to climb on and heat lights, etc. We put the cage in front of the window so she would have direct sunlight. Once she got bigger we took her out during the day and let her have the run of the house. I'm a night owl and don't go to bed until very late. Mother always started falling out about 10:00. She slept on the foldout couch during the visit. It had always been my routine that once Tom went to bed Rex Anne and I would spend a few hours working in my office. I tried continuing that routine during Mother's visit. I'd get her into bed and then Rex Anne and I would go to work. But after the first few nights Mother started complaining. She said, "How come I have to go to bed but she doesn't." That was funny; she was jealous of an iguana. So, then I had to put both Mother and Rex Anne to bed; when Mother went to sleep I snuck Rex Anne out of her bed and took her to work with me.

By the time Mother spent the winter with us Rex Anne had passed. But by then we had Ruffles and Buddy. They were both sweethearts (except to each other) and very lovable. Mother had her own room, although she did have to share it with the iguanas during the day. That room was full in the sun all afternoon with the bed right up to the window. Both iguanas loved that room, but Buddy spent the most time there. He would just climb up onto the bed and lie on the windowsill and look outside. Mother was a little surprised at first. Buddy didn't care whether Mother was already on the bed. After awhile Mother started petting and talking to him. She never tried picking him up; he was big by then. I'm sure she missed having a pet, although she had no memory of the dog she had to leave behind.

December 4, 2009

Winter is really hitting the south. We are having record lows, in the 20s. It is snowing in southern Texas, Alabama, and Mississippi. I was browsing around on the internet today and saw an advertisement for a snow thrower. I thought, what's a snow thrower? I went in further to check it out and it was just a snow shovel! When did they start calling them snow throwers? But really, that's not a correct term. When the shovel starts throwing snow by itself then you can call it a snow thrower. In the meantime, it's a person using the shovel to throw the snow. I used many a snow shovel growing up in Minnesota. We all used those shovels. There were no snowblowers back then.

December 6, 2009

Today I was getting my Christmas cards ready to mail. As I was putting on the Christmas Seals I was thinking about one of the visits I made to Mother when she was in the assisted living place. David brought along a stack of Christmas cards for Mother to sign. Mother had always loved sending out cards and would spend a lot of time picking out just the right ones (as I found out the year she was with me and it took her 30 minutes to pick out one box). David had a long printed list of names and addresses for the cards. He would hand one to Mother and say, this is for…You need to sign it Mom, or Grandma, or Sally, depending on who the card was going to. Mother would study the front of each card, open it and read the inside, and then would always say, who is this for, how am I supposed to sign it? It was funny, because she did the same thing for each card. It was slow going and it had to be frustrating for David even though he was always very patient with her. I don't know how many years he did that for her, but eventually she wasn't even able to sign her name, sending out cards altogether stopped at that point. It was the same way with Christmas presents. David did the shopping and then told her who got what. I did that for her when she was here. This is for…this is for…And her response was always, okay. David did the birthdays the first few years also. He has really done a lot for her. Thank you David.

December 9, 2009

I had a dream last night that I was in a huge building. It was like a warehouse, but I knew that at one time it had been a store. The woman who owned it was now dead. There were a few young women sitting at a table and I knew that they were the deceased woman's family. I was also a part of the family. A lot of the items had been removed from the building. The remaining items were scattered throughout. I talked briefly with the women. They didn't seem happy to see me. I started walking through the building looking at the remaining items. One of the women followed me. She was probably in her late 20s with longish dark brown hair. She didn't get really close to me, but I was always in her sight. They didn't trust me and were afraid I was going to take something. And they were right. I knew that I would probably slip something small into my pocket if the woman wasn't looking. I felt that I was entitled to receive at least something; they shouldn't get it all. I felt that they were being selfish. However, I was planning on asking their permission if I found something I really wanted and couldn't slip it in my pocket. But first I wanted to look at everything that was left.

I walked slowly down the aisles and among the shelves. I came upon a small display of Native American items. I remember a cream colored Indian woman statue. I didn't look too closely at the items because I knew I'd be able to come back to the area. I continued walking and saw a section with children's items, including a tiny, pink plastic stove that was tucked onto a shelf. Next I reached a display of jewelry in a glass counter. There was a box-like display case sitting on top. I just glanced at the jewelry and kept walking. Everything seemed kind of musty. There was no dust however, it just seemed like everything had been sitting there for a long time. And the place felt very empty. I reached the rear of the building and could see what looked like huge rolls of old, dark carpet sitting on shelves. This is where the dream ended.

This dream must be about Mother. The warehouse type store would be the different areas or sections of her mind. There is lot of emptiness but there is still a little in there. Were the different areas small glimpses of old memories? What does the group of young women represent? Are they guarding what's left of her mind, the remaining memories? Why are they guarding them? And why don't they trust me? Is it just self-protection? When Mother is enclosed in a world all her own is she having small memories? And she wants to guard them so that they won't disappear like her other memories? Maybe she's afraid if she shares them they won't be all hers, maybe she feels like that's all she has left of her old life and she doesn't want to give them up. I think the part where I'm planning on taking something is my trying to get some type of memory out of her when I visit, but she's not going to share them willingly. I don't think she can, I think she's unable to do this on her own. When I'm with her I need to be patient and see if I can get anything.

The parts of her memory in the dream were interesting. Childhood toys, Native American items, and jewelry. And way, way back was household items; the rolls of carpet. Although the only time she had carpet was when she lived in Ken's house, so it must just represent her house, or her home with Ken. I wonder if I can use those memories. For example, if I bring her a small Indian doll would it bring forward her affection for Native American items? Would a piece of jewelry bring some type of memory? Maybe the dream is telling me that she would like to receive these things as gifts. Maybe she needs to feel special enough for someone to give her a gift. It's interesting how my dreams of Mother often take place in some type of store. I wonder what the relevance is. I know that the different rooms in a building represent the different areas of the mind, so I'm guessing these dreams are my way of getting into Mother's mind. What is going on in there?

December 11, 2009

I was eating a bowl of cottage cheese for lunch and it made me think of the cottage cheese sandwiches Mother used to eat. They're actually pretty good. Sandwiches we had as children are so different than the sandwiches we eat now. When I was growing up Mother always put butter on our sandwiches first, and then whatever else was going in. Even peanut butter sandwiches had a layer of butter. When I moved to the south that was never even heard of, no one spread butter on their sandwiches. We used mayonnaise, or mustard, or nothing extra. I had forgotten all about butter on sandwiches until Mother spent the winter with us. Making her a sandwich she made sure the butter was there. It made me think of the really weird sandwiches we had eaten when I was young. There were the cottage cheese and butter sandwiches, brown sugar and butter sandwiches (the sugar stuck to the butter of course), cheese and butter, grilled (in butter) peanut butter, and I guess whatever was lying around the kitchen would go in a sandwich.

December 12, 2009

I got an email from David today. He went to see Mother yesterday and they were having a Christmas party with music and even Santa Claus. He said that Mother is doing good. I imagine she was in a festive mood with that party going on, and a visit from David. I am really missing her.

December 14, 2009

I was wrapping Christmas presents today. I'm such a perfectionist – Mother's fault. She taught me at a very early age the art of wrapping. The paper has to be cut exactly right to have completely straight edges; the design has to be centered. The corners have to be folded just right. Ribbon has to be applied just right, no just sticking on bows, although you can apply a bow after applying the ribbon first. It was fun learning from her. I remember one Christmas while I was probably in grade school; I had taken a nap and upon waking I wandered into the kitchen surprising Mother and Nancy wrapping a present for me. Mother was gluing glitter onto the package in the shape of the letter J. She was so mad when she saw me; I had ruined her surprise. I immediately turned and left the room feeling so guilty.

Doing the Christmas shopping growing up was always complicated. Usually the entire family would go to Target and Mother would take us kids into the store and shop for Daddy and then Daddy would take us into the store and shop for Mother. That stopped at some point, I don't remember when. After Daddy died we were on our own of course. Mother had to do double duty for a while. One year, after I started driving, Emily and I realized we didn't have a present for Mother. It was already Christmas Eve afternoon and we felt so guilty. We rushed out to any store we could find still open, which was a drug store. We didn't have very much money, and we knew we couldn't ask Ken for any money, and we were too embarrassed to ask Mother for money to buy her a present; especially at the last minute like that. So, Emily and I pooled our money and went in search of what we could get. We ended up buying her a large bottle of cheap perfume. I don't know if Mother liked it or not, she never would have said anything to hurt our feelings. Emily and I vowed to never let that happen again.

December 21, 2009

I mailed Mother's Christmas present today. I bought her a nice bottle of body lotion and a box of tissues. Usually I have flowers delivered for each holiday; David encouraged me and Emily to do that. The flowers rarely lasted more than a day or two, so it was only a momentary happiness for her. We asked if Mother needed anything, but David would always say no, then if she did need something he would buy it himself for his gift to her. But on my last visit I saw that she didn't have any lotion or tissue. I wrote her name on each and hope for the best.

December 24, 2009

It's Christmas Eve. I've always tried to keep the same ritual as we had when I was growing up. We always opened our presents on Christmas Eve and then our stockings Christmas morning. We drove to Minnesota every other Christmas for many years after we were first married, and after the boys were born. The last Christmas we were there it was 40 degrees below with a lot of snow. The trip up was really bad. The car didn't want to stay running. Tom finally put a piece of carboard in front of the motor to keep it from freezing and we had to keep pouring coke on the windshield to get the ice off. Mother and Ken had two garages for their vehicles. One was out back and contained his big wrecker truck and his fancy Chrysler car. The garage built onto the house contained Mother's truck. We'd had to bring our two dogs along, but Mother wouldn't let them in the house (one was a Basset Hound) so they had to stay in Ken's garage. He had heat in there. Our car had to sit outside. The morning we were planning to leave for home our car wouldn't start. It was after all a southern car. It wasn't until several days later when the temperature warmed up to 0 that our car would finally start and we could get out of there. I guess that scared us a bit and decided not to go in the middle of winter again. I sure did miss our Christmases together though. We did go one year after Mother had moved to Crosslake and we all spent Christmas at David's house.

December 25, 2009

Merry Christmas! Last night as I was trying to go to sleep I was having a lot of Christmas memories. We always had a huge tree that Daddy would cut down in some north woods. Us kids and Mother would decorate the tree after Daddy put it up in the stand, strung the lights, and set the big star on top. It was so much fun to revisit our ornaments every year. I'm the same way now; every ornament has a meaning to it. Mother had a small group of ornaments; fragile ones that she would hang on the tree herself. I don't remember what all of them were, but I remember angels and a delicate gold French horn. Once all the ornaments were on we would throw tinsel all over it. Mother would always wait until we were done then go and rearrange it so that it looked like the tinsel was dripping from the tree instead of sitting in globs. We didn't always have the tree in the same spot, but one year it was set up in front of the picture window and it was so large that when Daddy was sitting in his chair he couldn't see the television. He finally cur a tunnel through the branches so that he had a clear line of sight.

Years ago I started gathering up all of the old 8 mm tapes that Daddy had made over the years and had them put on VHS tapes (now I'm going to have to put them on DVDs). He loved to record and then he would edit and splice; he put a lot of work into them. Watching the old movies was hilarious. There was no sound of course, and he had to use a large light bar so that we were always squinting from the brightness. We were always sitting in front of the tree, wearing our new clothes; us girls in dresses, white anklets, and patent leather shoes. I was often crying. Even then I hated having my picture taken. It's a rare photograph if I look good in it and in those old Christmas movies I often had some type of weird frizzy perm going on.

On Christmas afternoons we always went to Grandma and Grandpa's house down in Minneapolis. Grandma Ruth's Christmas tree was always decorated in blue and silver; even the lights were all blue. Grandma always had a full Christmas stocking for us. Maybe that's why every year I fill a stocking for everyone; because it's so much fun! Grandma would fix us a huge dinner. Everyone got a chocolate Santa Claus, except me, I got a white one. Bummer. I came across an article recently on white chocolate. In the making of chocolate it is boiled and the fat is skimmed off. White chocolate is that skimmed off fat and sugar. Sounds yummy, doesn't it? It was funny looking back at the old movies. Putting them together we noticed that Grandpa wore the same blue plaid flannel shirt every Christmas. It must have been his 'Christmas Shirt.'

This morning Tom and I exchanged our gifts and opened the stockings we fill for each other. The kids all arrived in the afternoon and as soon as everyone was gathered in the living room they all opened their stockings. Tom and I sit and watch thinking, did they like that, did they like that? We love watching the smiles as they dig deep into the stockings to see what's in the very bottom. We opened all of our presents and had a very nice dinner. I love spending this time with my family.

After everyone had left I was thinking of Mother. Everything is so different now. We had always talked to each other on the phone on Christmas and I really miss that. She loved Christmas also and always tried to make it special for everyone; not an easy feat with our large extended family. Christmas has no meaning for her now and that's sad.

December 27, 2009

I had this dream last night. I was outside in what seemed to be a city. There were other people around, but I was alone. I don't know what any of us were doing. I was kind of focused on the sky and didn't see anything on the ground, although I could see some buildings. It was dark out, the sky lit up by stars. Out of the corner of my eye I saw a shooing star moving from right to left. I was excited and focused in on it. I moved my position a little so that I could see better. Then I saw another star moving the same way. Then I saw numerous shooting stars all across the sky. I realized that something unusual was going on and as I watched I saw that the stars were all moving to the center of the sky and that they were forming a picture. The scene was beautiful and awesome.

I moved again so that I could see the star picture better. It was in a box-like shape and the stars were moving across the sky taking their place in the picture. I was trying so hard to understand what the picture was but couldn't make out any particular images. The stars just seemed to be in a dazzling design. By now all of the people around me were watching the show. As I was trying to make it out a couple of the stars came flying out of the design hurtling towards the ground. One hit the ground near us and it landed with a vicious crash and we all realized it was a rock. By then all of the stars were suddenly raining down on us. Everyone dived for cover. Some ran into the buildings. Some jumped in parked vehicles. I was holding a large umbrella, probably because I wanted to watch closely to what was going on. There were big rocks coming down everywhere, some were crashing through car windows. As the people ran some were hit on the shoulders and their backs. Those people were all wearing heavy coats, so they weren't really hurt. That was the end of the dream; everyone was heading for cover except for me.

This dream makes me think of Mother for some reason. Maybe I've been having such good feelings about her new state of mind, that she seems so okay, in her 'own little world.' But maybe it's a false sense of good feeling. Maybe she's not okay, maybe she's crashing. The people were wearing heavy coats, which shows that's it's probably wintertime. It's now the end of December so I've been thinking about our next trip up there which is planned for January (winter). Will I get up there and find her in a state of chaos? Maybe the dream is about Tom – maybe he's going to back out of future trips and I'll be crashing back to earth, my plans dashed to bits. I don't know. It's like I'm all excited and then suddenly everything changes to bad.

This dream could be representing Mother's life. Before starting on this journey Mother was special, she brought joy into this world. She's still special, but once she descended into total dementia a lot of the people in her life disappeared; like they were running for their lives. To be honest, most of the people in her life ran. That's not only sad, but it's also shameful. I know that shooting stars can mean a brief moment in life that has passed.

December 28, 2009

It's only 7° in Minnesota today and they're expecting 20 inches of snow. Yikes! I remember visiting Mother one winter in Crosslake. She really didn't mind getting snowed in. One day on that visit she got out a toboggan for all of us to play with. She showed us how she did it. She put the toboggan at the top of the hill and climbed on, and then her big, yellow Lab, Kelly, climbed on and sat down between Mother's legs. Mother put her arms around Kelly, pushed off, and the two of them went flying down the hill. It was so funny. Mother brought the toboggan back up the hill and we played with it all afternoon. The boys loved playing in the snow; they sure didn't get it at home.

December 29, 2009

I got a letter from Delomia today. She was able to meet Mother several times before moving back to Kansas. The two of them really connected. It was kind of surprising because Mother had never been too thrilled with my friends in the past. She actually referred to one of my friends as scraping the bottom of the barrel. Delomia's age is in between Mother's and mine so maybe that makes a difference. The summer Mother came down for two weeks Delomia hung out with us a lot. Delomia and I had been going to a lot of metaphysical classes and we took Mother along to a couple of them. I remember one was a self-help class on manifesting your life dream or something like that.

We all sat around in a circle on folding chairs, with our motivational speaker. I don't remember a lot about the class except that we were to write down our life dream on a little piece of paper and then meditate on it. After the class Mother showed me her paper and written on it was, "Second Childhood." I asked what it meant and she said that was the name of the business she wanted to start. And boy did she. She went home and started sewing. She made her own little cards with her business name stamped or handwritten on them, usually with a small doll graphic. They were cute. She had a very successful business, selling mainly in a local shop, but also personal orders. She was very happy. Unfortunately the sales were only during the summer; everything pretty much shut down in the winter. Of course Mother then sewed all winter so she'd be ready for spring.

The last time Delomia saw Mother was when Mother was living with us that winter. Mother had been complaining about her shoulders and knees hurting. I said it was because she just sat around all day; that she needed to get some type of exercise, even if it was just walking. She started walking. One day I had been in the backyard and when I went back in Mother was gone. I started getting a little frantic and then Tom arrived and I asked him to drive down the street and see if he could find her. Sure enough, she had started just walking down the street. Tom brought her back telling her that she had really worried me. She admitted to him that she knew it would. I kind of went off on her and said if she was going to leave the yard she <u>had</u> to tell me.

She stuck to the yard after that. She walked around and around and around. Delomia arrived one day while Mother was walking and they walked and talked together around and around the yard. It was worth it though. When Mother arrived at my house that October she was on a walker, when she left in February she was completely upright on her own two feet. Mother was very proud of herself and I know David was really impressed. Job well done. She's never been on a walker since although now she's no longer completely upright.

December 31, 2009

It's New Year's Eve, and there's a full moon. Tom and I did our usual New Year's Eve celebration, which is nothing. When we were a lot younger we would go out and celebrate but we eventually lost interest in that. We're not drinkers. Now we're lucky if Tom is still awake by midnight. I have no memories at all of what we did when I was growing up. I guess we did the same thing I do now. I'm sure Mother and Daddy probably went out. I remember how sometimes during the holiday season all of the neighbors would get together at someone's house and have a big party. I have some of the old home movies to prove it. I had been looking at them one day and was able to remember everyone's names. It was funny seeing all of the (young) parents having fun, laughing, all dressed up, sometimes wearing little tiaras, always with a drink in one hand, a cigarette in the other, and drunk on their butts.

I don't remember my parents drinking very often, I know they did on Christmas Eve when Grandma Ruth and Grandpa came over. After all of the presents were opened they set up a card table and started playing gin rummy or something. They had mixed drinks. One time someone left a spoon on the counter and I picked it up and popped it in my mouth. Yuk! I know now that it was whisky. Many years later we discovered that Grandpa was an alcoholic, that he spent a lot of time in bars, and that sometimes Grandma called Daddy late at night and asked him to go and find him and bring him home. What a surprise to learn that, parents sure keep a lot of secrets. I'm sure Mother and Daddy drank at different neighborhood get togethers. We had a liquor cabinet in the basement that at some point had to be locked. Not to point fingers but I believe it was discovered that Nancy and David had been getting in there. I remember one of them filling the bottles with water until they were the correct level.

Drinking, however, was not a frequent occurrence in our house. That all changed when Mother married Ken. Not only was he an alcoholic (he was a happy drunk), but she drank quite a bit also. He drank scotch, she liked wine. Even when she was with her next husband, Bob(2), they did a lot of drinking. One year the boys and I flew up there for a visit. On the plane they served us a box lunch that contained a sandwich, chips, an apple, and a cheap bottle of wine (for the adults). It was a very interesting flight because among the passengers were several famous wrestlers. The boys and I recognized them immediately. At that time people would put the food they didn't want in the front seat pockets. As everyone was leaving the plane the wrestlers scooped up all of the apples and I scooped up all of the bottles of wine. That evening Mother and Bob cracked open the wine. The next morning after I got up I saw that there were still a couple of glasses with a little wine in them. When Mother and Bob got up the first thing they did was finish them off. In no way did Mother have a problem with drinking; she basically only drank when she was around those men. Once she was alone again she rarely drank, maybe an occasional glass of wine in the evening. I guess you could say she was a social drinker. Ken's drinking led to his early death, which devastated Mother.

January 2, 2010

I got a letter from David today thanking us for their Christmas presents. He said they'd had 12 to 15 inches of snow for the holidays. A cougar had been spotted about a month and a half ago for a couple of days in Champlin. That's where Mike lives and we drive through there to get to the motel in Anoka. Then the cougar, or a different cougar, was spotted in Stillwater, the second one in the area in the last three years. I don't know how far the two towns are from each other; David always thinks I know where everything is in Minnesota. It's neat thinking you might spot a cougar while driving along although I'm not sure I'd be too thrilled if I lived in the area. David sees a lot of wildlife himself of course working for the Transportation Department.

January 3, 2010

I sent David an email tonight telling him we're still planning on coming up this month, but there are a couple of things we're watching. Tom hasn't worked in a while and he's hoping that now that it's a new year construction will pick up again. Everything has been completely dead all winter. We don't have any money, so the entire trip will have to go on a credit card anyway. We're also watching the weather; not in Minnesota – cold is cold – but ours. It's been snowing this evening. Still, I'm prepared to pack at a moment's notice.

January 4, 2010

This would be the perfect time to go to Minnesota. Tom doesn't have any work. But now they're predicting that a huge Arctic Blast is coming our way. We really can't take the chance of driving in the middle of a big storm, or of getting stranded somewhere. Our safety has to be our first concern.

January 5, 2010

Even if we did go to Minnesota we really don't have the proper clothing. They don't sell the really good winter clothing down here. It's better than it used to be. When we first started taking the boys up there we'd have to buy clothing for them when we got there. We couldn't even find gloves and mittens here. One year the boys only had little cowboy boots and they froze. I still try to find insulated boots when I'm up there. None of my jeans are very heavy; the material is always very thin in women's pants. I used to buy myself boy's jeans when we made the trip because they are so much heavier. Why is that? Why are women's jeans thin but not men's? We can't find sleds and other snow toys here either. The last time I was up there in winter was a couple of years ago with Tommy and the kids. We went to a place and bought sleds and saucers, etc. for the entire family.

Scott called, he's getting snow. The entire South is getting hit. I told Tom to make sure the generator is ready. He went and got a supply of gasoline. The generator isn't very big, but it'll pull the refrigerator and a few other things: a couple of lights, coffeemaker, Chelsey's heating pad, a small electric heater. I checked the flashlights and batteries. We never know what's going to happen.

January 6, 2010

It was sunny today but very cold with the wind gusting at 15 – 25 mph. This evening it started sleeting. Walking outside is crunch, crunch, crunch. I got an email from David and he said the only weekend he won't be home this month is the 23rd. We'll work around that.

January 8, 2010

When Tom got up this morning it was only 10 degrees, but our high for the day was a whopping 18. We have to leave the water running at night. Our houses aren't as insulated in the south either. We are cold, cold, cold.

January 9, 2010

I was watching the weather channel and they showed a video of Ft. Snelling and Minnehaha Falls. The Falls are a solid curtain of ice.

January 10, 2010

Things are calming down now. I guess the Arctic Blast wasn't so bad after all. Today was in the high 30s.

January 11, 2010

It was in the mid-50s today, but the low tonight is only supposed to be 22° so we'll still have to leave the water running. Kelley called this evening all excited because she got her driver's permit today. Yikes, she's only 14. They were going to let her get a hardship license so she could drive herself and Zakary to school and after school activities, but the state just changed the law and now she'll have to wait until she's 16.

I remember when us kids started driving. Nancy was first of course. We all piled into Mother's car one afternoon with Nancy at the wheel. Her first lesson. She drove slowly down our street, but when we got to the end and the stop sign, she didn't stop. The car continued on across the next street and we ended up in someone's front yard. We weren't scared, she was moving so slowly; but I guess it scared her enough; she didn't get her license until she was about 30. She just took buses everywhere. By the time David was ready to drive Mother had traded in her car for a pickup truck with a stick shift. I suppose she taught him how to drive but I don't remember. When I was old enough Mother enrolled me in a driving class at the school.

January 12, 2010

There is a heat wave in Australia right now. Today's low was 93 degrees. Wow. It's only 40 here today. We have decided to leave for Minnesota Friday morning. I came across an article, written by Leah Zerbe, on the Rodale website today titled, "Low Vitamin D Linked to Brain Fog." It says that new research suggests that vitamin D-deficient older adults may have a higher risk of developing dementia or other cognition problems. A study looking at adults between the ages of 65 and 99 who were receiving home care, showed that the people living with dementia had lower levels of vitamin D than the other participants. After adjustments were made for age and sex, researchers discovered that vitamin D insufficiency and deficiency were associated with a twofold higher risk of dementia, Alzheimer's disease, and stroke. In another study of women, age 75 and older, they found a connection between deficient levels and cognitive problems, like memory difficulty and trouble processing simple math problems. A third study did not find a strong link between vitamin D levels and cognitive decline in a group of 1,600 older men. I wonder why there was a difference between men and women.

The article went on to say that though the importance of vitamin D to mental functioning needs further study, the vitamin has long been known to be necessary in helping our body absorb calcium for stronger bones. Emerging research is finding that the vitamin, which is a fat-soluble hormone, is vital to healthy functioning of many of our bodies' systems. In the past few years, there have been more and more studies suggesting that low vitamin D levels in the blood can cause health problems in children and adults. Studies have linked low levels of vitamin D, known as "the sunshine vitamin" because our body makes it naturally when sunshine hits our skin, to higher risks of certain cancers, of falling in older adults, and of diabetes, asthma, and a weaker immune system.

The article suggests people start taking vitamin D supplements. There is also a blood test that can determine if you have sufficient levels. I already take it; my doctor advised it many years ago. I don't take it as much in the summer, but I do in the winter. I doubt whether Mother ever took it and I'm sure they don't give it to her now. That leaves getting her out in the sunshine and eating foods with vitamin D. Some of these foods include fatty fish like salmon and mackerel, and fortified milk, juices, and cereals. I wonder which of these Mother gets. I wonder if her mind could get clearer if she did take the supplements.

I was watching the news on TV this afternoon and the guy said, "Why is it hard to breathe in cold weather?" I thought, yeah, why is it so hard to breathe in cold weather. I've always had that problem. In Minnesota during winter I'd always have to wear a scarf over my lower face when outside; especially at night. I focused in on the television guy and he described the condition as "cold-induced airway activity." It's also called cold-induced asthma. The lungs and bronchi get inflamed causing the airway passages to get smaller which results in wheezing, asthma, etc. Cold, dry air cools the bronchial tubes, causing the muscles around the bronchial tubes to constrict (producing bronchospasm). During exercise it's the rapid breathing in of the cold air, wearing a mask (or in my case a scarf) over your mouth and nose warms the air you're breathing.

It seems that you can also be allergic to cold weather, especially frigid cold air. It's got some fancy medical name. It causes a drop in blood pressure. It can cause itching, not due to dry skin but because it's an allergy. It can cause hives. In research studies an ice cube was put on someone's skin and hives came up. Treatment is taking antihistamines. At least I don't experience that.

January 13, 2010

I came across an article today on the benefits of potatoes. It was written by Amy Ahlberg, on the Rodale website. The article states that one baked potato with the skin contains 4.6 grams of protein and 4.8 grams of fiber, and is an excellent source of niacin, vitamin B6, and vitamin C. It's also a good source of iron, magnesium, and potassium. When researchers tested more than 100 potato varieties, they discovered 60 different phytochemicals and vitamins. Among them are flavonoids that are credited with boosting heart health and providing protection against prostate and lung cancers. Their skins also contain quercetin, which potatoes are rich in, has been shown to reduce blood pressure and help prevent strokes. Potatoes also contain plant chemicals known as kukoamines that aid in fighting hypertension. My earlier dream about potatoes may have also been giving me a message about staying healthy.

January 14, 2010

I had this dream last night. I was in a house, but I don't know whether it was mine. I was in a room that had a lot of stuff in it although I really couldn't tell what type of room it was. I was focused on the back wall. It was made of a rustic wood which gave the house a sense that it was a cabin. The wall only went up half way and the rest were windows. I was standing across the room (or maybe in the middle) looking out. There was a lot of greenery and a medium size tree right in the middle of my view. I saw movement then saw a jaguar start up the tree. It quickly moved around the side and into the branches, but I had clearly seen the jaguar's spots. I stood there in awe trying to see more.

Next I was entering another room. It was a small bathroom. On my left upon entering there was a free-standing sink and some other items. On the far wall was an old-fashioned bathtub sitting on top of a rather high platform. In the tub was a young dark-haired girl having a bubble bath. There were so many bubbles that I could only see the girl's head. On the floor looking up at her was iguana Buddy. He was the same size as when he died; big, 10 pounds. He didn't look too pleased. It was his bathtub, and he thought he should be in it, not the girl. I guess it was my house. As I stood there watching, Buddy walked over to a nearby step stool. With his body he started pushing it over to the tub. I was amazed at his cognitive reasoning; that he would be able to plan this out so well. I thought about what would happen when he got in the tub. Would the girl scream and jump out or would she laugh? I also thought how funny Buddy would look covered with bubbles. That was the end of the dream.

There were two major actions in this dream but no ending to either. In the dream the house/cabin looked really nice with the large window looking out on the trees and nature.

And a jaguar! I was so excited to see a jaguar. Right outside my window! According to my *Animal-Speak* book (by Ted Andrews), the symbolism of the jaguar is very interesting and parts of it are so much like Mother. The jaguar has over 500 voluntary muscles which creates an ability to do a variety of tasks. It is simply a matter of deciding and putting to use those particular "muscles" – be they physical, mental, psychic, or spiritual. As a whole, jaguars are loners (solitary) although they do associate with others they are most comfortable by themselves or within their own marked territories. They are drawn to those individuals who are likewise often solitary.

Mother used to be so active, always doing a variety of tasks—very multitasking; now she has become solitary and silent. The jaguar could also be a reference to developing clairaudience, to hear the communications of other dimensions and other life forms. Isn't that what Mother is doing? When she is in a half sleep communicating with someone who is not there and seeing things that are not there? The book also talks about a reflection of a reclaiming of that which was lost and an intimate connection with the great archetypal force behind it. It gives an ability to go beyond what has been imagined, with opportunity to do so with discipline and control. It is the spirit of imminent rebirth. Perhaps this is referring to my relationship with Mother. I hate to say an imminent rebirth could also be after death.

The other part of the dream is about the accomplishing of something difficult (using the mind first to figure it out) and reclaiming something – Buddy was trying to get to his bathtub, reclaiming it. The iguana is a reptile. Reptiles are cold-blooded. They need the warmth (of the sun) to help them survive – as Mother now needs help from our warmth. Reptile symbolism indicates a great sensitivity to the environments to which they are exposed. Mother has had to adapt to the nursing home environment. According to the lizard symbolism you will also see dramatic mood swings in accordance to what their environment is. The individual will often take on the tone and temperature of the environment. For example, if in a group that is cheerful and loving, they will display similar characteristics. Reptiles have a skin that is covered with tough scales. This is a reminder to keep your tough side outward. Some people will acquire this characteristic as they grow older or go through specific changes in their life. Such changes can be very dramatic—a kind of death/rebirth process, or they may be gentle assertions of new opportunities. A lizard's tail can come off, which may symbolize a need to become more detached in order to survive. I believe that Mother has had to become detached in some way in order to survive what she is going through.

The dream seems to be describing Mother in a symbolic way. And as with many dreams that come from spirit there is going to be humor involved. Although I'm still sad about the loss of Buddy and the loss of who Mother used to be, I can still laugh when I think of Buddy in a bubble bath and I can still have a good time with Mother; just in a totally different way.

   January 14, 2010
I called Nancy today and told her we are coming to Minnesota and said that I'd like to stop over and see her. I asked how Mother was doing and she said they had changed her room because she had gotten in a big fight with her roommate; she said Mother had never liked that roommate. I asked Nancy where Mother had been the last time she had visited her, and she said she had been sitting near the birdcage. I said, "The birdcage! How did she get there?" Nancy said, "She walked I guess." I said, "They let her out by herself?" She said, "Let her out?" I said, "Well, the birdcage is out on the bridge." She said, "There's one in the unit." I said, "Really? I've never seen one in the unit. Where is it?" I could tell by her voice that I was starting to irritate her. She said, "They just moved it next to the hallway. It's always been in there." I said, "But where?" She kind of mumbled something and then said, "I don't remember where it was exactly." I knew she was done with me on that subject.

January 15, 2010

We're on our way to Minnesota. It rained all the way through northern Missouri. I had trouble staying awake. Iowa had a lot of snow on the ground and the temperature really dropped. We stopped for gas in Iowa and I stepped to the side to smoke. Sure enough, I started wheezing when the frigid night air hit my throat. I had smoked earlier during the day and didn't have that problem. The wheezing wasn't enough to stop me from smoking of course. Back on the road with the heater going and sipping coffee it didn't take long for my breathing to go back to normal. We're spending the night at the Appletree Inn in Indianola. It's a nice place but tonight the bed feels hard.

January 16, 2010

Today was sunny and clear, but cold. There is a lot of snow here in Minnesota. We arrived at the nursing home at 3:15. It was too cold for Tom to sit outside so he headed inside with me, armed with several books, and his pockets full of change for the vending machines. When I got to Mother's unit I found her sitting in the middle of the dining area, sound asleep in a chair. There were no tables or chairs near her; she was just out in the open by herself, although there were other people in the general area.

I pulled a chair up next to her and sat down. Then I started patting her arm saying, "Mother, Mother, Mother, Mom, Mom, Mom." Nothing. I stroked her cheek and she flinched but didn't wake up. I started again, "Mom, Mom, Mom," and then finally said, "Mommy." She woke saying, "Yuk." She looked at me and I smiled, then laughed and said, "You don't like being called mommy?" "No." I realized she was in a bad mood. The scowl on her face was a good indication. I said, "Would you like to go to your room and lay down for a nap?" "No." I could tell she was mad. She said, "You're not doing this right!" I said, "Tell me, how should I be doing it?" "I'm not going to tell you that!" I said, "Well, I want to do it right." She just ignored me, her arms folded tightly over her chest. I tried to make conversation but every time I said anything she'd say I was doing it wrong. "I heard you have a new room." "You're not doing it right." I wondered what I should be doing differently.

The staff were again bringing in the residents and placing them at tables. One nurse was passing out snacks; she had a bag of popcorn and would pour some out on a napkin sitting on the table. She asked a woman if Mother could have some and then said, "or is she level 2 (maybe 3)" and the woman said that Mother already had pudding. I asked Mother if she was hungry and she said, "No!"

There really wasn't much staff; just the one nurse and a male nurse. The others were all behind little carts fixing meds. The nurse asked me if I'd like for her to move us to a different place and I said no, it was okay, that Mother wasn't talking to me today. The nurse replied, oh, it's one of those days; and as she passed Mother she patted her on the shoulder, making Mother flinch of course. I was sitting where I could see the clock and I thought I would give her one hour to get unmad then I'd go to her room for a few minutes and then try again.

There was a woman sitting way at the other end of the room and she was making loud noises, like a kid playing with a toy airplane. Mother said, "I feel like screaming when those birds make that noise!" "You don't like birds?" "No!" I knew she wasn't talking about the birds and that was just the best way for her to express herself. I asked if she had seen David lately and she said, "Not for quite a while. He's been really ugly lately." That was funny. The nurse brought a man in a wheelchair and placed him at the table nearest us. She called him John. She wheeled him up then left. John didn't want to sit there and let everyone know it very loudly. He tried to get up and the nurse came and sat him back down. He said he wanted to go back to his hotel room and the nurse told him that he couldn't because it was being cleaned; as soon as they finished cleaning it he could go back. She left again and soon John started backing his chair up. Since he had his back to us he didn't realize that he was heading straight for us. When he got close

Mother started kicking the wheel on his chair. The nurse came over again and moved him back to the table.

The man tried getting out of his wheelchair again and an alarm on his chair went off. The nurse came over again, turned off the alarm, and left. He started backing up his chair again and once again Mother started kicking the wheel. She was so angry. He tried getting out of the chair again and the alarm went off. The nurse came over and turned it off. She lifted him slightly and settled him in his chair; the cushion had gotten screwed up. She put him back at the table and left. All of a sudden alarms were going off all over the place. There were now alarms on the backs of all the wheelchairs and if the occupants got too far forward the alarm sounded. That poor nurse was running all over the place turning off alarms and readjusting people.

At another nearby table two men and a woman were sitting, in wheelchairs. Mother seems to be in the minority here, not being in a wheelchair. That's something to be thankful for. One of the men, I think his name is George, suddenly bent forward in his chair (setting off the alarm), almost laying across his own lap. I realized it was the same man from my last visit doing the same thing. Again I thought how that would really hurt my back to do that. The nurse sat him back up. That happened a couple of times and I realized that he had actually fallen asleep. The nurse finally rolled him closer to the table so that he couldn't fall so far forward. After awhile he woke up and continued on with his day.

Mother was wearing dark green corduroy slacks, a blue, green, and pink checked blouse, and the same powder blue fleece jacket she was wearing my last visit. Her hair is shorter again. Way too short; it looks like a man's haircut. It looks horrible. She would hate it if she could see it. Her color was good tonight. I'm really surprised because last time she looked so tragic with stark white skin. But today her cheeks were rosy. Her nose was a little red, but even her hands looked healthy and no longer the pasty white. I was really worried about her during that last visit. She had a light brownish colored polish on her nails; they looked freshly done, no chipping yet.

A man and woman from a local mortuary entered the unit wheeling a stretcher that had a brown cover fitted over it. I thought, oh, my God, someone has died. It was strange that there was no reaction from any of the residents, but the rushing around turning off alarms nurse looked a little agitated. The couple just stood there waiting for direction until one of the other nurses went over to talk to them and then they left. The first nurse said very quietly as she rushed past, "They must have gotten the wrong directions."

I had been there almost an hour when I noticed that Mother's posture had changed. Her arms were no longer crossed over her chest; one was in her lap and the other was on the arm of the chair, her hand on the side of her face. Her expression had changed; it was softer, and she looked like she was going to cry. Did she finally realize who I was; at least that I was someone familiar? Was she afraid I might leave, because of her attitude, or was she thankful that I didn't, that I had waited her out? Whatever, I was glad she was no longer in that foul mood.

The man started backing up his wheelchair again but the nurse got there first and stopped him, saying there were people sitting behind him and that he was about to run into them. She kept standing him up, straightening his clothes and his cushion, then sitting him back down. She left but this time she put his chair brake on. He started scooting his chair backwards again only this time he started going in a circular manner. When he got facing our direction he apologized for almost running into us. That was very nice. The nurse came again and moved him to the other side of the table with his back facing the wall. He started yelling, saying he didn't want to sit there, but she explained that this way he could see everyone, and he was okay with that. Mother said, "Is he crying?" Her entire personality had shifted. I said, "No, he's just talking loud because he's hard of hearing."

Her eyes started closing and I said, "You're not going to sleep are you?" She opened her eyes and smiled at me! I said, "Would you like me to walk you to your room?" "Yes." I helped her to her feet and we began walking, hand in hand, towards her hallway. There was the large birdcage in the sitting area that Nancy was talking about. I wonder where it had been before. The carpet was missing in the hallway. Mother and I took note of the floor at the same time. Mother said, "Isn't it pretty?" I said, "They pulled the carpet up. I guess they're going to put new stuff down." I had to lead her the entire way, to the hallway, and then to her room. We went into her room and I helped her sit on the edge of the bed, she was happy and smiling. The switch in her mood was incredible and it was so nice to see her smiling.

On her nightstand was a framed photograph of her, David, and Santa Claus. I remembered David telling me recently that when he arrived for a visit one day last month they were having a Christmas party. I picked up the photo and handed it to her saying, "Wow, look at this picture." She took it from me and was looking at it. I asked who the people are and she said she didn't know. I said, "Well, this is you, this is David, and this is Santa Claus. Do you remember seeing Santa Claus?" She shook her head no. I pulled Chelsey from her bag and held her in front of Mother saying, "Here's Chelsey." Mother looked none too pleased, so I just put Chelsey on the bed, put her blanket over her and she hunkered down. I said, "I have a present for you." I had bought her a small Bible and I took it out of the bag and handed it to her. She took the Bible and was looking at it. I had placed the ribbon in Psalms because I feel that if you just want to pick up the Bible and start reading that is a good place to start. I opened it for her and asked if she would read it and she said yes. I knew she couldn't and wouldn't but that's okay, I just wanted her to have it. I don't know where her big Bible ended up.

While I was in the store buying the Bible I saw a beautiful cross made out of small nails wired together. I love unique crosses so I bought it and I was wearing it today. It was kind of an experiment to see if Mother would notice it. I was wearing a yellow, cable knit sweater and I made sure my long hair was always pulled back so that the cross would always be visible. The cross has a long cord on it so that it hangs down to the middle of my chest – very visible. However, Mother never mentioned it, nor did I even see her look at it. She didn't seem to need to hold anything in her hands this time, although she did grab the corner of her blanket briefly and said, "Isn't it pretty?" There was a white towel lying on her bed and I picked it up to move it and said, "Here's a towel, you know what that means." She said, "What?" I said, "It means you're getting a bath tonight." She didn't look very pleased.

I opened the drawer of the nightstand looking to see what was in there. The box of Kleenex I had given her for Christmas was there, but the bottle of lotion was nowhere to be seen. I found her dentures and asked her if she wanted to put them in and she said no. She looks so much healthier than the last visit. The calendars from the last two years were in there so I pulled out last year's and asked Mother if she would like to look at the pictures. Nancy has those calendars made using photographs of Crosslake; all of the different seasons, etc. I took the Bible from her and put it in the drawer then put the calendar in her hands and we began looking at the pictures. We've done this before, but she had not seemed interested; today she was. She looked closely at each picture. I kept up a commentary…here's your house, do you remember it? She always says yes, like she recognized everything.

When we finished that calendar I took out the one from the year before and we went through that one the same way. Then I took out this year's calendar and we looked through that one also. She was particularly interested in any picture that had her dog in it. In one picture I didn't even see the dog until she pointed it out because the dog was in the shade. One picture really caught her attention and she said, "I really like this one." It was a picture of her! It was a September picture and she was outside surrounded by autumn colors. I said, "Who is that?" She said she didn't know. Obviously there was something familiar about the woman even if she didn't know it was herself. While she was still holding the calendar I looked in the drawer for the pen so I could sign it. Since she had recently changed rooms everything in the drawer was kind of jumbled and I couldn't find the pen. I got up and went over to the closet and looked to see if the pen had got set in there accidently. No pen. I turned back around and Mother was gone! I looked out the doorway and there she was boogeying down the hall with the calendar in her hand. I called out, "Mother!" She turned around and looked at me (she knew her name). I said, "Where are you going?" "I don't know." "Come back." She did. I dug a pen out of my purse, signed the calendar and put it back on the wall. I said it was about time for her dinner. I hugged and kissed her and told her that I loved her and said I would walk her back to the dining area.

When we got to the dining area I sat her down in a chair at a table. But before I could even take a step she jumped back up and grabbed my hand and we began walking back out of the area. We went over and looked at the birds for a minute and then sat down in nearby chairs. From there we could see almost the entire unit. We sat there for a moment then Mother pointed to an area in front of the nurse's station and said she could see something on the floor. I couldn't see anything and said that all I could see was a shadow on the floor. Mother seemed really agitated and said, "I feel like there's something wrong here." She was now totally aware of herself and her surroundings. It was so strange to see. She continued on saying, "I feel like I don't belong here." She seemed confused, like she couldn't figure out why she was there. I tried to explain to her what was going on saying, "Right now; this is where you need to be." She said, "I feel restless." I said, "That's because you don't have any friends here. When you were in the assisted living place you had a lot of friends. But you haven't made any friends here." Did she think she didn't belong there because at that moment she was completely lucid and didn't believe she should be in a nursing home?

Evelyn, the irritating woman, came over to us. She was wearing a bib in preparation of dinner. While we were sitting there I watched the staff go around the dining area putting the cloth bibs on each resident. We tried to ignore Evelyn and she patted me on the shoulder then walked away. Mother said, "Why does she do that?" I said she probably doesn't have any family. I asked her if she was hungry and explained that Evelyn was wearing the bib because it was almost dinner time.

Once again Mother said, "I feel like there's something wrong here." I said, "Well, there is a hole in the ceiling." There seemed to be renovations going on with the missing carpet, the moved bird cage, and now a hole in the ceiling. It was a place where they had moved the ceiling tiles and I could see what looked like ventilation tubing, etc. I pointed to the hole and said, "Do you see it?" "No." I said, "Well, come with me and I'll show you." I took her by the hand and we walked over to the hole. "Do you see it now?" "No." I moved so that we were right underneath it. Looking up and pointing I said, "Do you see it now?" "No." I realized she just wouldn't turn her head upwards. Once again, I wonder of her neck hurts although she's never admitted it.

We walked over to the other side of the dining area and found a couple of empty chairs. Most of the residents were at tables waiting for dinner. As we crossed the area Mother waved at a white haired lady in a wheelchair like they were good friends. She did that before when I was visiting with David. She must be lonely, she's always by herself. After we sat down we could hear a woman yelling loudly about something. Mother asked, "Am I like that?" That surprised me. I said, "No, your problem is your gray brain cells, they're affecting your memory." We started to joke about her lack of memory; it's something we can do when she's in a good mood. She always laughs knowing what we say is true.

There was music playing in this area. We started paying attention to it, trying to figure out who was singing. I said,

"Pat Boone?" I heard a woman nearby say, "it's Andy Williams." I looked over and saw that it was the activity director, a very pretty lady with long blond hair. Mother was really tuned into the music and started to quietly sing along. I was amazed and just watched her. The woman came over (I wish I knew her name) and said that the other day she had polka music playing and Mother was singing and dancing to it. I said, "She was dancing?" The woman said yes. I started talking about how she and her second husband, Ken, went dancing every week. She asked if Mother knitted and I said, "Yes, she had knit quite a bit. She made sweaters, hats, mittens, scarves; she made them for everyone except me. I lived in the south, so I guess she thought I didn't need them." She said she had knitting things out on the table the other day and that Mother was looking at the items, but she wouldn't touch them. She said they try to find familiar activities for them. Then I had to ask again, "She was actually dancing?" "Yes."

The lady started asking me about Mother dancing with her husband and asked where they went. I couldn't remember the name of the place; I think it was out by one of the lakes. I said this entire area used to be cornfields and dirt roads. She said, really? She said she wasn't from here. I said, oh yes, when I was growing up Boone Ave. (which is the road the nursing home is sitting on) was a dirt road and none of this area was here; it was all cornfields. I thought about how people used to go parking on this road. David and I would go riding around in his car and he'd do donuts on this road, a couple of times ending up in the ditch. Fun times. We had lived just a few blocks away.

I said that Mother used to sew a lot also; she made doll clothes; Barbie wardrobes, Cabbage Patch Doll clothes (which were popular at that time) etc., for extra money. After she retired she also started making stuffed animals, cornhusk dolls, etc. She was well known for her mini teddy bears. All this time Mother was really listening to everything I said like she couldn't believe she had done all of those things; she kept saying, "Really?" I talked about how the grown-ups all played cribbage when they got together. I remember when she was married to Ken they had a large cribbage table. I guess that's how to explain it. Instead of a board sitting on a table it was a board on it's own legs. Mother tried teaching me how to play one time, but I wasn't really interested. To me it was an older person game.

The lady left and Mother and I started joking again about her lack of memory. I said, "Do you know who I am?" "Yes." "Who am I?" She seemed to know who I am but not my name. It was the same thing with herself. "Do you know who you are?" "Yes." "Who are you?" She just couldn't come up with her own name. I said, "You actually have two names – Shirley and Sally, and you answer to both." She laughed and nodded in agreement. It's funny, I noticed that the Jamaican staff call her Shirley, but the American staff call her Sally. It doesn't seem to confuse her though. She started singing along to the music again. The lady came over to the table near us and changed the CD on the player. Mother got upset and said, "Oh, she's taking it away!" I said, "No, she's just changing the music." Mother started singing along again, quietly, but I could hear that she knew the words. She was tapping her fingers on the arm of the chair. I'm amazed how she can remember the lyrics to songs fifty or more years old but can't remember her own name (or mine).

A woman in a wheelchair rolled herself up and got as close to Mother as she could, toe to toe. I recognized her from my last visit who was trying to get our attention, Mother immediately started tensing up and shutting down. She was getting angry. That quick her mood changed again. I said, "Would you like to move?" "Yes." I got Mother up from the chair and we started walking, she really seemed restless. I said, "Are you ready for dinner?" "Yes." I walked her to an empty chair at a table and asked if she'd like to sit there. She said, "Don't start that!" She sounded very angry. I said, okay and walked to another table. "Would you like to sit here?" "Don't you start that!" Yikes, what was that all about, maybe someone sitting at the table? We continued walking and one of the nurses said,

"Hi Sally." Mother said, "Hi!" The nurse continued, "Do you want to sit here?" And off Mother went, happy as a clam. I can't figure her out. I quickly gave her a kiss and said I'll be back tomorrow.

I left the area and made my way back downstairs. As I was checking out I saw that I had been there 2 ½ hours. Tom was pacing the vestibule and it was already dark out. We drove to David's house. David and I talked about Mother. I asked him about her changing rooms recently and he said he had gotten a phone call from the nurse and she said that Mother and her roommate had gotten into a big fight and Mother was about to punch the roommate, so they thought it would be better to just move Mother out of there. I've never seen Mother interacting with her roommate at all so this is a behavior I haven't witnessed. I told David about snack time and how the nurse said she was level 2 (or 3) and that she'd already had pudding. David said that for some reason they had put Mother on a soft diet. He didn't know why because she's been really healthy. He said that he often has to feed her although yesterday they gave her a sundae and she was able to eat it.

David said that at Christmas he had gone to visit and Emily had sent flowers, and David asked her who had sent them and she said, "Janet." That's amazing that she came up with my name like that. Poor Emily, she just isn't able to visit Mother as often as she'd like. That's why I always try to bring her name into our conversation when I'm there and show her Emily's photo. I like to get Emily's name into Mother's mind. I asked David about the mysterious birdcage and he said it had always been in there, but he also couldn't remember where it had been sitting before they moved it into the visiting area. How strange. I told him about mentioning the towel to Mother and you know what that means, and he said, "Really? She usually bathes on Sunday." Today is Saturday. I said, "Maybe it's because she changed rooms." She's now on the other side of the hallway.

After we had dinner we had coffee and watched television for a while and then Tom and I left for the motel. We knew there was a motel down the road from where we usually stay that has a pool and a great free breakfast. We had found a discount from our insurance company for the motel so we decided to check it out. Tom went inside and said he had a 20% discount and the clerk said, "Well, I can rent you a room, but it'll be $85.00." Tom said no thanks and we came back to the Recency where it's only $55.00. I said next time we'll try it with no discount and see how much it is. Discounts, we have discovered over the years, are really a farce. We've tried different things and usually get the same answer, "The discount is already in." Yeah, right.

As I sit here tonight, waiting to get sleepy, I think about Mother and Ken and their weekly dancing. When they first started dating they went dancing every Sunday night. She'd often be drunk when she got home, which always pissed me off. I'd never seen her drunk before then and she'd have to get up early in the morning and go to work. I never could go to sleep until she got home, and I had to get up early the next morning and go to school. And there's just something about hearing your Mother in the bathroom puking. Years later, on one of our visits they talked Tom and me into going dancing with them. Tom and I weren't big on dancing, especially the polka, but we went. Ken got me out on the dance floor once; I was really whining about it, I didn't know how to polka and whatever else I could come up with. He said that was okay I didn't need to know how to polka he would take care of it. He started flying me around the dance floor and when we got right in front of the live band he stomped on my foot as hard as he could. I screamed but no one could hear me over the band. He thought that was the funniest thing and laughed about it all night. He wasn't a mean man; he just liked to have fun. Mother really loved him.

One time, after they got married, their night of dancing didn't turn out so well. Ken had gotten so drunk that Mother had to drive them home. Mother was helping him through the house to their bedroom when he fell. His head hit the corner of the dining room and hall wall when he went down. He was a big man and his head left a big dent. Emily and I were already sleeping but Mother yelled for us and we ran out. Ken was trying to get up and Mother told me to hold him down. Blood was gushing from his head and I jumped on top of him, straddled his chest, and started holding his arms down. I was probably 17 at the time. I was wearing a slinky nightgown, bright orange I believe, and he settled right down. I was hoping he was drunk enough to not remember that. Emily got dressed while Mother got her truck back out of the garage and then we hauled him up. There was a pool of blood on the floor and Mother told me to just leave it and she would clean it up when they got back from the hospital. Mike was living with us at the time and she asked me to wait for him to come home and tell him what happened. They got him outside and into the truck and headed for the hospital. I cleaned up the blood (after putting on a robe); you can't leave a pool of blood on the floor. Can you imagine walking in and someone says, "There's your father's blood."

I'm also thinking about the dolls Mother used to make. When Kathy adopted two little Korean girls I sent their photographs to Mother and she made them each a doll in their own image, they were beautiful. I wonder whatever happened to those dolls. I haven't seen Kathy in years. Mother made me two Native American dolls, a male and a female. They are about 7 inches tall, have felt clothes, and even have beaded necklaces. I treasure them, and they are proudly displayed near my bed. Mother's creativity, and skill, was unbelievable. Now it is gone.

The staff at the nursing home really puzzles me. Except for the activity director I never recognize anyone. Although today when I was sitting in the dining area a young black male nurse did a double take when he saw me and then said hi. He obviously recognized me. The male nurses are either black or Jamaican (all young). There are no white males. However, the females include white, black, and Jamaican. The men are now wearing the purple scrubs instead of all white. Maybe they were being mistaken for doctors. The kitchen staff seems to be Hispanic. So, does the staff change every two months or what? It must be difficult for the residents that just when they get used to someone, someone they can finally recognize, and then the staff changes. Then they're right back to being with total strangers. They need familiarity.

January 17, 2010

This morning we met David and Dorothy at Lundee's for a late breakfast before going to the nursing home. I like to get there right after Mother finishes lunch. As I checked in at the front desk I saw the smoking lady get off the elevator and head for the front door. The temperature was in the 30s. It was clear and sunny and really didn't seem very cold, we were walking around without our jackets. If we were at home we would have been freezing to death, but it just seems different in Minnesota.

When I got inside Mother's unit I could see a lot of residents sitting scattered all over. It's Sunday so maybe they were expecting visitors; usually there aren't any. I began walking through the dining area, looking for Mother. There was a woman sleeping in a chair that I thought might be her but when I got closer I saw that it wasn't. As I continued to walk I looked over at the sitting area and saw her. She was sitting on the edge of the chair, hands clasped between her knees, and she was watching me! Wow, I knew she recognized me. I walked over to her and said, "Are you waiting for me?" She said no. Then she started crying. It broke my heart. I knelt down, put my arms around her and said, "What's wrong, why are you crying?" She didn't say anything. I said, "Are you feeling lonely?" She said, "It's not that I'm lonely, it's just these people!" I said, "It'll be alright. Really, it'll be okay." I just wish I knew why she doesn't like the people here. I wish she was capable of explaining it. There is such an incredible sense of loneliness about her. I asked if she'd like to walk down to her room and she said yes.

As we walked down the hallway she looked at the floor (with the missing carpet) and said, "I wonder what happened here." I said they tore it up so they could put new stuff down. When we got in her room I sat her down on the side of the bed and then once again sat on the floor in front of her. That position works well for both of us; she can look straight at me. Her roommate was in her bed sleeping. I took Chelsey out of her bag and held her up, "Here's Chelsey. She came to see you. Do you remember Chelsey?" Mother gave a quick nod and that was it. I put Chelsey on the bed, threw her blanket over her and she hunkered down. Today Mother was wearing dark slacks and the light green sweatshirt that has little images around the neckline. I was wearing a blue and white sweater with a snowflake design. I could see Mother focusing in on it and she said it was pretty. Funny how she notices the designs on my clothes but yesterday she couldn't see the cross. I'll have to experiment some on my future visits. I took the Bible out of the drawer and handed it to her and asked if she had read from it last night. She said yes, but I know she didn't. We looked at her photographs again – the one of her, David, and Santa Claus and the one of her, Emily, and David. She still doesn't remember who the people are. I asked if she would like to look at the pictures on the calendars and she said yes. It was basically a repeat of yesterday, she seemed interested in all of the pictures, especially the dogs. When we got to what she said was her favorite yesterday she had the same reaction, "Oh, I like this one." I said, "Who is it?" And she said, "Me!" I said, "That's right, it's you."

I could hear a radio playing outside of her room somewhere, not music, but a man talking. Mother said, "What is that?" I said it's a radio. She looked puzzled so I said someone has a radio going. After finishing with all of the calendars we started looking at the cards she had received. She's got so many cards. They are lined up on a metal strip on the wall and there are stacks of them in the drawer. Most of the cards are from me but there are others, and there are even some that are not hers; they were made out to other people, some even had letters written in them. I don't know where they came from. Maybe they just came with the room. We went through them all. I would put one in her hands and she would look at the picture on the front. After a moment I would put the next picture on top until she had so many in her hands that she couldn't hold them all. Then I took that pile and started a fresh one. She looked at all of the pictures but the ones that got a smile out of her were the ones that had animal pictures on them, either a real photograph or just a drawn picture. That's why I mostly buy children's cards. After this long of time I have trouble finding new cards and end up sending several of the same pictures. I don't think she notices. There was also a very old photo of Pepper, the cocker spaniel we had when I was growing up. The photo was taken right after Mother had given him a haircut and he looked so funny because it looked like she had shaved him. Mother looked at that picture for a very long time. I don't know if she felt he was familiar or what she was thinking; she didn't say anything.

After we finished looking at the cards there wasn't much to do and she started dozing off. I asked her if she'd like to lie down and take a nap and she said no. After a while, with her swaying back and forth, I asked again and she still said no. I said, you're about to fall over. She smiled and said she didn't like to sleep lying down. I asked if she wanted me to take her into the other area so she could sleep in one of the chairs and she smiled and said she didn't like sleeping in chairs. I said so you just sleep sitting up, swaying back and forth, until you fall over. She smiled and said yes. Most of this conversation took place with her eyes shut, I laughed and then settled in to watch and see what she would do.

She put her hands on the bed on both sides to brace herself better and her right hand went slightly under Chesley's blanket with her fingers resting on top of Chelsey's right foot. I saw the expression on her face change to one of puzzlement. She lightly ran her fingers over Chesley's foot for a moment and then she smiled, leaving her fingers on top of the foot. Chelsey didn't even move. After awhile Mother moved her hand to the edge of the bed, palm upwards. I put my hand in hers and she closed her fingers around mine. Her fingers started gently pulsing. I wonder what causes that; my fingers will pulse like that sometimes.

After awhile she said, "Did you hear him start up?" I said yes. She said, "Wasn't that fun?" I said yes. I had no idea what she was talking about of course. Was she hearing things again or had she been dreaming? Doesn't matter. If that's how she dreams I can see why she sleeps so much. It wasn't long before she almost fell over again and I asked her if she'd like to lie down and take a nap and she said yes. I hugged her, kissed her, and told her I loved her. She said that she loves me too. I helped her lie down, making sure the pillow was under her head, and told her that I would see her soon.

Walking out of the unit I again saw a group of residents sitting in front of a small television set watching a movie. As I walked out the door a Jamaican man walked out behind me. I started down the hall and he said, "How was Shirley, was she conversating today?" Conversating? I don't think I've heard that word before. Oh wait; I have heard that word, one day while watching Judge Joe Brown on TV. It went something like: "We was standing there conversating when suddenly he punched me the face." In answer to the man's question I said, "Yes." I continued walking and he said, "Do you buy her clothes? She has a lot of clothes." Now why did he say that? How does he know how many clothes she has? I don't think that he does her laundry. Is he trying to tell me that he dresses her? That's creepy. I believe that the female nurses should be dressing the female residents; men shouldn't be doing that. Same way with the bathing. I already know that men do bathroom duty. It just seems more dignified for women to take care of those personal needs for the women. No wonder Mother is so often pissed off. I know that my mood instantly changed with his remark. I feel the same way with hospitals. I know that if I were in the hospital I would not want a man bathing me. Men don't seem to care about that, but I'm sure there are a lot of women who would agree with me. I know David feels the same way I do. I remember him telling me how upset he was one day when a man took Mother to her room to change her sweatshirt because she was hot. Besides, Mother doesn't have that many clothes, she used to but now she may have a week's worth, and only one pair of shoes. Everything she has now will fit in one box; her possessions have been reduced to the bare essentials.

In answer to his question whether I buy Mother's clothes I said, "No, I don't live around here." I kept walking and he started to go into the kitchen, then he stopped and said, "Shirley is a sweet lady, but sometimes…" then his eyes got really big and I said, "I know." He went on into the kitchen and I kept walking. That's the first time I've left that place angry. Tom was waiting for me when I got downstairs. I signed out and as we were leaving Tom said there was now a big sign saying that new residents would not be able to smoke outside any more. They were going to let the current residents continue smoking but would just weed them out until it was completely nonsmoking. Jerks.

We stopped at Nancy's house for a short visit on our way out of town. We talked a little about Mother and Nancy told me how she had taken her to the dentist one day there in the building. When they got in the dentist's off Mother refused to open her mouth. I can just see Mother doing that, clamping her mouth shut tight like a child. Nancy asked how Mother likes Chelsey and I said, "Sometimes she does, sometimes she doesn't."

Tonight we are at the Best Inn motel in Chillicothe. The sign out front says Best Western but when I looked at the receipt it says Best Inn. That's strange. Last time we were here it was packed, but tonight we are the only guests. It's strange to see this big place empty. Still, Tom had to negotiate with the clerk to get the price down to $60. She finally said, "Well, if you tell me you're with AARP I can give you the room for $60." He said, "Okay, I'm with AARP." Unloading the truck Tom almost got us in trouble. He had grabbed Chelsey's bed and had it under his arm and then couldn't get the card key to work. We were close to the office and the clerk finally saw we were having a problem and came out. She couldn't get the card to work either and took it back to the office to reprogram it. I said, "Put that bed back in the truck." Even though he had the bed under his arm if someone had focused in on it they would have been able to tell it was a pet bed. Probably no one would even care that we had a tortoise in there, but you never know; we don't want to get kicked out. Chelsey is so cute in motel rooms. She cuddles in the bed with Tom until it's time for her bath and feeding. Then she cuddles with Tom again until I'm ready to go to bed and I put her in her own bed. In the mornings she gets to cuddle in the bed with me while I have my coffee. Funny because she won't cuddle like that at home. She lets us hold her for awhile in the evening but that's it. Time for sleep, we have a long day ahead of us.

January 18, 2010

Tom was up early this morning and went to the lobby for the lousy coffee they serve here. Can't motels ever have good coffee? At least it will wake you up. There was a lot of heavy fog throughout Iowa and Missouri last night. It was really wet. Back out on the road this morning it was still foggy. It stayed foggy until about noon. We had an uneventful drive back to Arkansas. It's so good to be home. I miss Mother already.

January 19, 2010

I had this dream last night. I was in a pharmacy looking at the items on a shelf. I had a portable radio with me and I turned it on and it started playing music. It was a song I knew, classic rock, and I started singing along with it. It was loud, but I was the only one in the store. I was having a good time, singing and collecting the items I needed. I went around the end of the long shelf and started along the other side. I noticed that all along the back wall there was a big glass window. The pharmacist (my actual one) was sitting right in front of me behind the glass, at what looked like a counter. There was an entire room behind him, where they kept the drugs, etc. He seemed to be doing some paper-work. We saw each other at the same time. He looked alarmed and jumped up and started to the side like he was coming out to where I was. I said, "Oh hi. I didn't think you'd be here today." At that he sat back down and smiled at me.

Later in the night I had this dream. I was in what was my car and seemed to have been pulled over by a female cop. She was young, late 20s, maybe 30, pretty, with long brown hair slightly curled. She was not wearing any kind of uniform. It's a little fuzzy now but she kept telling me that I wasn't supposed to be there (driving in that area) and I was arguing with her, saying that it was okay for me to be there. I kept trying to give her my driver's license, but she wouldn't take it. She kept saying that I had to prove that I belonged there. She was losing patience with me and wanted me to turn around and leave and I kept pleading with her. Then I said, "Wait, I have something!" I knew there was something in the glove box that had my name and address on it. I reached over, opened the glove box and pulled out a large greeting card and its accompanying envelope. I said, "Look at this; it has my name and address on it." The card was pink and white and I knew there was all kinds of writing inside that would prove I was supposed to be there. But when I opened it to show her it was completely blank. I sighed in resignation, completely frustrated. End of dream.

What do the dreams mean? As Tom and I were driving home from Minnesota we were listening to classic rock whenever we could tune into a radio station. Singing along to those songs always creates a soothing effect and lifts our spirits. Singing in the pharmacy is showing me that music is medicine. Music is now being used as therapy for many conditions. Just look what it does for Mother, she sings and dances to it. Looking at both points of the dreams they show how frustrated I am after a visit with Mother. I know she needs a certain diet. I know she needs exercise. And I know that she needs counseling; someone who can get her to talk about her feelings. But there is nothing I can do about it. I have no say whatsoever in any way. In the dream I try to prove that I should have a say – that I belong there – but I just can't prove it. Yes, I visit every two months. But that is meaningless to Mother's care. The pharmacist sitting behind the window in the first dream also shows my position in Mother's care; and my saying I didn't know you were here is my position with the staff. They don't know who I am. I can watch what's going on (behind the glass) but I can't interact with the staff (can't come out from behind the glass). It's frustrating.

January 21, 2010

I found an article in the newspaper today entitled, "Music touted as after-stroke therapy." The article was written by Randolph E. Schmid for *The Associated Press* and it says that words and music are such natural partners that it seems obvious they go together. Now science is confirming that those abilities are linked in the brain, a finding that some say might even lead to better stroke treatments. Studies have found overlap in the brain's processing of language and instrumental music, and new research suggests that intensive musical therapy could help to improve speech in stroke patients. People who have suffered a severe stroke on the left side of the brain and cannot speak can sometimes learn to communicate through singing. Music making is a multisensory experience, activating links to several parts of the brain. The ability to sing originates in the right side of the brain. People who are recovering from stroke or brain injury can work around the injury to the left side of the brain by first singing their thoughts. Then gradually, they can drop the melody, restoring their lost speech. Music can also improve the quality of life for dementia patients. The ability to engage with music remains intact into the later stages of dementia. Music therapy can help to recall memories, reduce agitation, assist communication and improve coordination.

January 22, 2010

I just couldn't go to sleep last night. I wasn't able to quiet my mind. I tried to lull myself to sleep by thinking about how comfortable my bed is. And that bed is sooo comfortable. We've had it forever. It actually came from a thrift shop when I was pregnant with Scott. The frame is iron and it has the old style springs. I felt myself sink down into the softness, deeper and deeper. I wondered if Mother had ever slept in the bed and I let my mind start flowing back over the years; they say you should never give up your own bed to a guest but there are always exceptions. There was one time she slept in it. She and Ken had come for a visit. The boys were very young. We only had two bedrooms and I didn't want them to have to sleep on the couch, so Tom and I did instead. The house was a rental but it was pretty nice, we just didn't have a lot of furniture. We also didn't have air conditioning (no money for either). And it was summer. I remember that I had long orange plastic curtains (cheap) on the bedroom window and the next morning I saw that Ken had tied them in a knot in an effort to get some air in during the night. I had some new orange towels which I had placed in the bathroom. Mother told me later that Ken had gone in there and when he came out he had little orange towel fuzz stuck all over his chin stubble. She thought it was funny, but I was a bit embarrassed; I didn't know I was supposed to wash the towels before you used them to remove the loose stuff. They were always very gracious about our poverty and my lack of knowledge about being an adult.

I came across an article on the internet today entitled, "Dementia Risk Drops if You Lower Your Blood Pressure." It was on the Rodale website, by Leah Zerbe. There had been a study about people taking blood pressure-lowering drugs. Tracking the data researchers discovered that people taking certain types of the drugs had a lower risk of dementia—as much as 24 percent lower for some people. Among people who already were living with Alzheimer's disease, those who took one type of blood pressure medicine had a nearly 50 percent lower chance of being admitted to a nursing home, and a 17 percent lower risk of death when compared to patients taking other cardiovascular drugs. Mother doesn't have Alzheimer's, but there are similar symptoms. And, of course, the study doesn't say which drug was the one. Mother has had high blood pressure for a very long time; however, I don't know whether she was still taking the medication while in Crosslake. She takes it now I believe. Obviously, she hasn't been taking the one because since all of this has transpired there has been no improvement in her dementia.

In a separate study also illustrating high blood pressure's effect on cognitive functioning, researchers found that even slightly elevated blood pressure can damage small blood vessels in the brain, leading to damaged white matter. This, in turn, shows up on MRI scans as lesions that are associated with dementia. Researchers found that the women they studied with high blood pressure at the beginning of the study showed significantly more white matter lesions when scanned eight years later, compared to the women with normal blood pressure. The biggest concern, says the researcher, is that even moderately elevated blood pressure was associated with damage in the brain. This damage can lead to an increased risk of stroke, disability, and dementia. "It's life-shortening," said the researcher. What this second study shows is that blood pressure-lowering drugs seem to slow cognitive decline in people diagnosed with both dementia and Alzheimer's—perhaps by preventing high blood pressure's damage to blood vessels in the brain.

The article also listed some ways to bring down your blood pressure to reduce the risk of dementia:

Get your blood moving. The researcher says that if you don't get blood to the brain, you're not going to think very well. Anything that promotes blood flow to the brain is probably going to be good. One of the benefits of exercise is getting the blood pumping and delivered around the body. When your heart is pumping blood and you're pushing yourself a little bit, you're stretching the blood vessels, including the ones that keep your brain healthy. People with dementia get less blood to the brain.

Eat a cool diet. A diet loaded with sugar, fat, and salt is a recipe for inflammation, and one that seems to raise the risk of dementia. It is suggested eating a mostly plant-based diet, supplementing with omega-3-rich hempseed protein powder or flax seeds. To lower your blood pressure and inflammation eat whole, organic foods as much as possible, and erase processed, packaged foods, and much takeout from your menu.

Get your D. Many people are deficient in vitamin D. The vitamin is found in few foods, but our body creates it when the sun hits our skin. Vitamin D is involved in so many of our bodies' processes, and studies have found a link between vitamin D deficiency and dementia. There is a blood test that can be done by your doctor.

Shield your brain. High levels of stress can increase inflammatory chemicals in your body that can contribute to the dementia process.

January 25, 2010

I found an article on the internet by Emily Sohn on discovery.com tonight about blueberries. It says: there may be a simple way to ease the memory lapses and brain slips that typically accompany old age: eat more blueberries. Results of a study of older adults who drank a couple of cups of blueberry juice a day improved their scores on a learning and memory task by 20%. Studies in animals have linked blueberries with brain function. The results of the study suggest that blueberries might just live up to their reputation as "superfoods." Among other health benefits adding blueberries to your diet could help slow the progress of memory decline and possibly even prevent memories from slipping in the first place.

One of the doctors in the study said that there is so much research now suggesting that fruits and vegetables are beneficial. The case for blueberries has been building for more than a decade. In animal studies, older individuals that consume blueberry extract improve their performance on memory tasks, sometimes to the point of being just as sharp as their younger counterparts. To explain how blueberries might bring about such impressive brain-boosting effects, other studies have zeroed in on a type of antioxidant called anthocyanins. These molecules belong to a larger group called polyphenols, which come in thousands of varieties. Polyphenols appear in virtually all fruits and vegetables and have been shown to reduce the risk of cancers and heart disease, among other benefits. In animals that have consumed lots of blueberries, scientists have spotted anthocyanins in the brain structures that are known to be involved in memory. There, molecules appear to work their magic by helping neurons communicate with each other, facilitating memory processing. Anthocyanins also make brain cells more resilient in the face of stress. The molecules might even act as a sort of mild toxin that prods the body to grow stronger.

The major question lingering from that research was whether any of it applied to people. To find out researchers recruited nine adults who were, on average, in their mid-70s. All participants had experienced some mild memory decline. At the beginning each participant took a series of learning and memory tests. For the next 12 weeks, participants drank three glasses of blueberry juice a day, for a total of between two and two and a half cups. The exact amount depended on body weight. During the last week of the study participants took the memory tests again. There was a 20% improvement. A similar test had been conducted previously with anthocyanin-rich grape juice, which turned up similar results.

While the number of subjects in the blueberry study was small, the results were encouraging. The findings raise hopes that blueberries could stave off Alzheimer's and other age-related neurodegenerative diseases. Plenty of details will have to be worked out such as how many blueberries do you need to eat to see any benefits? Does juice work better than whole fruit? For now, research suggests that blueberries will do more for older people whose brains are starting to fade than for younger people who are still sharp. So, how do I get blueberries into Mother?

January 28, 2010

There's a big winter storm heading our way. At noon today it was 20 degrees blow zero in Minneapolis. That sure was good timing on our trip up there two weeks ago. On the news they were talking about ice fog in Iowa. Tom said that's what we'd been driving through on our way home. I've never heard of ice fog. I think I'll look it up on Wikipedia. Okay, ice fog is a type of fog consisting of fine ice crystals that are suspended in the air. It was probably a good thing we were just passing through quickly.

January 29, 2010

My dishwasher is leaking. What a pain. We didn't have a dishwasher while I was growing up, we all washed dishes, and dried them. Not that any of us wanted to. Chores were a major hassle in our house. Mother devised numerous methods of dividing up the chores because no one wanted to do anything. We had to, of course, but we fought about it all of the time. Mother tried to make everything fair so that chores would be rotated. She went through a lot; such as charts, assignments, and I remember at least once putting all the chores on scraps of paper and making us draw them out of a container. Nothing worked. We just didn't want to do anything. Poor Mother! It's funny now, but she must have been so frustrated with us.

One night Mother did the dishes by herself. I was still sitting at the dinner table, refusing to eat my peas. We were a 'clean your plate' family. I couldn't stand the taste of peas. So, I was being punished. "You'll sit there until you eat them." I sat there and watched Mother wash all of the dishes. Then she dried all of the dishes and put them away. We didn't say a word to each other. I just sat and watched. It was quite relaxing actually. For both of us, because no one else could enter the kitchen; I was being punished. When she had finished, and the kitchen was spotless, she told me I could go to bed. Peas untouched.

Our weather is still bad. It sleeted this morning and snowed this evening. Mother is getting an ice storm. I wonder if she stands out in the vestibule and watches the snow fall. She used to love it so much, even loved to shovel it.

February 4, 2010

I mailed Mother's birthday present today. Another bottle of lotion. Hopefully this one will stick around.

February 6, 2010

I had this dream last night. I was in front of a computer watching a television program. It was a dance competition and Tom was going to be competing. I was really amused because I knew he couldn't dance worth shit. I was waiting for the dancing to begin. All I could see was an empty stage and I was wondering if Tom could dance any better now than he could before. The room I was in was dimly lit and the program was dimly lit also. I began to wake up but I pulled myself back in because I really wanted to see Tom dance. But I couldn't hold it and woke up.

I don't know what the dream means unless it's that I keep waiting for Tom to go back to work and he hasn't. He hasn't been working at all this winter. He has a little work lined up but he hasn't done any of it yet. Mainly because of the weather, he always says he'll do it next week, then the next week comes and it's either getting ready to rain or snow. When you're broke you're supposed to work when you can, no matter how difficult it may be. I am so ready for him to start dancing again.

February 9, 2010

Today is Mother's 84th birthday! The last birthday I spent with her was in 2007. Emily and I had flown in at the same time to be with her. Mother was living with Rebecca and her family at the time. We were staying at David's and the three of us drove up there for a surprise birthday party. Mother had been going to a Senior Citizen Center a couple of days a week and really enjoying it. A small bus would pick her up and bring her back. We got to the house before she did. I'll never forget the moment I saw her. I was standing in the kitchen talking to Rebecca and she nodded behind me; I turned around and there she was—beautiful snow white curly hair, wearing a knit hat – and teeth. I hadn't heard her come in and she was just standing there in silence, smiling. I gave her a big hug. Today I got out the photographs I had taken that day just so I could see her like that again. I miss her so much.

February 10, 2010

We are having the coldest weather in 15 years. There are snow storms everywhere. There is thirty inches of snow on the east coast. Scott has 6 inches at his house.

February 12, 2010

They're calling it the "February Fury." (Why does every storm need it's own name?) It's hitting everyone. In the Mid-Atlantic and Washington D.C. they got record snows of 30 inches. Dallas got heavy snow. We got snow here last night. Every state in the country has gotten snow during this storm.

Seeing pictures of the big snow banks reminds me of the heavy snows we'd get while I was growing up. I have a vivid picture in my mind of Daddy shoveling out the driveway. He was wearing a bright yellow parka. Of course we all had to get out there and shovel. This one particular memory however was of so much snow that once the driveway was clear we couldn't see the road over the huge snow banks we had created. Cars would have to creep out of the driveways to look for oncoming vehicles. Then it seemed like you'd just get the end of the driveway clear and a snowplow would come along and fill it back up. Ken, of course, had a snowblower for his driveway. I'm in awe of that much snow, especially when it is still pure white and sparkling in the sunlight.

February 15, 2010

Now they say we're having a La Nina winter, the winter equivalent of El Nino. The wind is still blowing hard. I guess there's a "Clipper" going on. There was a 40 car pileup in Kansas City as a result. It's now heading east. The temperature is 20 degrees below normal. Looking outside and watching the weather I think about walking to school every day in elementary school. We all walked to school, no matter what the weather was doing. There was not one mother in our neighborhood that was willing to step outside and drive her kids to school. Back in those days we had to wear dresses to school so in the winter we had to wear slacks underneath until we got to school and then take off our layers of clothing before class. It was ridiculous really. We walked seven blocks I think; in blizzards, in rain, in freezing cold. And if we got to the school a little early they made us stand outside until the appointed minute. I know with my mother she couldn't wait to get us out the door so she could get ready to go to work. I never made my kids go through that. We learn from our parents.

February 19, 2010

I have come across some additional information about osteoporosis. They are now putting out warnings on the effects of long term use of osteoporosis medications. A woman wrote to a doctor (Peter H. Gott, M.D.) in the newspaper and said she had developed necrotic bone (which technically is the death of living tissue). She had been diagnosed with dead bone in her jaw. She had developed a large torus palatinus on the roof of her mouth. Her oral surgeon was convinced that it was caused by taking certain osteoporosis medications for seven years. The bone becomes exposed and sometimes will fall out on its own, or it is removed surgically. According to the doctor, the torus palatinus is a benign bony growth known as exostosis located in the middle of the hard palate in the roof of the mouth. It doesn't require treatment unless it becomes so large it interferes with function or dental placement.

There is also a warning about consuming phosphoric acid, such as Coke. The active ingredient in Coke is phosphoric acid. It will dissolve a nail in about four days (or the ice on your windshield in about one minute). Phosphoric acid also leaches calcium from bones and is a major contributor to the rising increase of osteoporosis.

Here's a fun fact. Is your index finger shorter than your ring finger? That could be a sign of osteoarthritis. Here's a tip. It's easier to look from the back of the fingers. Mine seem to be okay. The definition of osteoarthritis is: arthritis of middle age characterized by degenerative and sometimes hypertrophic changes in the bone and cartilage of one or more joints and a progressive wearing down of apposing joint surfaces with consequent distortion of joint position usually without bony stiffening; also called degenerative arthritis, degenerative joint disease, hypertrophic arthritis. Yup, that's crystal clear. That's what I get for using a medical dictionary. And what do they consider middle age these days? It used to be 40 or so, but nowadays who knows. I personally consider 60 to be middle age.

February 21, 2010

Tom is in Texarkana this weekend for one of his motorcycle races. I was thinking about the time I was riding somewhere with Daddy. We had pulled up to a stoplight and next to us was a young woman on a scooter. Daddy said, "Don't ever get on a motorcycle." If he only knew. I figured I'd probably never be on a scooter, but motorcycles were a different story. Not long after that I was riding my bike around the neighborhood after dinner. I came to a group of kids standing in the street in front of a house. Naturally I had to go over and see what was going on. One boy told me that someone had just bought a motorcycle and was giving everyone rides. I got in line and when it was my turn I climbed on behind the teenager's back and held on. I loved it. Going back home I didn't say a word about it to anyone. I knew I had been far enough away from my house for anyone to see me. Years layer before the boys were born I rode with Tom all the time. One day we were driving through downtown and stopped at a stoplight. There was a bus bench next to us on the sidewalk and an old woman sitting there yelled angrily at us, "Hippies!" We weren't, but it was still funny.

I got an email from David today and he said that he had stopped by on Friday to see Mother and she had asked him if Janet had come with him. David had said she couldn't make it this time. He said that had surprised him. Surprised him? That surprises the hell out of me. Wow. Talk about creating a really good feeling. It's been more than a month since I've seen her. Of course I suppose she could have just received one of my cards in the mail so my name was on her mind. I think I'll just believe that she remembers me and would like to see me.

February 23, 2010

I was cleaning the living room today and hidden in a corner I found a Christmas nutcracker. I suspect one of the grandkids had been playing with it. This particular nutcracker was one of Mother's. I actually gave it to her. Over the years she had gathered a large collection of them, from small to very large. Every Christmas she arranged all of the nutcrackers across her fireplace mantel; from the tallest on one end to the tiniest on the other end. I have some of her collection, but not all of them, which I put out at Christmas. Some of them are in the original boxes and Mother wrote on them where they had come from. When I saw that I thought that was a great idea, my ornaments all have a little story behind them. I should start taking photographs of my ornaments and then write down the story behind them, that way the tradition can live on. I wonder what the boys were doing with this nutcracker. They had spent a few nights with us and early one morning Ben actually got me out of bed yelling from the living room, "Grandma, can we use this?" I went in there and he was pointing at a rather large nutcracker. I didn't really want them to use it but my sleep fogged brain couldn't come up with a reason not to. I said okay and trudged back to bed. I really didn't think it would work, thinking he was going to try and crack the hard shell nuts. But when I got up later there was a pile of broken peanut shells on the floor. I said, "I see it worked," and he said, "Well, only on the peanuts." So, the hiding nutcracker I found in the corner went into a closet with all of the other Christmas items I find after everything has been packed away. Perhaps I'll remember to get the stuff out next Christmas.

February 25, 2010

We're expecting snow again tonight. This evening we were watching the cross country ski events on TV. Skiing is something I've never done. It's funny really, growing up in Minnesota and we never skied. When Mother retired to Crosslake she started cross country skiing. I remember she was so proud of what she was doing and was really having fun with it. She usually just did it around her house, but in the dead of winter she was pretty much the only one in the general vicinity so she could ski all over the neighbor's place when she wanted to. She also had some friends that she skied with, and most of the surrounding area empties out in the winter so they could go pretty much wherever they wanted to. I would have liked to have joined her with that. In one of the letters she wrote me, when she moved into the assisted living place, she said she especially wanted to get her skis so she could use them when winter arrived. She had written: "...there's plenty of room outside for me to use them and it'll be fun to ski again, no hills of course but I didn't downhill anyway, just cross country." That didn't happen. I wonder where her skis are now.

March 5, 2010

Kelley is spending the night with us. She went in to take a shower and a couple of minutes later she came running through the house into my office wrapped in a large bath towel. She was out of breath and was holding a razor in her hand. All excited she said, "Can I use this?" It was an Intuition razor. It was something new and had lotion built in or something. I got it free and had never used it. I said, "Sure you can use it." She loves looking through my stuff looking for something new or different. A while later Tom yelled from the living room, "Kelley is bleeding to death!" I went out there and Kelley was sitting on the couch with a handful of band-aids and cuts all over her legs. I said, "I thought that wasn't supposed to happen with that razor." She said, "I was trying to do it real fast." I just shook my head, hoping I wouldn't get in any trouble when she got home. She's been shaving her legs for years.

Kelley's blossoming into womanhood is so different than mine had been. One day in grade school all of us girls were herded into one room and shown "the movie" about reproduction and menstruation. I didn't understand any of it and all I remembered afterwards were pictures of flowers blooming. After the movie was over nothing was said and we were all sent back to class. When I got home that afternoon Mother was waiting for me. She had said, "Well, did you see the movie?" I said, "Yes." She said, "Do you have any questions?" I said, "No." And that was it. She was obviously relieved that I hadn't wanted to talk about it. I don't know what her problem was, she'd already been through it with Nancy. But Nancy and I had totally different personalities. Nancy was the oldest and she was always independent and outspoken. I was quiet and embarrassed really, about everything. During that time I was waiting for Mother to guide me into womanhood but she seemed embarrassed about everything also.

March 6, 2010

It's in the 60s today and so nice. There are ladybugs swarming everywhere, along with robins. We have seen the skunks and we can hear the frogs singing at night. There is clover blooming and soon we'll see dandelions. I love dandelions. My parents hated them. There were no dandelions allowed in our neighborhood. They made us dig them up every year. We didn't want to but didn't have a choice. We'd each get assigned to a different part of the yard, was given a bucket and a yard tool, and for each full bucket they gave us a nickel. It was hard work for sure. I love seeing the bright yellow dandelions in my yard.

March 9, 2010

It's been a long winter but work is finally starting up a bit. Mother had to work nearly my entire childhood. I hated her having to do that. Logically I understood that with four kids both of my parents needed to work. When she married Ken I was really hoping she wouldn't have to. Ken had a very successful business with his gas station and later his towing business. But that wasn't to be. She still worked. Later she was able to just work part-time. There were some rare times as a child when she hadn't worked. Coming home from school and seeing her waiting for us was the best feeling. That was a big reason why I didn't work after the boys were born. I worked occasionally for extra money but on the whole I was at home. I wanted to be there when they got off the bus, available during the day for whatever, and be able to participate in after-school activities. They say you learn from your parents. Watching my mother greeting us after school, doing housework, baking, sewing; that's what I wanted to do as a mother. Mother wasn't able to stay home full time but I was.

March 10, 2010

There were tornadoes in the state today. We had warnings all day. This evening things got really rough all around us. We were watching TV, watching them track the tornadoes getting closer and closer. We watched as one traveled over our town and then hit a town about 15 miles from here. It was bad, very bad. Our little spot out in the country has remained pretty safe. Tommy has more trouble right up the road because they're on a mountain. Still, we take these warnings very seriously.

March 11, 2010

The phone rang this morning while I was still sleeping. I answered, still in a grog, and a woman's voice said, "Janet?" I said, "Yes." She said, "Did you get blown away last night?" I said, "No." She said, "I saw it on the news and I was worried about you." The voice was really familiar but I couldn't put a face to it. I said, "Who is this?" She said, "It's your sister!" It was Emily. Smile. We talked about the storm and of course I apologized for not recognizing her voice. We talked about Mother and I filled her in on all of the changes and about my visits. Later I was sitting outside with Chelsey and I was thinking back on our conversation. Emily had talked about having a Facebook page and about how it worked. She was trying to get me to set one up but I'm really not interested in doing that. She was also talking about the little things that bothered her about it. There's a farm game that people play and she started getting messages saying that someone's cow got loose and Emily said she couldn't care less if someone's cow got loose. I thought that's exactly what Mother would have said. And then I thought, "That's it! Emily sounds exactly like Mother used to." No wonder I didn't know who it was. The voice was familiar because it sounded like Mother, but I knew it couldn't be Mother, so I didn't know who it was.

I had sent David an email yesterday asking him if he'd be home this weekend because Tom said we may get to go up there. I got an email back from him this afternoon saying he'd be home all weekend although the weather may be a little wet. He asked me if the big storm had gone through our neighborhood yesterday afternoon. Wow, Arkansas really hit the national news. Later this evening David sent another email telling me to look up the LaQuinta Inn in Brooklyn Park. He said it's right on Boone Ave. and right off the freeway between David and Mother's places. It's only $59 a night. I jumped online and found it, joined their rewards club, and printed up a map. That will be nice. I wonder how long it's been there, David's never mentioned it before.

March 12, 2010

Things have changed. Tom got some work so we won't be leaving this weekend. I sent an email to David telling him, saying we'll be aiming for the end of next week. He sent an email back saying the next Saturday night he and Dorothy are taking Alexsis and Steven to the Holiday Inn for the night. They have a big indoor water park. David always has all those hotel perks because he travels all the time so they'll be staying for free.

March 14, 2010

I am moping around today. I feel so guilty about not going to Minnesota last weekend. I'm really missing Mother.

March 16, 2010

Tom said we are definitely going this week. Yea! I called the LaQuinta and made a reservation for Saturday night.

March 17, 2010

I had this dream last night. I was standing in front of three tall glass fronted cabinets. Inside I could see shelves full of items. Included were some Valentine articles that were on sale because Valentine's Day is over. I was scanning the items looking to see if there was something I wanted. Some of the items were ceramic and I wasn't interested in them. Some of the items had little signs that said 18% off. I thought that was a strange discount. I kept looking and then right in the middle I saw some small, colorful, metallic religious stickers. They had the 18% off sign. I thought I would like to have some of them. The main colors were purple and gold. As I was standing there a woman and her daughter came in. They were both blond and the girl looked to be about 10 years old. I was looking into the middle cabinet and they walked over to the one on my left. The mother had a key and she unlocked the cabinet and pulled the glass door open on the top half of the cabinet. I thought, "I didn't realize they were locked," and I wondered if they would give me the key or if I'd have to go and ask for one. The mother and daughter were talking to each other but I wasn't paying any attention because I was thinking about the key. I asked the mother if I could use the key and she handed it to me. It was a strange key—it was built into a handle and had a square plastic sheath on the key part. I pulled off the sheath, put the key in the lock and was glad that it fit. I then focused in on the couple. The mother said, "So you don't see anything in there?" The girl shook her head no and they left. I knew they were talking about seeing something paranormally. I glanced in the cabinet and it looked to contain old dishware. I wondered what they were expecting to see.

Next I was pulling a kitchen stepstool (the one in my kitchen) over to the front of the cabinet I had been looking into. There was a lot of stuff stacked in front of the cabinet that was blocking my way and I was trying to maneuver the stool close enough to reach into the cabinet. Zakary was now helping me.

Next I was outside. There were several very long tables set up with people sitting at them. I don't remember this part of the dream very well. The people were all different ages, looking like families sitting there enjoying a picnic. I didn't recognize any of the people. I think I went over to a little girl who was sitting near the end of one of the tables and said something to her. That's where the dream ended.

I'm sure that once again this dream is about Mother and me. The Valentine reference must be our love for each other. At first I was just looking for a good deal. The only thing I was interested in were the stickers and I was thinking that I could maybe use them in the grandkid's scrapbooks. Interpreting the dream I can take all of the symbols together. I have love, religion, a mother-daughter relationship, and families. There is also the paranormal. The paranormal is actually the spirit world. I think this dream is showing me that I should discuss religion and spirit with Mother. In the dream the cabinets were locked and the mother had the key. In past dreams Mother's and my roles have become reversed so I could say that I unlocked the door to the spiritual world for Mother. The girl couldn't see anything paranormal in the cabinet so perhaps it's up to me to bring it out in the open—to let it be seen. I need to bring up the subject with Mother. She may already be thinking about it, but is keeping it to herself, which would explain why the key was in a protected sheath. It may be a difficult task shown as my having difficulty getting into the cabinet and ultimately having to use a stepstool (and Zakary). Bottom line—I need to discuss the spirit world with Mother. I already gave her the Bible but I need to go further. I'll be seeing her soon so when I have her alone I'll see if she knows who God is, etc. And maybe I can find some of those religious stickers to put on her cards.

March 18, 2010

When Tom got home from work today he said we may be going to Minnesota tomorrow. He has to go into town in the morning and check things out before he'll know for sure. He said if we don't go tomorrow we'll go on the next day (Saturday) for sure.

March 19, 2010

Tom called about 10:00 and asked what I was doing. I said, "I'm packing." He said the trip is on for today and he'd be home soon. I had a lot of the packing done when he got home. Packing is not as simple as it used to be because we have to pack for Chelsey also. For her we have to pack her bed, a cooler for her food, her plate and water bowl, and her bath towels. Chelsey is all about routine so everything has to be just right. Once packing was finished and the truck all loaded Tom had to move his backhoe to another job site before we could leave town. During the winter the motor on his big truck blew up. That was the only truck that could pull the trailer for the backhoe. The truck was so old that the motor couldn't be replaced and as of now we don't have the money to buy a new truck. So, Tom has to drive his backhoe from site to site. And, of course, someone has to drive him to and from the backhoe. It's slow and inconvenient and is really a hassle, but what can you do. It's not so pleasant for him either; it's pretty cold driving that thing around in winter, plus all the drivers that yell at him and make hand gestures.

We arrived at the backhoe and the man there suddenly had more work for Tom to do. "It'll only take 10 minutes." I left him there and drove into town and parked near the site where he was going to bring the backhoe. And I waited, and waited, and waited. About 30 minutes later he finally rolled up. The man knew that Tom wouldn't charge him for this extra work so had all kinds of little things for him to do. It happens all the time—you see a backhoe sitting in front of you and you start seeing all the different things it can do to make your life easier, so you say something like, "Before you leave can you move that small pile of gravel from there to there?" Tom rarely says no; he's a nice guy and everyone knows it. On the way out of town Tom had one stop to make—to see if he could get a check from a job he had done. But, nope, no check; what a surprise. Really, it's gotten so that we're surprised when we do get paid in a timely manner.

A quick drive through McDonalds and we were heading out of town. We were bringing some stuff to David and it took up a lot of room in the back seat. Once we got all of our stuff in there was no room for Chelsey. We had to put her bed in the front seat with us. That was a first. The bed is really soft, it has a cushion and a little baby blanket, and a large heating pad with a flannel cover that goes over the top of it. Chelsey loves to burrow under or up to something, anything really. The heating pad doesn't completely cover the bed; I leave the front open so she can look out and won't get overheated. Today I put her in and she stayed right in the front. She snuggled up to the side of her bed, resting her head against it. If she doesn't rest her head on something it vibrates from the motion of the driving; it's funny to us but not so much for her. She rode that way all day. I knew that the only thing she could see was the sky and tops of the trees, along with Tom and me of course. She seemed really comfortable and it was nice being able to see her awake all day. She'll ride in the front from now on.

I called David and told him we were on our way. I asked him if they are still taking the two grandkids to the Holiday Inn tomorrow night so they can play in the water park. They are. David said he had seen Mother today and she was doing good. He told me again about his visit to Mother last month and how she had asked if he had brought me with him and how surprised he was. He said the nurse told him that Mother needed new socks. They had to throw all of hers away because they all had holes in them. They gave her a pair to wear in the meantime. Her socks have holes in them because she never wears shoes. The nurse said she had told Nancy about Mother's need for new socks and Nancy had said, "Tell my brother; he's number one." Woooo…not nice Nancy. David said Dorothy was going to buy some socks tomorrow and take them to the nursing home before they went to the hotel. I told him that if she didn't want to go up there I would take them on Sunday. He also said that all of the figurines on Mother's nightstand were gone.

Tonight we're at the Best Western (or is it the Best Inn) in Chillicothe. I have to go outside to smoke. The weather has turned cold and the ground is wet although I didn't see anything coming down. The weather man said a winter storm is coming through this area. I started running Chelsey's bath and the drain didn't work right. The water was draining out at an alarming rate. I told Tom he'd either have to hold the drain closed or fix Chelsey's food. He said he'd hold the drain. I fixed the food then went to get Chelsey out. The tub was full of turds; some quite large. I couldn't believe Tom had kept his hand in there the entire time. Chelsey had gone to the end of the tub to get as far away from them as she could. I cleaned out the tub then got in the shower. While the water was draining out too fast for Chelsey's bath it was draining too slowly for my shower and pretty soon three little turds started floating around. I rarely fill out a customer satisfaction card but I did this time. Why can't motels keep their drains working properly.

March 20, 2010
We woke up this morning to three inches of snow on the ground. We grabbed an Egg McMuffin at the drive-through and headed out of town. As we drove through Missouri we started seeing cars that had slid off the road during the night. Their tracks were plainly visible in the snow. Each vehicle had a yellow crime scene tape wrapped around it. We figured the police did this after checking it out so that all of the other police driving by would know that it had been done. The roads were clear but everything was kind of slushy. There was snow flying off a lot of the vehicles driving down the highway. We passed an eighteen wheeler and it threw muddy water all over our truck. It was cold but sunny all day. Chelsey decided that one day of traveling in the front of her bed was enough and she went right to the back and we didn't see her again.

We got to the nursing home a little after 4:00. There were no parking spots in front of the building. There must be a lot of visitors on Saturdays. I had Tom drive back around and then just let me and Chelsey out at the door. There were new signs scattered around saying it was now a smoke-free facility. I checked in and a nice woman about my age was working the desk. As I got off the elevator on the second floor the residents in that area were already being served their supper. I walked across the bridge and at the end, passing by the rehabilitation and therapy area, I could see that it was completely full. I've never seen so many people in there at one time before. In the last hallway leading to Mother's unit I got behind an elderly woman who was walking very slowly. There was a younger woman with her (daughter?). As I reached them the younger had the older move over to the side so that I could pass them. When I got to the unit I pressed the button on the wall unlocking the door and as I started to go in I held the door for the two ladies. The younger woman said they were only going as far as the door. Okay. They were just out walking. That's a good thing about Mother, she has no problem walking.

I entered Mother's unit and began scanning the area. I was a little later than usual and there were a lot of people in there. I quickly saw Mother walking past the dining area. She was walking next to a nurse but I don't think they were actually walking together. She was bent over more than my last visit, but she didn't seem to be leading with her head any more. I went over to her and said hello. She looked up at me immediately but continued walking. She makes eye contact with me a lot more now also. I began walking next to her. I knew she had a specific destination she was heading to so I just followed her lead. We got to the end of the dining area and she grabbed onto the arm of a chair. I said, "Would you like to sit down?" She didn't say anything but started to drag the chair away from the table it was at.

Just then a black woman sitting at a nearby table started making the strangest noise very loudly. It was like, "nananananananna." It was very high pitched and kind of musical. Mother grimaced and I asked her if she'd like to move to a different area but she said no. She was dragging the chair and I asked her if I could move it for her but she said no. She pulled the chair over to the wall and then sat down. I got another chair and placed it as close to her as possible and sat down facing her, but so that she could see the entire area clearly. The woman started the noise again and I thought it sounded like a bird trilling. We were sitting quite close to her and I could see that when she made the sound her head would go up, stretching her neck out, and she looked like a bird that was trilling. She was also asleep. There was another black woman at the same table. She was awake, but never seemed to look up or out of her immediate space. She was wearing a small knit hat, covering all of her hair. Both women were in large, high backed wheelchairs. The chairs were really padded, including the arm rests. There are very few black residents in this unit.

I was very surprised when Mother started talking right away. She seemed very excited and said, "How did she know...?" and quickly looked out at the dining area and then back to me. I said, "I don't know." Then again "How did she know...?" She had a look of amazement on her face. "I don't know," I said, getting the same expression on my face. Mother was smiling. She said, "How did she know that I know?" "I don't know." Then, "She was right out in the open..." "Really?" She never finished a sentence so I didn't know what she was talking about but I was game. She nodded her head and said, "Right out there in the middle... How did she know? She was right out there in the middle..." I said, "Where?" "Out there in the middle of the...diamond. Did you know that?" I said, "No, I'm glad you told me." "So am I." She was acting like we were girlfriends chatting and I was enjoying it.

Occasionally a staff member would bring a resident into the area, but other than that the only staff there was the activity director and a young lady that was with her. I've never seen her before but she seemed to know everyone so I guess she's a regular. They put some polka music on and Mother got right into it. She started tapping her fingers on the arm of the chair, tapping her foot, and humming. After awhile she said that she should know the words. I said it's because they are only playing the music, no singing. I noticed that the black woman with the cap was tapping her foot also, although she seemed to be totally concentrating on her hands in front of her on the table.

At the table on the other side of the black woman a man and a woman were sitting in wheelchairs. The activity director came over and placed what I think was a puzzle in front of the man. The pieces were extra-large. The woman reached out and tried to pick up one of the pieces and he snapped at her, "Don't touch that!" She drew back. He was trying to fit the pieces together but was getting frustrated and the activity director came back over to help. She called him George. She walked away and began giving magazines to some of the women at the other tables. I looked back at George and he was asleep. Someone brought another lady in a wheelchair over to the table and placed her directly opposite George. A black male nurse walked over and woke George saying he needed to take his medicine. He asked George if he wanted some water and when he said yes he left, coming back with a small plastic glass of water and handed it to him then walked away. The new woman started reaching across the table trying to pick up a puzzle piece. George snapped at her to stop. She wouldn't. She reached out again and he said something that I couldn't hear. She said, "If you don't stop that I'm going to kill you." He said, "You're not big enough." She said something else and he picked up the glass and threw the water on her. Mother was watching also and said, "What did he do?" I said he threw his water on her. Mother's eyes got really big. The woman just sat there for a minute then wheeled herself over to the activity director and her aide. She sat there for a moment and then the aide noticed that she was all wet. The aide called her Donna and said, "What is that all over you, you're wet?" I couldn't hear what Donna said, but then the aide said, "He threw water on you?" The aide looked at the director and said, "George threw water on her." I noticed that one of the women with a magazine was now slapping it up and down on the table.

While all of this was going on Mother and I were talking. Mother was wearing light gray sweat pants, the white top with the little flag designs on it, her navy blue pull-over sweater, white socks, and no shoes. Her nose was really red and the sleeves of her sweater looked like she had been wiping her nose on it. She used to always have a tissue in her pocket. Her nail polish was red and severely chipped. I said, "I hear you've been looking for me." She said, "I have? Who told you?" I said, "David did. So here I am." She said, with a smile, "So, here you are." I don't remember everything we talked about but she was very animated and kept getting a range of expressions on her face, such as excitement, awe, puzzlement. I made sure I also got the expressions on my face and I smiled a lot so that she would keep smiling. I realized that her hearing is exceptional. I even tested it by speaking very quietly and she had no problem hearing me.

Donna wheeled her chair back across the room and parked herself right next to George. He said something to her and she started yelling, "Help! Help!" The aide came over and asked what was wrong. Donna said, "Make him stop doing that." She backed up her chair somewhat and was sitting there waiting. The aide then said, "You're blocking the door and someone is trying to come in." She started to move Donna's chair but it wouldn't budge. She said, "Oh, the brakes are on." She finally got Donna's chair moved and then looked at the person still standing out in the hall. She said, "Push the button on the wall, then open the door." Mother said, "What's going on?" I said she was blocking the door and someone is trying to get in. The door opened, and I should have known, in walked Tom. Only Tom wouldn't know how to open that door. I said, "It's Tom." Mother said, "Who?" By then Tom had spotted us and walked over. I told him I would get him another chair but he said no. I tried to get him to sit in my chair but he wouldn't do it. We were sitting right next to the wall and a recessed window (although the blinds were closed) and I moved over and sat on the window sill and told him to sit down. It's a little rude for someone to visit standing up, towering over the people sitting down. He sat down. He said he'd had a hell of a time finding us. He'd had to ask directions several times. He'd only been up there the one time, on our first visit. I asked how he had looked for us. He said he had asked using Mother's name and she was looked up in the computer. I said you could have just asked for the memory care unit. He said he hadn't thought of that. Tom loves to make simple things difficult; drives me nuts.

I was surprised he had come up. I guess he was feeling restless. He greeted Mother, although I'm sure she didn't know who he was, well, she doesn't know who I am, but at least she recognizes me. Tom said, "Your hair looks really good, Sally." She smiled and said, "Thank you." He said, "You look like the old Sally now, you didn't the last time I saw you." She said, "Thank you." He looked around and I told him he had just missed a big fight between George and Donna; Mother and I both laughed as I explained it to him. Alarms started going off around the entire area as people tried getting out of their chairs. As the aide ran around turning them off I explained to Tom about the chair alarms. The polka music was still playing and Tom said, "I actually know this song." I said, "Yes, it's roll out the barrel." He started singing it, "Roll out the barrel…that's all I remember…we're going to have a barrel of fun, that's all I remember." I said that's all I could remember too. About five minutes was all that Tom could sit there and he said he had to go but told me to take my time, no hurry. He said, "How do I get that elevator open?" My mind went what? Then I realized what he was talking about. I said, "You push in the year and then push the button, just read the sign." He said goodbye to Mother then walked towards the door and realized he couldn't get out. He turned and mouthed the words; how do I get out? I said, push in 3650, if they haven't changed it. I said it just loud enough for him to hear, we wouldn't want anyone else getting out. Just joking.

A nurse wheeled up a woman in one of those large wheelchairs and placed her at the table next to us with the black women. The woman was sound asleep. The back of the chair was tilted back somewhat and there were small square cushions holding her head from falling to the side. The woman was very pretty with brown hair and didn't look near as old as the other residents. She kept her right hand curled up while she slept. She didn't wake the entire time I was there, neither did the trilling black woman. Mother said, "I wish I could just go to sleep," and she kind of waved her hand at the room. I knew what she meant but I said, "You don't want to take a nap do you?" She said no. What she meant was that she wished she could go to sleep and sleep through all of this. I can understand her feelings.

It's like when you're really sick and you want to go to sleep and not wake up until it's all over. I feel so sorry for her, for what she's going through. She just seems so unhappy at times. Depressed.

Mother said, "I want to go home." I said, "You are home," and quickly changed the subject. A few minutes later she said it again, "I want to go home." I said, "There is only one thing you need to do to go home." She said, "Just one thing?" I said, "Yes, just one thing. You have to get your memory back. You have to knit those gray cells back together and get your memory back." She said, "Okay." I said, "When you do get your memory back I want you to call me on the phone and I will personally come and get you and take you home. Okay?" She looked at me and with a little smile said, "I forgot." We both laughed. I wish I knew what was going through her mind right then.

During this entire time a woman was walking back and forth throughout the area. She was tall and stood straight up and walked and walked. When she got to a wall or piece of furniture she came to a stop and didn't move. It made me think of one of those wind up toys, when they come to an obstacle their feet keep going up and down as they walk in place until someone turns them around; bump, bump, bump. I wanted to look and see if her feet were moving. After a minute she would turn and off she'd go in the opposite direction.

A woman wheeled a man up to a table off to the side. It was another one of those large chairs. The woman was pushing him up to the table when he started loudly howling, "Ow, Ow!" She said, "You did that yourself." I think his foot hit the table leg. The man was dressed in his pajamas and a robe. He had short hair and dark rimmed eyeglasses. You don't see a lot of eyeglasses around here for some reason. I had never seen him before. The woman was probably his wife who had come to visit. She had pulled him out and was trying it again and again he started howling, "Ow, Ow!" Again she said he had done it himself. A nurse came over and started to adjust the footrest and the woman said she thought it was too small for his foot. They finally got the man up to the table and put a large cloth bib on him for dinner. When I looked over there again he was asleep. He had just leaned his head back on the high back of the chair and that was it; his mouth was hanging wide open.

A man entered the unit and began crossing the area. Mother said, "He's old." I said, "Old?" She said, "Yes. Doesn't he look old?" He was wearing a blue, checked flannel jacket, had shaggy hair and a beard that was salt and pepper. He looked to be my age. I couldn't believe she thought he looked old. I said, "Old?" She said, "Yes, old, you know O L T?" I just nodded. At least she was making some complete sentences today. It really surprised me that she spelled it out even though she spelled it wrong. The man crossed through the area and entered a locked corridor. When Mother first moved in there that corridor had been open. There is an entire wing of residents behind that door.

After Mother moved to this nursing home Tommy, the kids, and I went up to visit her (she still knew who we were). We found out that she had taken up with a man who lives in that wing. On the first day we found her sitting with him in the visiting area. We went over to them and I tried to introduce myself to him but he was so totally rude that I instantly disliked him. The next day we found Mother pushing an elderly woman in a wheelchair down the now locked hallway. We tried to get her to stop but she wouldn't; it was almost like she was on a mission. I don't think she knew who we were at first. We followed her as she pushed the woman all the way down the hallway and then circled back around, struggling to get the chair around corners. When she got back to the beginning I was able to get Mother to park the woman in the visiting area. We sat down with her to visit. The grandkids were having a lot of fun visiting her; they hadn't seen her since she lived with us that winter.

As we were sitting there I saw the rude man enter the unit with a woman, both wearing coats. It was Thanksgiving. I knew that the man was married and figured he was with his wife. Mother didn't even look at him as he passed through, nor did he look at her. The couple went down the now locked hallway and a few minutes later the woman returned and left the unit. Then the man appeared and walked through the dining area. Mother was out of her seat in a shot and took off. I said, "Mother! Where are you going?" She turned around, without stopping and said, "I'll be right back." Well, she wasn't right back and finally I said to Tommy, "She's not coming back. Let's go find her and say goodbye." We found them walking near the end of Mother's hallway, hand in hand. We started towards them. They had gotten to the end and the man turned around and saw us coming and started taking her into the nearest room. I hurried and reached them and grabbed Mother's other hand. I explained that we were leaving and wanted to say goodbye to her. The man would not let go of her hand. I finally had to put my hand on her wrist and pull her hand out of his. At least I was stronger than him. We said our goodbyes; hugs and kisses, and then left. I was really disappointed. So I was glad when I found out that he had been locked in that corridor. But I wonder if she would be happy if she could still hang out with him; or would she have forgotten who he is by now. She needs someone to hang out with. I can't understand why she hasn't been able to make any friends.

More staff started arriving in the dining area. I saw that they were coming from the locked corridor. A kitchen guy came out pushing a food cart. I realized that the residents in there were fed first and now they were getting ready to serve Mother's group. A young black woman came into the area and Mother waved at her like a schoolgirl. The woman waved back. There were a lot of people in the area suddenly. I think the staff people I have been seeing at this time of day are probably the kitchen staff that comes in to help serve supper. That's why I don't see them before-hand. Men started bringing in carts of steaming food and setting up. A man came into the unit, Carlton, the chanting 'help me' woman's husband, and went over to where she was sitting at a table. I hadn't noticed her before. She was sitting quietly coloring. Actually, I haven't heard her chanting help me since she had the big yell out with the other woman. Carlton started talking with the activity director. I couldn't hear what he was saying but she told him there was some roast beef over there if he wanted some. He went and got a plate of food, sat back down and started eating. The activity director asked him if he had filled out the census yet; he hadn't. I filled mine out the first day and mailed it back. It only took five minutes. I wondered about the huge job it would be for someone to fill out the census report for this nursing home.

All of a sudden Mother said, "I have to go. Will you go with me?" I said, "Go where? It's almost time for you to eat dinner." A couple of women at the next table had trays of food set in front of them and Mother jumped up. I moved my chair over to the table that was right there and asked Mother if she wanted to sit there. It looked like she was going to sit down and I asked her for a hug first but she shrugged me off. She skirted across the front of the chair and took off. She went into the main dining area, with me following, and the black woman said she usually sits here. She greeted Mother and pointed to her usual chair and asked if she was ready to eat. It looked like Mother was going to sit down, but again she skirted the front of the chair and took off. I just stood there. The woman said Mother does that often. She said, "We just let her go. She circles the area a few times and then comes and eats." I said, "Yes, I've seen her do that." I could see Mother heading down one of the hallways.

I asked the woman if it was okay to visit in the evening and she said yes then said she'd ask the nurse just to be sure. I was sure then that the woman was there just for meals. We walked over to the nurse's station and the woman asked one of the nurses if it was okay to visit in the evening. The nurse was wearing white slacks and a short sleeved top that has a blue and white abstract design on it. As the nurse came over to talk with me the black woman started to leave and I thanked her for her help. I asked the nurse about visiting in the evening, saying that I'm from out of state and I never know what time I'm going to get there. She said they finish eating about 6:30. I asked what time they start getting them ready for bed and she said about 7:00. Wow, that's early, but I guess with that many people they have to. I said, so I have a window from about 6:30 to 7:00. She said she doesn't usually work this shift and asked who I was talking about and when I told her she said, "Oh, they save her for last. They want to tire her out first." I laughed and said, "Because she won't?" She nodded yes. I said, "So I have a window from 6:30 to 7:30." That was good information to know. I thanked the nurse and left the area.

I started towards Mother's hallway and could see her walking down the other hall. At least I don't have to worry about her getting exercise. I walked down to her room so I could sign her calendar. David had told me that all of her figurines were gone. I looked around and her nightstand was completely empty on top. I opened the top drawer and the only things in there were bottles of lotion and the box of tissues. The second drawer contained Depends, or something similar, and the bottom drawer was stuck and wouldn't open at all. I signed the calendar and left. As I was walking back down the hall Mother was walking up it. I said, "Aren't you going to eat?" She looked up at me but didn't say anything and kept walking. It looked like she no longer recognized me.

After leaving Mother's unit I made my way back downstairs and signed out. I asked the woman at the desk if they lock the front doors at night. She said they do but you can still get in. I asked what time they lock them and she said around 9:30. Tom had said he would be waiting for me in the vending area so I walked down there to get him. He was sitting at a table reading and sipping coffee from a small Styrofoam cup. He got up and poured the coffee out and threw the cup in the trash. I asked him why he threw it out because I was thinking that I would like to be drinking that coffee myself. He said he didn't get it out of the vending machine but from the lobby and that it was really bad. There's nothing worse than bad coffee. We left and headed down the road to the LaQuinta.

The LaQuinta was a couple of blocks from the nursing home. I could see how David could overlook it for so long. There was a row of brown buildings along this part of Boone Avenue and the motel just blended in. We always turned off before we got this far. Entering the lobby there were two people working the desk, a young woman and a young man. The man was on the phone talking to someone about a wedding. The woman started checking us in. I kept trying to give her the paper I had printed from the internet with our new reward club number. It had all of our information on it and it would have made it so much easier to read it right off there instead of making me give all of the information. I realized she was new here because she had to ask the man for help a couple of times and didn't even know how to enter the member's number. However, she was very nice and so was he. I asked if the pool was open and she had to ask him. He said yes it was open. I asked if it was heated and he said, yes, he checked that morning and it was 87°. How late is it open? 10:00. Tom asked if there were any nice restaurants in the area and the man gave him directions to a business area nearby. We asked for a smoking room on the ground floor and they said (it took both of them) the only one they had left was one with a queen size bed. I said it's the same price isn't it and they said yes. Okay then. I asked if I would get a membership card in the mail and the man said yes, it would take about six weeks. I know with the card they have express check-in and that will be nice. We got our keycards and headed out to the truck.

Tom said as soon as we unload the truck we'd go eat. He said he knew I was hungry because I hadn't eaten all day. He was right, I hadn't eaten since the Egg McMuffin right after leaving the motel this morning. I sometimes have a problem with food; my problem being I can't eat. I'm kind of like opposite of other people, if I'm nervous or anything like that I just can't eat, even looking at food can turn my stomach. I was having that problem today. I was all right for the breakfast but then as we went along I got a little queasy. Every time we stopped today Tom ate; I tried and would walk the place looking for something I could eat but couldn't find anything. I couldn't even drink coffee.

We started to unload the truck and I told Tom we didn't need to get everything right then, just what we could carry and we'd do the rest after we ate. We carried in Chelsey and a few other things. The room was nice although it was a handicap accessible room; it had the railings in the bathroom, etc. We took Chelsey out of her bag and put her on the bed. She quickly made her way to the pillows and burrowed underneath. I said we could just leave her while we went to eat. I knew she wouldn't move. We went in search of a place and found the area the guy was talking about. We went past the mall and I just couldn't understand how it could be there. I was so lost; everything is totally different from when I lived there, I just can't get my bearings. We pulled into a Baker's Square restaurant. I'd never heard of the place, but the motel guy recommended it. Once inside it looked a like a Perkins. It had the display counters with fresh baked pies and cookies. Tom has a habit of always ordering the same meal – hamburger steak, but I like to vary mine. I ordered the chicken pot pie. It was so good, unbelievably good. I stuffed my face then when I couldn't eat any more gave it to Tom to finish. Looking over the pie menu I saw that they had strawberry rhubarb, my favorite. I got a piece to take with me.

Back at the motel we put on our suits and went down to the pool. It was packed! There were kids everywhere. Tom sat down on a lounge chair but I was going in. There were so many people that I had trouble getting in the pool as there was a young family on the steps that didn't want to move. However, I stood there until they made a path for me. Did they think I was going to jump in off the side? The water was cold; 87 degrees might be warm in Minnesota but those of us from the south want it to be at least 98 degrees. But, I was in and I was determined to swim if I could. There were so many kids playing though that I couldn't even get two strokes in. I made my way over to the side, in front of Tom, and a kid did a cannonball right next to me. Tom thought that was funny as hell, ha ha. I said I'm done, let's go. We went back to the room, me wrapped in towels, freezing. Tom said we'd try it again at 9:30, surely it would be cleared out by then. They had free coffee in the lobby so we got some of that. At 9:30 we went back, there were less people but I couldn't see a clear path where I could swim so didn't even go in. On our way back through the lobby I asked the woman if it was always crowded like that. She said it stays busy but there was a basketball tournament going on right now.

Back in the room I gave Chelsey her bath and fed her. Then I was ready for my shower. I had the water just the right temperature but couldn't figure out how to turn on the shower. How weird. I was standing there naked and couldn't turn on the shower. I gave up, wrapped a towel around myself and went to get Tom. He went in there and couldn't figure it out either. He went to the front desk and asked the woman how to turn it on. She didn't know and said she would send the guy over. We waited about 15 minutes and the guy showed up. It turns out there's a ring on the bottom of the water faucet, pull it down and walla, you get water. The shower was nice and when I was finished Tom and Chelsey were both asleep. I'm going to eat my pie then go to bed. I'm exhausted.

March 21, 2010

This morning I sent Tom down to the lobby for coffee and orange juice. We weren't going to check out until almost 11 because we were going over to David's first and he wasn't going to check out of the Holiday Inn until 11. The LaQuinta serves a free breakfast but I rarely eat breakfast. Tom came back and said there were so many people eating that they were out of coffee and orange juice. Instead he had cranberry juice and apple juice along with little muffins and some pastry. He always does that, gets food, even though the stuff usually goes uneaten. I was snuggling with Chelsey in the bed, nice and comfortable. Tom doesn't like just sitting in a motel room so he kept leaving and going outside. I finally started getting ready to leave and by the time I was finished Tom had the truck all loaded. He said he had walked around outside and in the back was a wooded area with a large pond and a lot of geese. There were also deer tracks in the soft ground. We checked out and he said come on I'll show you.

We started seeing the geese as soon as we got outside; Canadian geese. I'll never forget one time while with David and he was talking about what I thought he said were snogeys. I said snogey's? What are snogeys? Then very slowly he said "snow…geese." Those northern people sure talk fast. There were two geese right near the parking lot and standing on top of a small hill with a little frozen pond in between us. We had put the muffins and pastry in a bag and I took one out and broke it into pieces and started throwing it to the geese, trying to get them to come closer. Tom had the camera because I was hoping the geese would want the food so bad they'd eat it out of my hand. But they didn't; they just stood there and looked at me. We walked away and looked at the deer tracks and the geese came down from the hill to eat the food. Then all of a sudden there was a big whoosh of flying geese swooping down and they started fighting over the food. Unfortunately we were not in position with the camera. When we got back over there the only ones left were the two original geese but nearby was a small group of mallard ducks.

I began throwing food out again landing it on the ice this time, which would bring them closer. The geese came down to get it and as soon as their feet hit the ice it broke. They went after the food, breaking a path through the ice to get it. It looked so cold and uncomfortable that I felt guilty. We then walked behind the motel to the pond behind it. It actually looked like a small lake, surrounded by reeds. It was still frozen in some places. As we approached all the geese flew off, except for one, he stood his ground. I had the camera ready and took some shots of them flying off. Then I thought I'd like to get a good shot of the one bird winding up to fly. I trained the camera on him and started taking a few steps forward. He didn't move. Just stood there looking at me, with anger if that's possible. I took another step and he just stood there looking at me but started bitching in a loud voice. I kept the camera on him and told Tom to walk towards the bird and make it fly off. Tom went all the way to the edge of the pond but that bird wouldn't budge. Okay, you win.

We left heading for David's, getting coffee on the way. Alexsis and Steven were still there and I asked if they had fun at the water park. They are so shy and they just kind of murmured yes. I asked Steven if he had gone down the big slide and he shook his head no. I asked Alexsis if she had gone down and she said no, but that Grandpa had. Funny. Dorothy said the water in the pool was cold so she had headed for the hot tub. After awhile Steven got so cold that he was shivering so he climbed in the hot tub also. Dorothy gave me the socks she had bought for Mother and explained that she had gotten men's socks by mistake. They were diabetes socks, white with ribbed tops, I guess so that they won't fit tight. She said they should still fit her although they'll be very long. There were several pairs; hope they fit.

It was a beautiful sunny day, warm enough to sit out in the backyard. I wrapped Chelsey in her light blanket and put her on my knees right in the sun. She had her head sticking out looking at everything and Steven petted her a little. David and I talked about Mother. He said when he had been to see her the last time they had brought out root beer floats. Mother had tried to drink the root beer out of the spoon instead of the straw. David had had to show her how to use the straw. David is so patient with her. We were there for a couple of hours and had a good time but it was time to get moving.

We hadn't eaten yet so we stopped at Lyndee's for a late breakfast. As we were driving to the nursing home Tom said that while he was wandering around yesterday he found a shorter way to Mother's unit. He had parked in a back parking lot and the door was right on Mother's floor. I told him that I like the long walk because I'm a little nervous when I first get there and the walk calms me down and then after the visit I have so much on my mind that the long walk out helps calm me. He asked why I was nervous and I said I don't know why, I just am, I never know what to expect. Tom was able to park right in front of the building, which was surprising because it's Sunday and the parking lot should have been packed with visitors. Chelsey and I made our way inside. It was already 3:00.

When we got into Mother's unit I saw the same nurse as yesterday crossing the area towards the nurse's desk. She was wearing the same uniform as yesterday—white pants and blue and white top with the abstract design. I stopped her and handed her the bag of socks explaining they were for Mother and my sister-in-law accidently bought men's socks and if they didn't fit she should tell my brother and he would replace them. She seemed puzzled that I had given it to her and asked if I wanted labels put on them, which is what David told me to do. When I said yes she asked who they for and I said Shirley Thomas. I thought she would have recognized me from yesterday. She said I could try them on her and see if they fit and I said no, she probably wouldn't do that. She started to walk away with the bag and I asked her if she knew where Mother was. She looked around and saw a black nurse and asked her and she said Mother was walking the halls and pointed down the first hallway.

I sat down in a chair where I could watch her come up the hallway. She had her left hand on the railing and was walking at a good clip. She got to the end, never looking up, and had to cross behind a nurse's cart to get to the other hallway. I wondered why she didn't just go around it instead of maneuvering around the back, but I'm sure she has a tight routine on it. As she started down the second hallway, which is hers, I went over and started walking next to her. I said hello and she looked up at me but didn't say anything. I noticed that she was holding her right hand over her stomach. I asked if she okay and she said yes, with a puzzled look on her face. I said, "You're not sick are you," and she said no. I said, "Because you have your hand on your stomach." She said she was fine. I asked if she wanted to go to her room and she said okay. Her room is about half way down the hall. When I led her in she said, "Here again?" She didn't sound too pleased.

Once in the room she walked right over to her bed. There was a white towel lying on the end and what looked like a hospital gown. She moved them over and then sat down. I said, "Oh, a towel, you know what that means," and she said what? I said, "You get a bath tonight." I doubt whether she likes bath nights, I had a hell of a time trying to get her to bathe when she was living with us. David also had trouble when she was living with him. There was a large teddy bear with pink and red hearts on it sitting on the back of the bed; a Valentine's bear. I picked it up saying something like look at this bear, wow, it's nice. She didn't take it from me, which surprised me, so I just set it back on the bed. I took Chelsey out and held her up in front of Mother saying, "Here's Chelsey, she came to visit you." Mother cooed over her for a moment and then I set her on the bed and she made a beeline for the teddy bear. I covered her with her blanket and she hunkered down. The top of the nightstand was still empty; looking in the drawers they were the same as yesterday. I said, "All of your stuff is gone." She said, "Really?" I looked in the closet and found a tub full of stuff. I pulled it out and it contained all of her cards and the old calendars and that was it. There were no figurines, no stuffed animals, and even the Bible I gave her in January was gone. I said, "Who would steal a Bible." With her eyes wide open in amazement Mother said, "I don't know." At least her name and mine was written on the first page so maybe someone will return it.

I said, "I brought you a present." Her eyes lit up. When I bought the Bible I had also bought some rosary beads. I pulled them out and handed it to her. She said, "Oh, they're beautiful." She had them in the palm of her hand and I stretched them out so she could see what they were. I said, "These are rosary beads. You use them to talk to God. See the cross?" She seemed so touched and she fingered them lightly. We aren't Catholic but that doesn't matter. I love rosary beads and other religious objects. I asked, "Do you want to talk to God?" "Yes." "Do you talk to God?" "Oh yes." She had the beads cupped in one hand and was stroking the glossy light blue beads. I asked, "Do you want to walk with God?" She looked right at me and said, "No." "You just want to talk to God?" "Yes." "That's good." I would love to know what her prayers are.

I grew up Presbyterian. It was a newly built church with modern architecture, the walls built with red brick in a curving design. At first there were no pews, just folding chairs. As the church made money pews started being installed a few at a time. The children went to Sunday school at the same time the adults were at the church service. Mother worked part time at the church putting out the Sunday bulletins. She had to type up the service and then make copies. During the summer I sometimes went with her and helped. The copy machine was nothing like today's; it was big, clunky and an antique. It had a rounded hood that we had to open and ink up by hand with a roller. Once it was inked up and the first bulletin put in we had to crank a big handle to make the copies. Once the copies were made we had to fold every one of them and insert the middle pages. It wasn't easy; it took arm strength and patience.

Sometimes I helped out with Vacation Bible School, serving snacks and Kool Aid, reading stories, and playing with the kids. All of the parishioners had to fill out a pledge card on how much they were going to give to the church every month. One summer we received a bill in the mail from the church saying we hadn't fulfilled our pledge. There were times when money was very tight in our household and this was one of those times. Even though I was just a child I was very surprised that the church would send us a bill. They should have been helping us. It all ended when the parishioners actually fired the pastor. I didn't know you could even do that. When I asked why Mother said it was because they didn't like the way the pastor was spending the church's money. He kept buying enormous crosses for the building. I guess instead of pews. The church closed down soon after and eventually turned into a private boys' school. We never sought out another church. When Mother married Ken she started attending the Lutheran church he was a member of. Their wedding was held there. And after he died a tree was planted in his memory.

We started going through the stack of greeting cards. There are a lot of cards, mostly from me of course. I picked up the one on top, showed her the front then opened it and read the inside. When I got to who it was from I said, "Love, from…" And Mother said, "Janet!" That was funny and surprising. I handed the card to her and she held it and looked at the picture. Then we went on to the next card and when I said, "Love, from…"she said, "Janet!" We went through every one of them this way. After a few of the cards, as I was opening it she said, "I Love You Mom!" which is what I had started writing on the inside of every card. I was surprised that she could remember that. I was sitting on the floor in front of her again and I had kicked off my shoes. They were sitting near her own shoes and she pointed in that direction and said, what's that? I said, "Shoes." I wondered if she had seen something else. We were having a good time, almost like we were playing a game, both of us smiling and laughing. One time when I said, love, from…she said David. I was glad she remembered his name. There were a lot of Christmas cards that I hadn't seen before. They must have been on the wall last time I was there. I didn't take credit for all of the cards and when they were from someone else I said so. There were some from David, Emily, Nancy, and some of their kids; and some cards from Aunt Jane. There were also some cards that weren't hers at all, I don't know where they came from, but I took credit for them. There was also a packet of photographs. I've seen them before but always forget and open them anyway. I don't know any of the people. I showed them to Mother and asked if she knew who the people were and she said they were friends of Janet's. Doesn't she realize that I'm Janet? I think sometimes she does. It's all so strange.

There was also a large manila envelope that contained information about the nursing home from when she first moved in. I set it aside and at one point Mother said she wanted to see the card inside. I said, it's not a card but I'll show you. She seemed disappointed. I need to get her a big card. Cards are so expensive now; it's ridiculous. I have already bought her Easter card but Mother's Day will be coming up. I do have a reward certificate from Hallmark I can use. She looked so closely at all of the cards and I could see a pattern. The ones she likes best are the ones with drawn animal pictures. I thought she would like the actual photographs of animals more but she doesn't. She also likes glittery pictures. She was looking at my Christmas card and inside was a small picture of a snowman lit up with glitter. She wouldn't let go of it and put it right in front of her as she continued looking at the other cards. There is a volunteer (Mary I think) that has made a few cards for Mother. She hand makes them out of construction paper and stickers. They are so nice with shiny butterflies, flowers, and stuff like that. They always have a cheery message like have a happy day. Mother likes those also.

Mother's stomach kept grumbling and I kept asking her if she was hungry and she kept saying no. The first time I asked her if she had eaten lunch and she said, "I must have," although she had a confused look on her face. Now I have to worry about her eating. We looked through the calendars again. She acts like she remembers everything. I would say, "Here's your house. Do you remember it?" "Oh yes." "Here's your lake, do you remember it?" "Oh yes." "Isn't that a pretty sunset?" "Oh yes." She didn't seem as interested in the dog photos as in the past, or in the people. Some of the photos had Caroline in them but whenever I got to one of either Mother or Caroline I said, "There's you," and she'd say, "Yup." We finished the calendars and I started putting everything back in the plastic tub. Mother was wearing her light blue fleece jacket and she began taking it off, with some difficulty. I helped her and as we got it off she gave a big shiver. I said, "Are you cold, do you want it back on?" She said, "No, it was just at first."

She was wearing a short sleeved top and I guess when the air first hit her arms it was cool. I said I would put it in the closet. There was no empty hanger so I just laid it in there. When I turned back around she was standing at the door. I asked her if she wanted me to put lotion on her hands but she said no. I got the tub and put that back in the closet and when I turned back around she was gone. She had set the rosary beads down on the bed when we were looking at the cards and it was still there, in a very neat little pile. I picked it up and put it back in its box and then put it back in Chelsey's bag. I couldn't leave it there. If she had carried it with her when she left it would be one thing, but I know that by the time she got back to her room she would have forgotten, and it probably would have been gone. I'll give it to her again on my next visit, and she'll be just as happy.

I signed the calendar, picked up Chelsey and tucked her in the bag, and then left the room. As I stepped out I could see Mother passing her old room. There was a white haired lady sitting in the doorway in a wheelchair. She said something to Mother and Mother said something back although I couldn't hear what was being said, Mother had kept walking. I noticed a dark gold carpet had been installed. I walked down the hall, saying hello to the lady. I caught up with Mother just as she was entering the sitting area. There was a man with a shock of bright white hair sitting right inside in a wheelchair. Mother said hello to him as she passed. He didn't say anything but I noticed that Mother's voice sounded young, at least while saying hello to the man, it was the voice I remember from my entire life. I didn't try to talk with her any further; I knew she was done with me for today, as I passed through the unit I again thought that there were so many people in there. It looked like a lot more than in the past. I made my way back downstairs feeling very sad but feeling good about the visits. I signed out and began walking to the truck. There was a woman (the same one that always said hello to me) sitting in her wheelchair, wrapped in a blanket, smoking. There was a man with her as I passed. When I got to the truck Tom's window was open and he was sound asleep. I tapped him lightly on the arm and when he woke up I said, let's go.

I wanted to drive through Crystal again so we went that way. I wanted to look and see if the crystal ball was still there. We recognized the shopping center but the ball was gone. We continued driving and went through Robbinsdale. I've had dreams about that town for some reason. Mother used to do her banking there. I never could figure out why, why would she drive that far just to go to a bank. We got out of the cities and stopped for gas and coffee. Inside the convenience store they had racks of Leaning Tree cards and I found a cute one for Mother with a Chihuahua that had huge ears. As we drove through southern Minnesota I relaxed and thought about the visit. I realized that I didn't see Ray or the two women Mother doesn't like, Evelyn and Judy. I'm not saying they weren't there, just that I didn't see them either day. I also didn't see the large birdcage, not saying it wasn't there, just that I didn't see it. I couldn't stop thinking about that hospital gown laying on Mother's bed so I told Tom about it. I said could they really make her wear that gown to and from the bathing room? How humiliating that would be to have to walk up and down the hall with that on. Talk about no privacy.

Tonight we are at the Apple Tree Inn in Indianola. The weather was getting bad so it was time to stop. As we drove into town the main light of the motel was off. Tom said, "They must be closed." I said, "No, they don't look closed, just because the light is off doesn't mean they're closed, maybe they just forgot to turn it on. Go back and check." He turned around and went back and it was open. The motel has a very small, narrow lobby. The smoking rooms are through a door right next to the check-in desk. It's a challenge bringing the stuff in because you have to pass right in font of the clerk; especially bringing in Chelsey's bed. I can't imagine anyone objecting to a tortoise, it's not like bringing in a dog, but you never know. We once had to check out of a motel in Texas because the dog hair in our room caused me to be instantly so congested that I couldn't breathe. We've been staying here at this motel since the boys were really young and we made frequent trips to Minnesota. It's old, but still comfortable.

March 22, 2010

This morning when Tom got up he went to the lobby. He could smell the coffee as he walked in. There were also pastries and a waffle maker with a small cup of batter next to it. Tom brought me some orange juice. There was a small coffee maker in our room and I had brought my own Folgers coffee and bottled Mountain Valley water, along with packets of cream and sugar. I made a pot for us and then started filling our thermos bottle. It took four pots to fill the thermos and our insulated cups to take with us. While I was doing that Tom started loading the truck. He said that since we hadn't eaten anything the owner had started putting everything away in the lobby. There are a few tables along the wall, each with a red ceramic apple in the middle. As we were checking out Tom was talking to the owner, an Indian man with a heavy accent, and told him he should get his sign fixed, he's losing business. We were actually the only guests all night. He said the maintenance guy said they had to get someone from the government to come out first. I don't know what that means except maybe they needed an inspection or something. Whenever we stay here and are leaving in the morning the housekeeper is either vacuuming the lobby or cleaning the front windows, probably waiting for us to leave, which is never early.

Down the road a bit we stopped at a place for gas and getting out of the truck the pavement was a big sheet of ice. It was a challenge not falling on my butt crossing it. I walked towards the building and could see a car parked horizontal to the curb. As I approached a man got out of a pickup truck and began quickly walking towards the car saying, "Do you need help?" I looked to see who he was talking to and could see an elderly woman sitting on the ground next to the front car tire. The man had reached her by then. She had been checking the air in the tire. He took the device from her and started doing it. He asked her if she had fallen or was she just sitting on the ground to check the tire. She said she had squatted down to check the tire and then went down. The man was so nice. I was on the sidewalk smoking. She grabbed the front bumper and tried to get up and he stood, grasped her arms and helped her up, saying it had to be uncomfortable sitting there. And cold on the butt, I thought. When she was standing I noticed a cell phone lying on the ground so I went over and picked it up and handed it to her saying, "Here's a phone; it must have slipped out of your pocket." She took the phone, checked for messages, and then slipped it in her coat pocket. The man got the air hose and aired up her tire. The woman said that her husband usually does that but he was in Bethel Manor. I'm guessing that's a nursing home or something. That was so sad. The man finished and walked to the store and the woman got in her car and left. There are good people in this world. If the man hadn't been there I would have gotten Tom to do it for her. Hopefully there will always be a gentleman around when a woman needs help.

We stopped at a tiny town in Missouri for lunch called Malta Bend. There was a diner called The Waggin' Wheel and with that cute name we just had to go in. Posted on the wall was the daily special—goulash. I love goulash. When it arrived it was homemade (and just like mine) with a salad, and it was so good. After we ate we sat outside at a picnic table so I could smoke. A woman came walking down the street and through the parking lot and said, "It's the perfect day isn't it?" Tom was leaning on the front of the truck (in the sun) and said yes, it is. As the woman went into the diner he looked at me and started laughing because I was actually shivering. It was about 50° and I was sitting in the shade. It was warm to the Missouri woman but cold to this southern woman. The diner is a place we'd like to stop at again but it was one of those towns that if you blink, you miss it.

We had an easy trip home. There was snow in northern Arkansas. Fayetteville received 12 inches the other day, but we don't go through there. The snow we were seeing was up in the mountains. Northern Arkansas is so beautiful with the Ozarks. We love mountains. As we traveled south the temperature kept rising until it was in the 70s. We stopped at Taco Bell for dinner and coffee. When we entered I went to the counter to order our food and Tom went to the restroom. While I was waiting I happened to glance down at the receipt and saw that it had a senior discount on it. That disturbed me a bit. Just then Tom came up and I showed it to him. He said, "That's good. You asked for the discount." I said, "No, I did not ask for the discount." He said, "Well, she must have seen me walk in with you." That must be it, she says with a wink to herself. His hair is almost pure silver now with some black streaks. He's been getting the senior discount for years (even before he was the proper age) without even asking for it. I love getting the senior discount but I don't want people to think I look old enough to get it. It's a slippery slope. I've always thought the age for a senior discount was too low. When did it go from 62 to 55? We finally arrived home at 10:00. That was a long trip. I already miss Mother.

March 23, 2010

It was in the 70s today and beautiful. The ants have woken from their winter slumber and have invaded our kitchen. For some reason it reminded me of the spring we went up to Crosslake. The cabin had been shut up all winter long. When we got there Mother unlocked the door and was the first to enter. She came running back out and said, "fleas!" The cabin was infested. They had multiplied all winter. We had to go back into town and buy a can of flea spray and then went back and she had to spray her way in. Every year after that we arrived armed with spray. That's the problem with having dogs – fleas.

March 24, 2010

I was sitting outside with Chelsey today and thinking about how amazing it was that just a few days ago we were driving through a winter ice storm. We were enjoying the warm sun and I was thinking about those cars in Missouri that had slid off the road. It made me think of the time I had gone through an experience like that. Nancy had been in high school and the girl next door, Janice, had just gotten her driver's license. She was about a year older than Nancy. They were going up to the high school one evening for some program—crowning of the homecoming queen or something, and they said Emily and I could go along. I don't remember the program at all but on the way home the car went into a spin and we ended up backwards in the ditch. I'll never forget that spinning. It was pretty scary; we didn't even have seatbelts back in those days. A family in a station wagon stopped and picked us up to give us a ride to the nearest gas station. We had to climb over the back seat into the rear. I remember a young boy yelling at us for getting snow and water on the seat. But we were more concerned about climbing over the seat wearing a dress. They dropped us at the gas station, which was actually Ken's station although we didn't know him at that time. Ken was a big man even back then. He climbed into his huge wrecker and told Janice to climb in to go get her car. She said, "I'm not going alone." I said I would go with her. I remember when I began climbing up into the cab he had a big smile on his face and I could understand why she didn't want to go alone. He was a perfect gentleman though. Who knew that one day he would become my step-father.

March 25, 2010

I saw "Ba Bra," today at Kroger. Barbara is the elderly lady that had come to exercise class at the pool and then refused to get in. She was with her caretaker, Judy, with the accent. I haven't been to the pool in a while so I don't know if they've been back. I was a little ways from them and I know they didn't see me although I don't think they would have recognized me. Well, Barbara wouldn't have of course. I look totally different away from the pool. At the pool my hair is pulled back in a tight ponytail and I don't wear a speck of makeup, although there are some women who enter the pool made up; perfume, jewelry, everything. People do recognize me but I don't think Judy would. As I watched from a distance I could see Barbara walking a few steps behind Judy's left elbow as she pushed the cart. A female employee greeted them and said she was used to seeing her with her daughter. Once again I though how lucky Barbara is to be able to live with her daughter.

March 30, 2010

Today I have been wearing one of Mother's old T-shirts. It's a Minnesota Twins shirt with red paint all over it. I don't know what she was doing to get the paint on it, it could have been anything. She was always so independent, always doing something. I remember one year David said he was going up to the cabin to help Mother revarnish the outside log walls. I was thinking how much work that was going to be—and glad I didn't have to help with it.

It was funny how Mother always wore one set of clothes at home but then had to change if she was going somewhere. I always had to wait for her to put on her going out clothes; which was usually a white cotton blouse and culottes. I'm just like her now. Somewhere along the way I started doing the same thing. Well, actually, I remember exactly when it happened. It was when we first got an iguana. I spent a lot of time holding her (and the ones that followed) and she started making holes in my shirts with her sharp claws. The holes were tiny at first then kept getting bigger. So I kind of separated my clothes—these shirts have holes or got messed up in the laundry somehow, I can't wear them out, but I can wear them at home. Then it went to the pants I couldn't wear in public. Now I look like a slob at home and nice when I go out.

March 31, 2010

Last night I sent an email to David telling him about my visit with Mother that last day. I told him that Mother was walking the hallways when I got there so I was able to get her to go to her room. I said the big Valentine teddy bear with the red and pink hearts was on her bed. Looking in her drawer the only things were some bottles of lotion, the box of tissues, and a green plastic necklace. In the closet I found a tub full of cards and the old calendars. Everything else is gone. There were no small teddy bears, no figurines, no jewelry, no framed photographs, no picture of her parents. No Santa Claus picture of her and you. Even the small Bible I gave her in January was gone. Today I received an email back from David. He said, "Everything disappears over there. That's why I say don't send anything good because it is gone in no time at all. People donate stuffed animals and dolls and they just end up in different rooms all the time." He asked how our trip home was and said they are having 70° weather but by the weekend it will be back to normal, around 50. He also said that if I send flowers to Mother to let him know and he'd try and get the vase but most of the time he was too late. I doubt whether I'll send any more vases. Not that she'll care. So it goes in a nursing home.

April 2, 2010

I had this dream last night. I was in a large outdoor area. There were a couple of long tables with chairs. Trisha was sitting at the end of one of them. She was eating something from a plate. I knew the hospital was providing the food. I walked over to her. She handed me a clear plastic cup and said that I could have it; she wasn't going to eat it. Inside the cup was a piece of cake with about 2 inches of blue and white frosting on top. I took it and walked over to the other table, sat down in one of the chairs and began eating the cake with a plastic spoon. There was another young woman sitting at the same table eating something also. We were the only people in the area. I reached the spoon in along the side of the cup all the way to the bottom to get the cake. The cake was so delicious! I was surprised at how good it was. It was so moist and the frosting was very sweet. For each bite I put the spoon in down along the side. I was still eating when the scene changed.

Next Tom and I were in what was Tommy and Trisha's house. It looked like a mobile home because it was long and narrow. I think they were having us over for dinner. I missed part of the dream but I remember during the course of time I was going back and forth through the house. From what I could see the kitchen was on one end and a bedroom on the other end. There was a bathroom off the hall next to the bedroom. Although it was their house Tom and I were alone. I think Tommy and Trisha had just left. As I walked through the house I saw that there was a radio on in the bathroom. It was sitting on the edge of the tub, facing the open doorway. It was playing loud music. After a while I wanted to turn the radio off so I walked back to the bathroom. The light wasn't on but I could clearly see the shape of the radio. It looked like a mini boombox with the rounded ends. I walked over to it, reached out my right hand and tried to find the knob. I couldn't find it so I went back to the doorway and started feeling for a light switch. While I was doing this the music was blaring loudly.

I couldn't find the light switch but saw some switches on the wall in the hallway. I walked over to that and as I reached towards it I was blasted with a powerful energy. It knocked me backwards into the bathroom doorway. I bounced back into the hallway and the energy threw me to the side. I bounced back and it threw me to the other side. The energy then started bouncing me back and forth. I was terrified. I could see Tom in the kitchen. It looked like he was clearing off the kitchen table which was up against the same wall as the hallway. The energy was bouncing me violently but I wasn't being hurt. I started screaming for Tom but nothing was coming out. I was screaming, "Tom! Tom! Tom!" I screamed it over and over as loud as I could. When no sound came out it put me in a panic. Tom finally saw me and as he came running towards me I became aware that I was dreaming. I started yelling, Wake up! Wake up! Wake up!

I finally woke with a jerk. I could feel that my entire body was asleep, there was a small tingling all over, but that lasted for only a moment and then I could move. My heart was really racing. It was beating so fast that I was afraid I was going to have a heart attack. I started chanting, it was just a dream, it was just a dream, it was just a dream. My heart gradually slowed down to normal. I went over the dream in my mind so that I could remember it in the morning then let myself go back to sleep.

At first I thought this dream was telling me that I have a medical problem because it was Trisha and the hospital providing food. But as the dream went along there were some symbols that pointed in a different direction. First of all, everything seemed white. Trisha was wearing a white nurse's uniform, the tables were white, the cake was white. In the house the walls were white. In the bedroom I could see a big white fluffy quilt on the bed. In the bathroom the toilet, sink, and tub were all white. White often represents the spiritual world.

The radio had an antenna coming out of the top. An antenna can also symbolize the spiritual world. The radio was in shadow which can symbolize the spiritual world that is hidden – that is not clearly seen. So now I can see that I need spiritual help. And I do. I am so stressed right now. I am tight with stress, my body aches. I am stressed with two different things. Mother, of course, I am constantly stressed about her. The other is our financial situation. Tom is working now but people are still not paying. We have a stack of unpaid bills. I am so quick to tears. I see something really good on TV and my eyes tear up; I see something bad and my eyes tear up. I am right on the edge.

So now I can see that the energy that grabbed me is spiritual energy. I could almost see white clouds at the ends of the bounce area, like white energy—spiritual energy. The spirit world was giving me a good, hard shake. Looking at what happened when I woke up I can now see this as a warning dream. If I don't reduce my stress level there could be consequences, physical consequences. But how do I do that? It's right in the dream. Family. Easter is in a couple of days and baseball season is starting soon. And three birthdays this month. I need to immerse myself in the comfort (blue in the cake frosting) and enjoyment of my family. And I have to trust that Tom will be able to handle the financial situation. I have to relax and know that everything will work out. And try not to worry about Mother so much. The cake being in a plastic cup shows that stress relief can come in a cheap way, free even. The plastic cup was clear, meaning I should be able to see the remedy clearly; which I do now.

April 3, 2010

We were at Zakary's baseball game this evening. It's always so much fun watching the kids. Today brought back memories of when I used to play softball. I can't remember how old I was, maybe eleven or twelve. We wore dark pink cotton blouses. I was really the worst girl on the team. I always got put out in left field and had to run for the balls. I couldn't hit the ball to save my life. Except for one time, everyone was shocked, including me. The ball went straight to the pitcher and she easily threw it to first base. I think I could have been a better player if only the coach had worked with me even a little bit; but she never did. She spent all of her time working with the pitcher and the catcher. We were undefeated. Mother was at every game. We didn't go to the games together but I could always look into the bleachers and see her sitting there. Whenever a team won they got to go to the nearby root beer stand and get a large frosty mug to drink. I still remember the smell and the taste. Something funny happened one time. The girl bringing out the root beer was real pretty with dark brown hair and pointy breasts. I know it's something that a girl my age shouldn't notice but it was unavoidable. On this one day she was wearing a white, tight, knit sleeveless top. She was carrying a tray loaded with mugs to one of the boy teams. It looked heavy. When she set it down she bent forward and her breasts neatly slid into two of the mugs. As all of the boys roared with laughter she turned red (I'm sure I did also) but she didn't say anything and with a small smile on her face she turned and walked back to the stand.

I had played at an even earlier age; Emily and I both. Maybe third grade, or second, I can't remember. I know we had a lot of fun. One of the neighbors was the coach. He had a bunch of little kids of his own. He was really nice and all of us kids loved him. I don't remember anything about the games but I remember him. However, the next winter he went up to the north woods deer hunting and he died in his cabin of asphyxiation. As Mother was telling us about it I thought about his wife and kids and wondered how they were going to get along without him.

That was something I had to worry about years later after Daddy died when I was 14. Mother came home from work one day with a cigar box full of money. She said the people who had worked with Daddy had taken up a collection. For the first time I had the thought, are we going to be okay? But she brought us through it. Life continued on; there was even a wedding for Nancy that winter.

April 4, 2010

Today is Easter. It was a beautiful, warm, sunny day. All of the kids were here this afternoon. Easter was a real big deal when I was growing up. In Minnesota it was still cold on Easter so our egg hunts were indoors. We didn't get boiled eggs, just candy. And back then the candy wasn't wrapped individually in plastic. Chocolate eggs were wrapped but that's about all. In preparation Mother would get our Easter baskets out of the attic and we would make sure everything looked good and that the grass was just right. Mother and Daddy, of course, would hide the candy before they went to bed the night before. On more than one year David woke me up really early and together we would find the bulk of the candy then go back to bed and wait for the family to wake up. And, of course, we were able to find the most candy during the hunt. Not nice, I know, but what can you do; I adored my big brother and would do anything he wanted me to. He knew all the Christmas present hiding places also, well, so did I after he showed me. After breakfast we would go to church wearing our brand new Easter clothes. After church it was to Grandma's house we would go. We'd have a ham dinner, another Easter basket, little chicks, white chocolate Easter bunnies (or maybe almond bark).

April 5, 2010

I sent David an email today telling him about our nice weather and that Tom is back to work but not every day. I told him about our Easter yesterday and asked him how his was. I got an email back saying that their Easter was nice. David cooked out on the grill and it was warm and sunny. He said that he had stopped to see Mother today on his way home from work. She was in a good mood but fell asleep about 25 minutes after he had gotten there, so he left. He said no one sent Mother flowers for Easter this year. I guess he didn't either. He continued, saying that he thought that if he brought her flowers he'd put them in a small plastic milk bottle because they have a bigger mouth and then it can disappear.

April 6, 2010
I sent this email to David today: "Funny you should say that about putting flowers in a milk bottle. Tom and I had just been talking about bringing her some flowers in a coke bottle, then it wouldn't matter if someone stole it." Great minds think alike (someone said).

April 7, 2010
Today is Tommy's 38th birthday. Boy, do I feel old. I have been receiving newsletters online from LaQuinta but they weren't showing our stay last month. I went to the website and it didn't show our stay either. At LaQuinta when you stay ten nights you get a free night so this has to be taken care of. I sent them an email and they sent me a link to the website telling me how to take care of it. I'll have to make a copy of our receipt and a copy of our reward card and send it all to them. Looking at the receipt I saw that the girl typed in our address wrong and our member number didn't even make it onto the receipt. I'll have to write a letter explaining it.

I was watching a program tonight on the Sci Fi channel called "Destination Truth." The team goes out to different locations around the world and investigates strange sightings. Tonight they were somewhere in a different country paddling a canoe, in the dark, in heavy rain. All of a sudden mosquitos were swarming all over them. They began freaking out and I laughed, thinking, 'That's just like Minnesota at dusk.'

April 8, 2010
I was sitting outside with Chelsey today and there was a large, dirty cloud sitting in the sky. I kept looking at it and then realized it was a pollen cloud. When it got pretty near us we went inside. Several years ago I got hit by one of those clouds because I didn't know what it was. It had just gotten extremely windy and I saw something coming

towards me. I had run for the house but as I got to the door it had hit. I was pelted by all kinds of crap that was riding in that wind. It makes me wonder if Mother has always had allergies. She sure had all the symptoms. She was never far from her nasal spray bottle and she would cough and cough and sneeze and her eyes would water. She never went to the doctor for this, just bought over the counter medication. I wonder if that stuff is hereditary.

April 12, 2010

I saw our first hummingbird of the year today. We already had a couple of feeders hung. I was telling Tom about it and he suddenly started spouting out hummingbird information like he was an expert. Among other things he said that hummingbirds are the only birds that can fly backwards and that they beat their wings in a figure eight. Let the games begin.

Tommy called me this afternoon and said that Zakary has a dentist appointment and he might need me to take him. Zakary is going to have to have his wisdom teeth removed in preparation of braces. I remember going through that; it was awful! I was older than Zakary when my ordeal started. Zakary is only 12. Mine started with having my eye teeth removed. Mother took me to an oral surgeon's office where they put me under in the chair. Next thing I knew I was waking up in a recovery room, lying on a couch, Mother sitting nearby. To this day I don't know how I got in there, and of course I never asked Mother. Some time later they said I had to get my wisdom teeth removed. They put me in the hospital for that. I was probably 15. Waking up afterwards, in the hospital bed, I saw that Mother had brought me an artificial, bright orange, sunflower plant. I was so touched by that. I wonder whatever happened to it. After leaving the hospital my face was so swollen that I could barely get a spoon between my lips. I was so miserable. Many years later Mother told me that they had done the surgery in the hospital because I had been a bleeder. I thought, "That would have been a good thing to tell me a long time ago." Didn't she think I might need to know that information?

April 13, 2010

Tonight Tom had gone outside and then he called me out and said, "Look." There were several fireflies in the trees. There were so many fireflies around when I was a kid. And before we moved out here, in the other house, we had quite a lot. When we first moved here there were a lot also, but they seemed to disappear. Researchers have said that they are dying out because the world is becoming so lit up and that fireflies need the dark. So, when we saw several tonight it was exciting because it means they are repopulating. It's all darkness around our house but our neighbors have large outdoor lights. As a child we were like all the other kids trying to catch them in jars, etc. Now we just watch them and marvel at their wonder and beauty.

April 14, 2010

On the news tonight they said that researchers have discovered that Alzheimer's patients who have a good (joyful) experience holds on to the good feeling for a long time afterwards even if they don't remember the experience. I hope that's true for Mother. I like to think that she feels good long after my visit. Does she have a smile on her face all day? Is she in a good mood all night?

April 15, 2010

Obama was on TV today, visiting the Space Center. It brought back the memory of that great first moon walk in 1969. At the time I was working at the nursing home. I had worked all day and was completely wiped out when I got home. I lay down on the couch, still in my uniform, and went to sleep. Mother woke me up saying, "They're about to walk on the moon. I know you don't want to miss it." She was right.

I was looking through a magazine tonight and came across an article entitled, "Googling stimulates grandma's brain." The article said that it's good for the elderly to perform searches on the internet, as it keeps the brain healthy. When researchers asked people 55-78 to spend one hour a day using Google to explore a variety of topics, brain scans indicated increased blood flow to various parts of the brain. According to one of the researchers, the important thing is that keeping the brain active in new activities "preserves cognitive skills."

When Mother was living with us I tried to get her interested in the computer. I thought it would be good for her to receive emails from people and I could send messages for her. I started out with just colorful flowers on the screen and called Mother in to look at them. I figured getting her to look at the flowers, and other pictures, would grab her attention somewhat and we could go from there. However, I couldn't get her to even look at the flowers. It was like the computer screen was completely blank. David tried the same thing when Mother lived with him and got the same result.

April 16, 2010

There was a doctor on TV today talking about rhinorrhea and automatic rhinorrhea. Rhinorrhea is excessive mucous secretion from the nose. Automatic rhinorrhea is when your nose runs while eating. It has something to do with the salivary glands. I think Mother has this, or at least did. When she was here every night at dinner at some point she stopped eating, pulled out her hanky, and blew her nose. Every night. It was a little disconcerting because she never left the table; she just blew her nose while we were all eating. Not too long ago David did the same thing. Afterwards he said, "I don't know why but every time I start eating, my nose starts running." Now we know; maybe I should tell him why.

April 18, 2010

Scott and his family were here today. TJ loves books and he gathered some up and had me read to him – over and over. Made me think of how Mother used to love to read. She had tons of books of all different subjects when we cleaned out her house, but her favorite was westerns. She was like Tom in some ways. They both love old movies and westerns. I like neither. David also loves old movies, although I've never seen him read a book. It was always funny when I'd go to visit Mother in Crosslake and David was there. They would sit in front of the TV and find an old movie (didn't matter how many times they'd already seen it), and it wouldn't be long before both of them were asleep in their chairs. Even if I woke them up they wouldn't go to bed. And there I'd be, the night owl, stuck watching a movie I didn't want to see. Maybe I should have gone to bed and see if they were still sitting there in the morning. I tried to get Mother to read a book while she was here but that didn't work. She could read however. We had her mail forwarded to her for awhile and one day she received a mailing from a nature conservatory. She read the entire thing and even shared some of the information with me. But, by the next day she would have already forgotten and she would read it again and share the same information with me. Then the next day she would read it again and share the same information with me. I don't know how long that went on before she lost interest in it.

April 22, 2010
I got an email from LaQuinta in response to the letter I had sent them about not getting credit for the night we stayed there. The email basically just says that they have posted our stay and apologized for any inconvenience etc. So, that's good that it's been taken care of. Now we only need nine more nights to get the free one.

April 26, 2010
I had to go renew my driver's license, and of course I waited until the last minute. I really thought it expired at the end of the month; not that that should have mattered. I went to one of the revenue offices and of course had to take the eye test, and of course I failed it. I always fail it; hardly anyone can see those tiny numbers and letters. But, for the first time ever the woman actually failed me. They never do that, they don't even check to see if you're right; as long as it looks like you can do it they pass you. Not today though. I told her I was having a bad allergy day. She didn't care. I don't understand that test at all. I could read every piece of paper on the wall behind her, just not the tiny numbers, they blur together; doesn't make sense. I'll have to

remember not to go back to that particular office. I'll just have to wait until Tom can take me.

April 27, 2010

I woke up this morning looking forward to the phone call I'd be getting from Mother today. She always calls me on my birthday. Then I remembered.

April 28, 2010

I was setting my chair up to take Chelsey outside this afternoon and as I came back up to the house there was a snake lying right next to the path. I gave a little start when I saw it. I must have walked right past it and not seen it. But, it was lying there quietly. I talked to it and it raised his head a bit and looked at me. It was a black snake with small white spots on his back, nothing dangerous. I continued into the house but went back out through the other door. I didn't even go get my camera. I love animals. Mother and I are just alike in our connection to animals. Some years ago she said, "Do you remember that baby giraffe in the zoo?" I said no, I didn't remember. She told me how one year when the boys were young we had all gone to the zoo together. At the giraffe enclosure there was a mother and her young one. I had put my hand over the fence and beckoned for the young one. The little giraffe came right over to me and I was able to pet her. Funny, I had no memory of that myself. I'm glad Mother remembered it.

April 29, 2010

There was a doctor on TV today talking about arthriosteoporosis. I can't figure out how to spell it, but anthro-or arthr- means the joints and then osteoporosis. The dictionary definition of osteoporosis is a condition that effects especially older women and is characterized by decrease in bone mass with decreased density and enlargement of bone spaces producing porosity and fragility. So, arthriosteoporosis would be osteoporosis in the joints. I think Mother has this, especially in her knees. When she was here she was always complaining about her knees hurting. The doctor had diagnosed her with lupus, which has since been disproved, but he gave her medicine for the aches and pains. Whenever she complained I told her it was because she just sat around all day; she needed to walk. She finally started walking. Maybe that's why she walks so much now. Perhaps that little piece of advice has stuck somewhere in her mind and she has come to realize that walking will make her feel better. I'm so glad she's walking, for whatever reason, because it's the only exercise she gets.

April 30, 2010

When Tom got off work today we went down to the other revenue office so I could renew my driver's license. It was raining so I thought maybe I'd be able to pass the eye test. The man was so nice and when he typed in my name there was a report of my visit to the other revenue office and how I had failed the eye test. I was so surprised, and so was the man. He said, "I can't believe she did this. Did she tell you that you had to go to the eye doctor?" I said no and explained that I had been having a bad allergy day. He asked if I had taken the eye test and I said yes and he renewed my license.

I don't know why they think passing the eye test will make you a better driver. I'm an excellent driver even though I can't pass that test. Mother, on the other hand, had exhibited some crazy driving over the years and it didn't have anything to do with seeing those tiny letters and numbers. The year Scott graduated from high school he wanted to go on a road trip with his new truck. So, the two of us went to Minnesota. We went to see Mother, living happily in Crosslake. After a few days we left heading for David's house. Mother was leading the way, in her truck, because she had business to take care of somewhere. We were on a two lane highway which was completely full of traffic. Mother was behind a truck towing a large boat and all of a sudden she pulled out and passed it, causing a driver traveling in the opposite direction to screech to a halt on the side of the road. A while later we were driving through Anoka, us right on her tail, when she zipped through a yellow light. We had to stop and then catch up to her. We came to another stoplight and I told Scott to stay right on her tail so we could get through the light with her. The light turned yellow and Mother stood on her brakes! We nearly hit her. When we got to David's house I said, "Mother! What were you thinking passing that boat?" She said, "I don't like driving behind boats." I said, "But you made that guy go off the road." She just shrugged. Maybe at a certain age people should have a different type of testing in order to renew their driver's licenses; not make sure they can see tiny numbers and letters, which nobody can.

I was reading a Redbook magazine this afternoon and came across an article on easing eye strain. The article said, "Text addicts, beware. Computer Vision Syndrome (CVS)—marked by headaches, blurred vision, and focusing problems—can strike anyone who spends two or more straight hours per day in front of a screen, from TVs and computers to cell phones and Kindles. That's because our eyes are designed to view 3-D objects, not flat images. Avoid CVS by following the 20-20-20 rule: Every 20 minutes, rest your eyes by looking at something 20 feet away for 20 seconds." Sounds like good advice. I wonder if I look away from the computer every 20 minutes and look at the TV for 20 seconds it will work.

There are tornados going across the state tonight. This time last year we had a particularly bad storm and lost our electricity. Looking out the window we could see up on the road a downed power line that was jigging with live electricity. It was quite a sight. Beautiful but deadly. We called Entergy to report it and it wasn't long before trucks started arriving. We were out of power for about three days. It made me think about when I was working in the nursing home. One evening tornados were on the prowl and the nursing staff started taking the residents to a small basement in the maintenance area. I was working in the kitchen and was a little concerned about my own safety but everything turned out okay. It makes me wonder about Mother's nursing home. What do they do with the residents to keep them safe? I need to ask David about that.

The tornados are headed towards Scott again.

May 1, 2010

I came across an article today about how manganese is good for the brain and the bones. It's from the Rodale website, written by Amy Ahlberg. It says, "Does your daily diet provide enough manganese? It's a good idea to double-check and ensure it does. Though it may not be as well-known as other nutrients, manganese happens to be essential for many of the enzyme systems within our bodies. The essential trace mineral is vital for brain function and for healthy bone, skin, and cartilage formation. It helps break down fat and carbs for energy, and it also helps activate an antioxidant enzyme called superoxide dismutase (SOD) which protects cells from the damaging effects of free radicals. And though true deficiencies are rare, lots of people consume less than the 2 to 5 milligrams of manganese that's recommended for daily intake."

The article also states that manganese is part of the molecules known as mucopolysaccharides, which form collagen, the connective material that builds bone and cartilage. Within our bones, a mesh of collagen creates the framework on which calcium, manganese, and other bone-hardening minerals can take hold. In combination with copper and zinc, manganese helps protect against bone loss; while a deficiency of any one of these nutrients is bad for bone health, studies show they work better at preventing the brittle bones of osteoporosis when ingested together. And osteoporosis sufferers do sometimes have low blood levels of manganese, suggesting a possible deficiency of this mineral.

In addition to keeping bones strong, manganese also helps our bodies utilize certain nutrients—biotin, thiamin, vitamin C, and choline. It also helps the body maintain normal blood sugar levels and synthesize cholesterol and fatty acids, and it aids in maintaining healthy nerves. Also, it's thought that manganese may play a role in producing thyroxine, a thyroid hormone.

Foods that are great manganese sources include pineapple, raspberries, nuts and seeds, green leafy vegetables, shellfish, whole grains, brown rice, legumes, wheat germ, cocoa powder, and maple syrup. I wonder how I could get these foods into Mother. I read somewhere that a lot of elderly people and nursing home patients are malnourished because they don't get enough nutrients in the food they are eating. I wish I could go in there and talk to the nutrition people in charge of meals and ask what they serve and tell them what they should be serving and why. Of course I can't do any of that. I feel so helpless. But, they may already have all this information and do serve really healthy food. I hope so. I can bring the fruit to Mother but that doesn't mean she'll eat it.

When Mother was down here she tried magnesium supplements after being diagnosed with osteoporosis. Magnesium is similar to manganese, both being a metallic element. I had taken her to a health food store to find something to strengthen her bones, probably calcium, and the woman working there got all excited about helping her. She said she just had to have the magnesium. We were looking at the package and the dosage and stuff and the woman said that Mother should triple the dosage since she already had osteoporosis. I didn't think that was a very good idea but Mother was hanging on her every word. We bought a large bottle and Mother started taking it at night. A couple of days later she came to me and said she just couldn't take it any more—it was giving her bad diarrhea. I said okay. Since then I have done a lot of research on herbs and supplements and you really have to be careful about them. You certainly shouldn't double or triple the recommended dosage. There is so much involved with them, so many things you shouldn't do, like mixing them with prescription medicines or with each other. It gets very complicated. It's better to get the nutrients from food.

I did some research on magnesium at naturalnews.com. Magnesium is a necessary nutrient for the function of virtually all systems of the body. Adequate levels are crucial for the brain, cardiac and muscle function, and is needed for bone health. Magnesium can also alleviate gastrointestinal discomfort and disease and regulates healthy blood levels. A deficiency is directly linked to causing insulin resistance, which in turn can lead to diabetes, high blood pressure, and other chronic health conditions. The body's magnesium supply is stored in the bones, and magnesium also acts as a co-factor with both calcium and vitamin D to maintain and strengthen the bone structure. Magnesium is considered a powerful detoxifier as well, especially since the body's "master antioxidant," glutathione, requires magnesium in order to function properly. Heavy metals, environmental chemicals, pesticides and herbicides, and various other toxins are greatly inhibited from taking hold inside the body when magnesium is present. Wow, what a great nutrient!

Processing foods cuts into the amount of magnesium that is in food. In some cases, the nutrients are completely eliminated from the food when it is processed. The biggest example is sugar; there is no magnesium in sugar because it is taken out of the food during the refining process. I guess we should be using raw sugar instead. Why take supplements when we can get nutrients the natural way. Some foods that contain magnesium include: okra, sunflower and pumpkin seeds, almonds, black beans, cashews, and spinach. There are plenty more I'm sure. I hope Mother is getting magnesium rich foods. I know she can't eat nuts, of course, with no teeth but hopefully she's getting it in some way. I don't know if osteoporosis is genetic but I'm definitely going to make sure I get enough magnesium.

May 2, 2010
Today I was putting my tomato plants into my new garden. Scott and Ruth had given them to me for my birthday, along with cucumbers, squash, and cabbage. It actually didn't take me very long. Tom was really surprised when he came home and it was all done. I was using a bamboo mat to sit on. I started seeing the mats a few years ago and thought they'd be good for gardening. Growing up we used

mats like these at the beach. Mother always had a large one that she used for sunbathing. I rarely saw her swim, and I don't ever remember her wearing a two piece suit. She was really beautiful. She had coal black hair and bright blue eyes. I always wondered how she had black hair but none of us kids did. Even in old photographs when she was growing up she had dark hair.

Later, I was sitting outside with Chelsey and I saw her look at something on the ground near us. I didn't pay much attention; she's always looking at something, especially the birds and squirrels. A short time later I started to get up from the chair for some reason and saw a baby snake lying in the grass next to us. It was on the other side of Chelsey so I guess she saw it coming and it must have flowed under the chair to the other side. Too bad Chelsey can't talk so that she could have warned me that I was about to step on a snake. But, I saw it in time, and I was very good, I didn't try to pick it up.

May 4, 2010

Mother's Day is next Sunday so I bought Mother a card today. I tried to find a really big one but couldn't. So I picked out one that has pink roses and butterflies and a lot of glitter. I like how it says, "I love you" on the front.

I found an article today, again on Rodale, about the benefits of walking. One of the benefits is that it is good for the mind. It says, "It can save your mind. Italian researchers enlisted 749 people suffering from memory problems in a study and measured their walking and other moderate activities, such as yard work. At the four-year follow-up, they found that those who expended the most energy walking had a 27 percent lower risk of developing dementia than the people who expended the least. This could be the result of physical activity's role in increasing blood flow to the brain."

Another benefit of walking is that it can reduce stroke risk. "Walking briskly for just 30 minutes, five days a week can significantly lower your risk of suffering a stroke."

According to University of South Carolina researchers after studying 46,000 men and 15,000 women over the course of 18 years, those with increased fitness levels associated with regular brisk walking had a 40 percent lower risk of suffering a stroke than those with the lowest fitness level." I wonder why they studied so many more men than women. There is definitely a history of strokes in our family. Mother had the major one and some small ones. Her mother had a series of mini strokes. I like to walk, but I don't like to walk briskly. I like to take my time and stroll. I don't really like to get my heart beating too rapidly, but I guess that's what you're supposed to do. That's how you get the increased blood flow to your brain. Having asthma might have something to do with my hesitation. I can get short of breath easier than other people. Of course I know that getting my heart working harder can actually benefit my lungs also.

May 7, 2010

I had this dream last night. I was at the computer getting ready to play a game. I clicked on a button to bring it up and instead of the game a page came up that said, "You have no cubes or spheres." In the middle of the screen was the black outline of a cube. Along the outside edges of the screen were small black words. I didn't read any of it but I knew I was supposed to choose something. Instead I clicked in the lower right corner of the screen to bring up the next page. The page came up but it contained black images of cars. It also had black writing around the edges. I clicked on one of the car images and the next page came up. In the middle of the screen was the car I had clicked on and next to it was the word "Affinity," which was the model name of the car. Then Tom was there and he said, "Why did you choose the Affinity?" I said, "What's the difference? It's just a car." He said, "Why did you choose the Affinity?" I said, "Why all the questions? I just want to get on with it." End of dream.

As soon as I woke up I thought, this is how Mother must feel when someone starts talking and asking questions and she has no clue as to what they are talking about. In the dream I was frustrated and didn't know what was going on. I just wanted to skip the bullshit and get on with it. Is that what she goes through when someone starts asking her questions, especially about her past? I know whenever I ask a question I can see her try to stop the flow of thoughts going through her mind and then try to concentrate on my question and then there's just a blank where that memory should be. That would absolutely be very frustrating. And that's why whenever someone asks, "Do you remember…" she just says, "oh yes." So much easier for her. When I start asking a lot of questions she always gets a confused look on her face, then she gets irritated, and then she gets angry, like "what difference does it make?" And the Affinity? Affinity can be a relationship or a similarity. I would imagine that sometimes Mother feels like she's in a box (cube). I know I sure would if I had to wander the same space over and over. She must be so bored.

Well, it's been less than a week after putting the vegetables in the garden and rabbits have moved in. We hadn't seen our rabbits in a long time and were wondering where they were. They're back! We have two adults and one young one. They're cottontails. I wonder if they could smell the vegetable plants. There's no vegetables yet but it will be interesting to see what happens; with the raccoons also. I wonder if Mother had rabbits. I think we saw an occasional rabbit growing up but I don't remember if Mother had any in Crosslake.

May 9, 2010

Today is Mother's Day so all of the kids were over. I was talking to Trisha about Mother and showing her the photographs I dug out to take to her. Trisha suggested I find some old photos of us kids. She said more often people with dementia will remember things from the past like that better than more recent events. I thought that was a good idea and I will dig through the old photographs again.

May 19, 2010

Tom wasn't working today so we loaded up the bicycle he gave me for my birthday and his bike. Zakary was out of school for some reason so we went and got him and his bike and headed into town. There's now a fancy bike path we wanted to try out. My new bike is so nice. It's an old fashioned style Schwinn. It's pink and white and the brakes are on the pedals instead of the handlebars. I absolutely hate hand brakes. After years of riding I still can't get adjusted to them. I feel like I don't have proper control.

I used to ride all of the time as a kid. In the summer we lived on our bikes. One year Mother and Daddy gave me a beautiful new bike for my birthday. I don't know how old I was—grade school for sure. I loved that bike. It was big and a pretty blue. There was a small rack on the back fender (Emily rode on that quite often). I didn't even need a place to go on that bike; I would just ride it around the block, and around the neighborhood; around, around, around…all day long. One day Nancy and David came up to me and asked if Nancy could borrow the bike, that they wanted to go up to Crystal and she didn't want to ride her bike (maybe it had a flat tire). I said, "Oh, no, you're not taking my bike." Nancy got all sweet with me, probably made a bunch of promises, and finally talked me into it. They left and I sat in the house in a sulk waiting for them to get back. They finally arrived. David was on his bike and Nancy was walking, with a very guilty look on her face. She said they had left the bikes outside of a store and someone had stolen it. I threw a fit. I screamed and yelled and cried and demanded that my parents replace it. They wouldn't do it. They said I could have Nancy's bike. I said I didn't want Nancy's cruddy bike. I really think they should have made Nancy save her allowance and somehow make extra money and make her replace my bike. But nothing happened. And I never had another bike again, not until I was in my forties.

May 11, 2010

Tonight we went to see Trevor's 8th grade band concert. He is so good on that trumpet. They played a medley of Beatle songs. The ninth graders played the theme to Star Wars and the Pink Panther. We had a lot of fun watching them. We never played fun songs like that when I was in band. We played boring stuff like The Blue Danube.

After I left home Mother sold my clarinet in a yard sale. I didn't find out about it until years later. I was in town and went to visit Nancy in a new apartment she was renting. As she was giving me a tour she opened her closet and proudly showed me what had been one of my favorite dresses. It was red, smocked at the top, and had pleats all the way around it. Nancy explained that after I left town she, Mother, and Emily went through all of my stuff and took what they wanted. Most of the remaining items were sold. That really hurt my feelings. Mother was upset that I left (and I was traveling light) but when Nancy left home all of her stuff stayed in her bedroom until she could retrieve it. I know that because I moved into her room and was told not to touch any of her things. Only my body moved in, not my stuff which had to stay in the room I shared with Emily.

Some time after that enlightening conversation I was visiting Mother and she pulled out a few of my things that she had saved. I can't remember everything but some of the items had been in a scrapbook. She said she had removed the items and then kept the empty scrapbook for herself. She gave me the stuff which was mostly photos, bowling scores, and beer labels. I chucked them all in the trash. She did save a small corner vanity table that Ken had given me. I still have it. I had actually wanted to keep the clarinet. Oh well.

May 12, 2010

Tonight I was washing dishes and looked up to see a frog on the outside of the window. The light from the kitchen had created a smorgasbord of insects for the frog. It looked so funny sprawled across the glass.

I've always loved frogs. We used to find tiny frogs and toads in Crosslake during the summer. We'd build a little pen for them so that we could keep them. But every time by the next morning they were either dead or gone. I was visiting Mother one year and David was there at the same time. One afternoon I was walking along the shore with David and Rebecca when she found a tiny frog. She was so excited. David told her to throw it in the lake to see if it could swim. Always trusting her daddy Rebecca tossed the tiny frog in the lake. A fish promptly came up and ate it. I know Rebecca and I had the same look on our faces – eyes and mouths wide open in a stunned expression. She said, "DAD!" He just laughed. Lesson learned.

May 14, 2010

We got a call from Trisha this evening saying that she had taken Tommy to the emergency room because he was choking on a piece of meat. Again. There's not much worse than seeing your child lying in a bed in the emergency room. Last time we went through this the waiting room was packed with people, standing room only. Tonight the waiting room was completely empty and we were quickly led to Tommy. I said to the nurse, "I can't believe your waiting room is empty, it's usually packed." She said, "Shhh! Don't jinx us. Anytime someone says that it fills up. It was full earlier and once before that." Maybe it was empty because it was really storming outside. The lightning was quite impressive. Only the real emergencies show up during bad storms.

Tommy was propped up in a sitting position in the bed. Medicine was dripping into his vein intravenously trying to dissolve the meat lodged in his throat. He was very pale. He was also hooked up to a monitor showing his blood pressure, temperature, and heart rate. His blood pressure was so low: 108/77. I said, "Tommy, you've got to learn to cut your meat up into smaller pieces." He said, "I did, Mom, but I was eating dry brisket and the doctor said that brisket without some kind of sauce on it was absolutely the worse thing to eat."

Tommy and Trisha had met up at the restaurant so Tom took Trisha back to get Tommy's truck which they had left in the parking lot. Sitting beside Tommy as things got quiet I could hear the drips of the medicine, the low beeping of the machine, and the deepening of his breathing as he fell asleep. I thought about how Grandpa had died as a result of choking on a piece of meat. I remember Mother talking about it years later. Grandpa had been in a nursing home in Crystal after breaking his hip. At dinner he started choking and the choking caused him to have a heart attack, which killed him. Mother was so sad when she told me about it, years after it had happened. She's been through so much, losing all of her family.

They decided to admit Tommy to the hospital overnight so they can run tests on him in the morning to find out what's going on.

May 15, 2010

Tommy called me himself from his hospital room this morning. He said the meat had gone down during the night. He was waiting for the doctor; they were going to put a scope down his throat to see what was going on. Tom was already there. He had picked up Kelley and Zakary from a friend's house where they had spent the night and had then taken them to a fundraiser they had to participate in. They didn't want to go to the fundraiser but they didn't have a choice. Tom left the kids at the hospital then came back home and got me. By the time we got back there Tommy had already had the procedure and was in the recovery room. Trisha said the results showed that he has a hiatal hernia. The hernia causes acid reflux and this has caused, over time, ulceration of his esophagus which is what's catching the food causing him to choke. The technician said she found something "weird;" something no one else has, something they've never seen before. They did a biopsy on it, just because. Treatment will be a prescription medicine for eight weeks and he can't eat any dry food, only moist food that will slide right down. The worst food is chicken breast, along with pork chops and steak; bread has to be eaten with gravy. The doctor said that the one thing everyone should remember is to take small bites and chew thoroughly, saliva helps it go down. At the end of eight weeks he goes back to the doctor. Boy, what a challenge that will be for him.

Trisha was trying to catch up with her paperwork on a laptop and we waited together for Tommy to get back to his room. They had to wait until he could stay awake. When he finally arrived we asked how he was feeling and he said he was starving. The nurse came in and said they wanted to watch him a little while and then he'd be able to leave. She asked if he wanted something to drink and he asked for a Pepsi. As we watched him drink it Tom and I had the same thought, "I bet the acid in that is great for his throat." Tom and I left and took Tommy's truck to his house. It was still parked in the ER lot. When we got there Tom started loading motorcycles. Crazy, the boy spends the night in the hospital and then gets a scope put down his throat, yet no one's about to miss the motorcycle races tomorrow, except me, I stayed home. When Tommy was finally released everyone packed up their gear and they left. The races are about 200 hundred miles from here. I'm sure Trisha will be doing all of the driving, today anyway. Tommy hasn't been racing this year, but the kids are, and Tom, and Scott. Tommy called me on his way out of town and said that he was feeling fine and had eaten potatoes (with gravy I'm sure) and coleslaw. It doesn't matter how old your kids are, they're still your babies and you worry half to death when something happens.

Now I'm worried about Mother; with no teeth is she able to chew her food properly? What do they feed her anyway? I would think that they really have to keep a close eye on the residents in that unit. That's probably why there are so many of them at mealtimes.

May 16, 2010

I called David this evening and told him we might be heading his way in a few days. I'm so anxious to see Mother. I'm very excited. I really miss her. I told David that I wanted to take Mother out to Lakewood cemetery to plant the urn. Mother did that every year about this time, right around Memorial Day. After she went down David and Dorothy took over.

I had just gotten home from shopping and put everything away when the phone rang. I answered and a young man with what sounded like a middle eastern accent asked to speak with Janet. I said, "This is Janet." I could hear a bunch of noise in the back ground but he didn't say anything for a moment and then he said, "What did you say?" I said, "this is," getting a little irritated. Then he said, "Janet…" He pronounced it strange; the name should just flow off your tongue; it's hard to explain, but he put the emphasis on the et, sounding like Janit. By then I was even more irritated because he was addressing me by my first name. He said, "Janet. I represent Green (something), and you have the opportunity to invest in a process that turns waste energy into green energy. So, Janet, do you know about waste energy?" I said, "I'm not interested." He was still talking of course when I hung up. I sometimes let them talk awhile, just to kind of waste their time. It's funny, once they realize they've got past the first sentence they start talking real fast thinking they have a sucker on the line; but once they start asking questions I'm out of there. If they make the mistake of asking me how I am I'll say something like, I'm unemployed right now, I don't have any money, and…, they get off the line really quick. Over the years Mother got talked into getting credit cards from phone calls like that. "Don't you want to help the animals?"

May 18, 2010
The trip is on! I called LaQuinta and made a reservation.

May 19, 2010
In between the laundry and packing I went through a box of old photographs picking out some to take to Mother. I couldn't find any of the real old ones where we were young children because they're all packed away in the storage building. Maybe I can find some of those photos by the next visit. But I did find a few from when we were teenagers. There are a couple of Ken; one of him on his motorcycle, and one of Mother on the motorcycle. A few of the photographs are of Mother's parents at different ages, and a couple of Aunt Laurie. There are several of Mother at different ages in Crosslake; in the canoe, with her dog, etc.

I was so sad after going through all of them, close to tears about what we have lost. She was always smiling and happy in those photographs, all of her grandchildren and great-grandchildren, fishing, playing with the dogs, friends, making a snowman. She definitely had a full life, a good life.

May 20, 2010

It started storming during the night. It had been thundering and lightning for hours but the actual storm didn't hit until about 3:30 am. There was a thunderclap so loud that it brought me out of a deep sleep; then the rain started; heavy rain. A while later there was what sounded like a loud crack of thunder. It nearly brought me out of bed in a panic when the room lit up. It wasn't thunder though but lightning hitting a nearby tree. The storm was raging.

Tom got up early and took the truck to Sears for an oil change and minor tweaks. When he got home he said he wanted to wait awhile before leaving until the weather settled down. It was still raining hard and he said people were driving all crazy. We just took our time getting ready and finally left about 1:00. The sky was quickly clearing. The Christian bookstore had small Bibles on sale for $5.00 so we stopped and got one for Mother; to replace the first one that has disappeared.

Driving through Arkansas the storms were over, the sun was out, with just a few wispy clouds. Everything looked refreshed. When we first arrived in Missouri the sky was filled with huge white clouds in numerous different shapes then they started turning into one big cloud band. After awhile dark clouds started moving in and it rained on us off and on all day. There were so many dead armadillos on the side of the road and animals I could no longer identify. Later in the dark, I could see the live armadillos, eyes lit up peeking out of the greenery along the road looking to see if it was safe to come out. I noticed a lot of storm cellars in northern Arkansas and southern Missouri, but they were a ways from the house. That's just something I don't under-stand; why would your shelter be so far away. Also a lot of them were facing in the wrong direction. Tornados frequently travel in a northeastern direction and if a tornado is coming the wind could be blowing so hard that you can't get the door open. The door should be out of the wind (preferably right close to your house's back door). A woman was actually killed recently when she couldn't get into her cellar in time.

In Iowa there were big black heavy low hanging clouds. There was no thunder or lightning except once, which was spectacular. It lit up the sky in a horizontal zig zag bright purple flash. We stopped at a convenience store and browsing through the bottled drinks I saw that they had Sioux City Sarsaparilla. I thought, oh, I need to get a bottle of that for Mother, for our snack time at the cemetery. Tom was energized and drove all the way to Indianola. It was nearly midnight. We stopped at the Burger King drive-through and picked up a couple of Whoppers. And now we're at the Apple Tree Inn. Tom and Chelsey are asleep and I will be soon. It's now 1:45 am.

May 21, 2010
I really don't like staying in motels. I always wake up congested. My eyes are always sore and bright red from all the bleach in the towels and bedding. This place has to be the worse. You can almost see the bleach fumes and the smell of chlorine in the water is so strong that I have to bring my own bottled water. I think I'll start bringing my own pillowcase. I try not to have the blanket and bedspread anywhere near my face. I worked in housekeeping at motels before the boys were born and I know that those things rarely get laundered. They were supposed to be washed every month but I don't remember ever washing one. The beds always feel soft when I first get in but after awhile they feel hard as a rock. Every time I wake during the night I have to tell myself to turn over so I won't be too sore in the morning. I really need a soft bed. This place is at least quiet, but then we always have the fan going for a little white noise.

I heard Tom wake up about 8:00 but he just cuddled up and we went back to sleep. When he woke next it was almost 10:00. He said, "Time to get up!" I said, "Is the coffee ready?" "No." "Let me know when it's ready." This place has the regular coffeemaker so last night I set it up with our Folgers, all ready to be plugged in and turned on. We left just a few minutes before check-out time. As we left Tom said, "We need to hurry so we don't hit rush hour in Minneapolis." I said, "I don't think it will matter what time we get there." It was only 60° and cloudy. It drizzled off and on throughout Iowa.

We got on the Interstate in Des Moines. Modern rest areas finally. In Iowa, however, they are all non-smoking. It's crazy; it's all outside, just set up ashtrays. In southern Minnesota there were state troopers and city police stopping cars all along the road. It was strange seeing state troopers and the city police working the same area. We were going through Albert Lea and Owatonna at the time. After many miles we realized the stops were only on one side, the vehicles heading south. Then we drove past some construction going on and figured that's what they were doing—patrolling the construction area, people driving through it too fast or something. We had gray clouds all day, rain off and on, only in the 60s.

Southern Minnesota is so pretty. There are perfectly kept huge green fields, even right outside of the neighborhoods. We saw several dead deer on the side of the road. It's always sad for me driving past Northfield; that's where Daddy died. We arrived in Minneapolis about 3:00 and promptly missed our turn off. It just springs up on you so fast that you're not prepared. No problem, we just stayed on 35 knowing we could still get where we were going. We ended up going right through downtown and even went through the big tunnel.

We were close to the nursing home and I remembered we didn't stop and get Mother some fresh flowers. There was a small shopping area and we drove through it to see what kind of stores were in there. None sold fresh flowers; we did go in a small supermarket but no luck. I looked for some fresh raspberries and blueberries to take with us tomorrow but they didn't have any of them either. We went on to the nursing home and I signed in at 4:05.

I went on up to Mother's unit and as I walked through I didn't see her so I headed down the hall to her room. I was nearly there when I heard her voice coming from the room next to hers. I stopped and waited and out she came with a young, male Jamaican nurse, their arms around each other. I said, "Mother." When she saw me she got a big smile on her face and said, "Well hi there!" She let go of the guy and wrapped her arms around me. I was really surprised. I said, "You were in the wrong room." She said, "Was I?" I said, "Yes. What were you doing in there?" She said, "Oh, just looking around." I suspect she was using the bathroom. We started down the hall and I steered her into her own room. I sat her down on the bed and she reached her arms up to me for another hug. That surprised me even more. As I hugged her I told her that I love her and that I have really missed her. She said she had missed me too.

I noticed that her bed now had a brown covering on it. I said, "Where's your teddy bear blanket," and she said, "I don't know." I got to looking and it was underneath the brown covering. I said, "Here it is," and she said, "Isn't it cute," while stroking it. Still looking I saw that it was attached to the brown covering. Her roommate's bed also had a brown covering. How odd. I said, "I have some things for you," and she said, "Really?" I reached into the tote bag and pulled out Chelsey. I said, "First, here's Chelsey." Mother reached out her hands and said, "Oh isn't he cute?" I said, "She has come to visit you. Would you like to hold her?" "Oh yes." She started pulling the bottom of her shirt down, straightening it out. I said, "Hold up your hands and I will put her in them." But she kept pulling the front of her shirt down. I said, "Put your shirt down." She said, "I am." I said, "No, let go of your shirt," and I started pulling her hands off. She finally understood and reached her hands out. I placed Chelsey in them but she didn't really know how to hold her and Chelsey's head was pointing downward. We've been through this before. After adjusting Chelsey in Mother's hands I grabbed the camera and took their picture. Then I told Mother to pick Chelsey up higher and give her a kiss. But she wouldn't do that and started to put her down on the bed. I took Chelsey from her and put her on the bed next to Mother. She quickly started to take off and Mother tried to pull her up next to her leg. I took Chelsey's blanket and threw it on the bed and showed Mother how Chelsey would just hunker down underneath. I never know how Mother is going to react to Chelsey. Mother has always loved animals so I'm a little surprised when she doesn't want to have anything to do with her, but not today.

I sat down on the floor, kicking off my shoes. I took the Bible from the bag and handed it to her saying, "I brought you a Bible." She took it and said, "Oh, this is so nice." I said, "Do you like it?" "Oh yes." She opened the front cover and was looking at it like it was the best thing in the world. All she could see was the inside of the cover which was just two black pages. I reached over and opened it further saying, "You have to get inside to see anything. See? It's a Bible." She didn't seem to understand so I just left it at that. I pulled out the small manila envelope that contained the photographs and said, "I have some pictures for you." She said, "Oh good," and held out her hands. I kept ahold of them though so I could hand them to her one by one and explain each. I said, "These are pictures of our family when we were all a lot younger." She said okay and seemed excited to see them.

The first picture was of David, younger but still with a white beard and receding hairline. I handed it to her and she said, "And who is this?" I said, "This is David." I was surprised because I thought she would recognize him. "David," she said quietly while looking at it. I said, "He's standing in front of your house. Do you recognize it?" She said yes, but I doubt it. I took that picture from her and handed her one of Ken. She said, "Ohhh..." in a warm voice. I said, "This is Ken. You used to be married to him." She didn't say anything, just kept looking at the picture.

I'm sure she was feeling something. I quietly took that picture and handed her one of me, Tom, and one of her dogs. We were all sitting on the end of her dock. I pointed to myself in the picture and said, "Who is it?" She said, "I don't know." I said, "It's me!" She said, "Oh, it's Janet!" I said, "Yes and that's Tom." "Tom?" "Yes, and look, here's your dog." She looked and said, yes. I said, "You rescued that dog." She looked and said, "Yes, I know you did," then looking at me said, "didn't you?" I said, "You rescued her." She looked back at the picture but didn't say anything. She kept looking at the picture then said, "You always had such pretty braids." Braids? I never had braids. She then slid the photograph inside of the Bible. I said, "Oh, you want to keep the picture in there? Okay." I then handed her a picture of her parents. It was taken in their apartment near Mother's house after moving from Florida. They were elderly in the photo. I said, "This is your parents." She started rubbing her finger up and down her father's face and said, "Isn't he cute?"

I gave her a minute to look at her parents then took it and handed her a photo of herself. She was probably in her 50s, standing in her yard in Crosslake. She was wearing a short-sleeved white blouse and blue jeans. She always wore jeans when she was in Crosslake. I said, "And who is this?" She said, "You?" I said, "No, it's you." She handed it right back, not wanting to look at it. I then handed her a small picture of Ken sitting on his motorcycle. I don't know what year it was taken because she rarely put dates on her photographs, but it was probably taken in the late 60s. I said, "Here's Ken sitting on his motorcycle." She seemed to like the picture. I said, "Do you remember Ken's motorcycle?" "Oh yes." I said, "You used to ride it with him all the time." "Did I?" I took that photo from her and handed her one of her sitting on it. I said, "And here's you on the motorcycle." Once again she didn't want to look at it. I took that photo and handed her the next one. I said, "Here's your sister, Laurie. She's sitting in front of your fireplace." She studied the picture but didn't say anything. I said, "Do you remember Laurie?" "Yes."

I handed her a picture of her with Trevor and Ben. I explained they were my grandkids, making them her great-grandkids. The photograph was taken in December 2005, during our visit with her in the assisted living home. It was such a recent visit that I wanted to see if it would stir any memories; also we're thinking about bringing Ben with us on our next trip and I wanted his picture to be in her mind. I don't know if there was a memory but she sure got excited, especially about Trevor. She kept stroking his face saying, "He's so cute." Mother actually has a history with Trevor. When she was living with us I picked up Trevor from daycare every afternoon and brought him to the house until Ruth got off work. Mother and Trevor would get down on the floor and play together. Does she remember him or is it something else? She slipped the picture right inside the front cover of the Bible and kept the cover open so she wouldn't cover it up.

I then handed her a photo of me, Tom, and Ken. Tom was holding baby Tommy. Tommy had just been baptized in Mother and Ken's church. We were all dressed up, smiling, and standing very close together, a loving family. That picture was taken in 1972. I pointed out to her who everyone was and what was going on. She looked at it but didn't say anything. I then handed her one of David's high school pictures. There was no response. I handed her another photo of her parents in their apartment and said here are your parents again. No response. The date on the back of this one said July 1980. I handed her a photo of her self with Santa Claus. It was a more recent photo also; she had her pure white, silver hair and boy was she smiling. She wouldn't take the photo from me, wouldn't even look at it; she still had her eyes on Trevor. I finally put it right in her line of sight but she still wouldn't look at it. I took it away and handed her a photo of me holding baby Tommy. She smiled and said, "How cute." I handed her another picture of her parents in their apartment. Both of them were smiling right at the camera. They were standing next to a small decorated Christmas tree. Grandma's hair was in a poofy hair style. There was no response. I said, "That's one wacky looking hairdo isn't it?" She said yes. I took that photo from her. In between each picture she went back to the one of Trevor. She kept rubbing his face saying he's so cute.

I gave her a photograph of Emily. It was one of her grade school pictures. Mother got really excited, "Oh, she's so cute!" I said, "Do you know who it is?" She said, "You?" And I said, "No, it's Emily." "Emily?" I said, "Yes, but a lot younger than the picture you have of her on your wall." She said, "Really?" and looked towards the wall. I got up and pointed out Emily's picture. She couldn't seem to focus on the right spot so I got the picture down and handed it to her. She looked at it but was more interested in the other one. After a minute I put the picture back on the wall and sat back down on the floor. She kept stroking the picture. It was really like she recognized Emily, the little girl. Just then the same male nurse walked in the door carrying a chair. Mother looked up with a big smile on her face and said, "Oh, did you come to visit?" He said, "No, I brought a chair for her to sit on." Clumsy me, I tripped over my own feet getting up. His hands instantly reached out to catch me. I got myself in the chair and Mother was saying, "Come and look!" He said, "Is this your daughter?" Mother said, "Yes, she's my daughter but come and look at my other daughter!" Wow, I was so impressed by that sentence. He leaned forward and glanced at the photograph, backed away, and then said to me, "I'm Zachary." I said, "I'm Janet." Then he left the room. He is so nice, late 20s probably, dressed all in white with a name tag pinned to his shirt. Mother had already put the picture inside the cover of the Bible with Trevor's picture. She kept stroking Emily and saying, "Isn't she cute."

I gave her a couple of minutes to gush over Emily's picture then tried to hand her another picture of herself, but she wouldn't even take it from me. Her eyes were still on Emily. I moved the picture down her line of sight but she just wouldn't look at it. I handed her another picture and said, "This is you and your sister Laurie and your cousin Lois." She took the picture and I pointed out each person to her, "This is you, this is Laurie, this is your cousin Lois."

She studied it and then slipped it inside the Bible. I had two more school pictures of Emily, one from junior high and the other from high school, but Mother just ignored them. She was back to looking at grade school Emily, then back to Trevor. I handed her another picture of Tom and me still as teenagers. She wouldn't look at it. She took the picture of herself and Laurie back out and was studying it again. She ran her finger down herself in the picture and said, "Isn't she wearing a pretty dress?" I said, "Yes, she is." After a moment she put the photo back in the Bible. I handed her a high school picture of Nancy saying, "Here's Nancy." She took the picture and seemed surprised and said, "Oh, that's…" I said, "That's Nancy," and she said, "Yes." That was the only older photo I could find of Nancy at that time. I had another high school picture of Emily but she wasn't interested in it. I handed her another high school photo of David (probably the last picture of him without a beard) and there was no interest in that either. My last photo was of her parents again, only a lot younger. The photo was taken in October of 1973. She took the picture and I said, "Here's your parents." She said, "Yes, Mother and Daddy." I said, "They were in front of their house in Florida. Do you see all the flowers behind them?" She said yes, and then said, "That was so nice of them to come and visit." Which made no sense, of course.

That was an interesting experience. What was it about those particular pictures that was so captivating to her? She kept four pictures: one of me and Tom, one of Trevor, one of Emily, and one of her sister. I was surprised that she wasn't more interested in the photos of David. He has spent more time with her over the years than anyone else, especially while she was living in Crosslake. Maybe that's why; she spends so much time with him now that she doesn't need any photos. Looking at the photos she seemed able to grasp the concept of family. I know she recognized Nancy, who also spends a lot of time with Mother right now. But it was that grade school picture of Emily that made the biggest impact. For my next trip I will try to find some more photographs. I'll have to go in the storage building and dig.

I need to find all of our grade school pictures and see what happens.

While Mother looked at Emily and Trevor I put the other photos away. I opened her drawer and was surprised to see a pair of reading glasses in a flowered case. I said, "Mother, you have glasses in here. Where did they come from?" She seemed surprised herself and said she didn't know. I took them out. They had a thin turquoise frame and brown arms that had masking tape wrapped around them, her name written on one side. I said, "Do you want to put them on?" and I handed them to her. She reached her hand up but then looked like she didn't know quite how to take them from me. I slipped them on for her. She sat up real straight and looked at me in wonder. I laughed and said, "Can you see those pictures better now?" She said yes. I pulled out my camera and said, "Let me take your picture with your glasses on." She looked directly at me and I took her picture. I think today is the only time she has looked directly at the camera lens, usually she turns her eyes at the last second.

I asked her if she would like to go on an outing with me and David tomorrow. She got very excited and said, "Oh, yes!" I said that we wanted to take her somewhere where she can walk in the grass and sit in the shade and see a lake. I told her we'd be coming to get her right after lunch and she needed to be ready and to have her shoes on. As she continued looking at the pictures I went through her closet. The socks Dorothy bought were in there but there was also several pairs of colored socks. I bet Nancy brought her some after all. I decided not to leave the socks I had with me; she doesn't need them right now. I'll bring them back at a later time, this winter probably. I looked for the top I had brought earlier in the year and it was there with a name label sewed in. I took it out and showed it to Mother saying, "Here's the top I bought you. You should wear this tomorrow." She said, "Okay." She does have a lot of clothes actually. There was a winter jacket and a spring jacket. In the bottom there was a pair of brown moccasins. I was surprised, I hadn't seen them before. I didn't pick them up but I could see that they were fleece lined. They were probably slippers.

I took out the tub of greeting cards and went back and sat down. Mother was still looking at the pictures. I dug under the cards and looked to see if everything was the same as my last visit. Really I was just wasting time while Mother looked at the pictures. I took out the plastic storage bag containing her jewelry and began taking the pieces out one at a time laying them on the bed. Mother ignored them. The pieces were all costume jewelry of course, mostly Christmas pins. After awhile Mother said, "I'm ready to go home now." I put the tub back in the closet and when I turned back around she had laid the Bible on the bed and was heading for the door. I said, "Don't you want to take those glasses off?" She said, "No." I said, "Are you sure? Can you see clearly?" She said, "Yes." I said, "Look out in the hallway, do you see it clearly? Wait, let me go out there." I stepped into the hallway and said, "Can you see me clearly?" She said yes and started out the door. I said, "Are you sure you don't want to take them off?" She said, "Did you take yours off?" I said, "I don't have any. Look down the hallway, do you see clearly? Now lift the glasses, do you still see clearly?" She lifted the glasses and then said, "You're right," and she took them off and handed them to me. Down the hall she went. I went back in the room and put the glasses back in the drawer. The bottles of lotion are now missing. I signed the calendar and then wrote her name in the front of the Bible then slipped it into the bottom of the tub in the closet. I got Chelsey and put her in her bag, turned off the light, and left the room.

I started down the hall and could see a woman in a wheelchair sitting in the doorway of Mother's old room. Mother was just walking past her and the woman said something to her, Mother said something back, still moving down the hallway. I walked slowly and as I passed the woman I smiled and said hello. As Mother reached the visiting area a nurse handed her a small glass containing what looked like milk but wasn't. Mother kept walking, glass in hand. She merged into the mass of people and I made my way over to the nurse's station. A young nurse was standing there and I told her that my brother and I wanted to take Mother for an outing tomorrow and asked if they could have her ready. She said sure, what time? I said about 1:30, right after lunch. I asked if Mother is able to use the restroom by herself and she called over another nurse. It was the same nurse that I talked with on my last visit. She said that Mother needs assistance in the restroom but that she wears a pad. We talked about tomorrow and they said she eats lunch at 11:00 so I said we'd come get her at 1:00. I asked if someone would have her ready, including having her shoes on. They said they'd leave a note for tomorrow's staff and asked if there was something in particular I wanted her to wear. I said, yes, I'd like her to wear the blue and white top. Finishing, I left the unit not seeing Mother. I started my long walk back to the front door, signing out I saw that I had been there only one hour.

The front parking lot had been full so we had to park around the side. I made that long walk and found Tom sitting in his chair reading. We always carry a couple of camping chairs with us. I said, "Are you ready to go?" On the ground I saw several seed pods that we used to play with as kids. I said, "Look, helicopters," throwing some up in the air, watching them flutter down. I said, "We need to bring some of these home for the kids." I gathered up a handful thinking I'll get a bag or something and get some more tomorrow. We drove to the LaQuinta and checked in. We each took in an armload of stuff and Chelsey, and then went out back for a cigarette. We walked down to the pond to see the geese. Tom suddenly said, "Do you see that? A beaver is swimming across. I think it's a beaver." I had my camera because I only had a few shots left on the roll and wanted to use them, however, I forgot the long lens in the room. So now I have a few shots of the geese that I'll have to use a magnifying glass to see.

There was white stuff floating all over the place, in the air and covering the ground. I said, "Look at all that dandelion fuzz. It can't be dandelion, there's too much of it, look, the ground is covered with it. Could it be the geese losing their winter fluff? There looks like too much for that also. It's probably not good for me to be breathing that stuff." It's a mystery to us. We went back to the room to freshen up and David called on Tom's cell phone. He said he had just driven past the nursing home and looked for our truck but didn't see us so went on home. Tom told him he had just missed us. David said, "The pizza's on the way." We had made up a small spot for Chelsey between the bed and nightstand, which is where she went when we set her down on the floor. Throwing her towel over her like a cocoon she hunkered right down. We decided to just leave her there while we were gone.

We drove on over to David's and finally found that shortcut he always uses to get to the nursing home. We seem to take a different route every time and there's so much construction going on in the area that we get turned around easily. This route will be easy to remember. David has beautiful gardens all over the place. Approaching the side door I stopped to admire the flowers in the garden up against the house. He has huge flowering yellow lady slippers. Turning to Tom I said, "Look at all these lady slippers." He said, "Is that what they are?" Just then David came out on the steps and I said we were admiring the lady slippers. I said, "They're the Minnesota state flower." David said, "Well, they're almost the state flower." I said, "I thought they were the state flower." He said, "Well, the lady slipper is the state flower but these are moccasins. The lady slippers are pink and the yellow ones are moccasins." So, I had the whole thing wrong. The pink lady slipper is the Minnesota state flower. They are wildflowers, but also a type of orchid. I don't think I've ever seen the pink ones.

We went out to the backyard to wait for the pizza. They have a new patio set. It's real nice with a black wrought iron table and chairs. Dorothy started a fire in the outdoor fireplace which is enclosed wrought iron with black mesh sides and a door in front. I was surprised to see David's entire yard covered with the helicopter seed pods! David said they were from a maple tree. Looking we could see them hanging in bunches from the tree. I said I'd like to bring home a bag full for the grandkids. We walked out to a big garden in the back of the yard and he showed us around and talked about each plant. He definitely inherited Mother's green thumb, I can't keep a flower going for the life of me. We have to depend on wildflowers for our color and we have a lot of them, daisies, black-eyes Susans, Queen Ann's lace, and numerous flowers we can't identify, in every color.

Dorothy brought out a bag of marshmallows and some roasting forks and she and I dug in. I was so hungry. I hadn't toasted a marshmallow since the boys were little. Growing up we often made S'mores, mine without the chocolate of course. Every once in a while Mother let me have the chocolate and it was heaven. When the pizza arrived we went inside and ate then went back outside to enjoy the evening. It's still early in the year for mosquitos so it was really nice out there. After a while David and I went inside. He had come across some of Mother's papers and wanted me to look through them.

The papers were amazing. Actually, mostly they were her parent's old papers. There were numerous papers containing Grandpa's discharge from the army. Some of them were dated 1935, his discharge from the Army Reserves as an Office Supply Officer. I was surprised at that date. Mother was born in 1926 and that meant he was still in the army—the reserves anyway. Also, it said Camp Pike, Arkansas. Wow, I'd never heard of that. I'll need to do some research on Camp Pike.

There were also copies of Grandma and Grandpa's birth certificates. They were both born in Chicago and both of their parents were born in Sweden. The copies were dated 1967. I wonder why they had all these particular papers together. Was it for retirement benefits, or to draw Social Security?

Grandma and Grandpa owned some stock in a couple of real old hotels out west. They were old frontier hotels. Stocks weren't even available any more. In order to get some someone has to put their stock up for sale. It would be interesting to check them out if I could find the names and locations. I started hearing about them after Grandma and Grandpa died and Mother started receiving the annual dividends. They weren't worth much; out of the two she received about a hundred dollars a year. Among the papers was a letter Grandma had received from one of the stock companies in reply to a letter she had sent them. She was requesting that Grandpa's name be removed and that she be the sole owner. It had to have been after Grandpa died. The stock company said that the wording on the certificate had to be very precise stating that the names had to be listed as and/or, or she had to be listed as the beneficiary. There was a copy of the letter she had then written to them with a copy of the stock stating very plainly the and/or wording. Next was a copy of a letter adding Mother's name to the stock. Next was a copy of the letter where Mother had sold the stock in the amount of $4300. I'm assuming this was after Grandma's death, but maybe not. Grandpa died in 1981, Grandma in 1983. Next was a copy of the check Mother wrote to Aunt Laurie for half of the stock sale.

There were several geographical maps of the land in Crosslake that Grandma and Grandpa owned. They had owned the land where the cabin was sitting and an island, and Mother and Daddy owned the adjoining property where we spent our time camping out. I remember when the cabin was built, I was grade school age. Daddy did a lot of the work. Next was a contract for when Grandma and Grandpa sold their land to Mother and Ken.

While David and I looked at the papers we talked about our plans to go to the cemetery tomorrow, the flowers we needed and how many, etc. I was to get the colorful flowering plants and the potting soil, and David was going to get some ivy to hang down along the sides. He also had a favorite type of grass that stands straight up for the middle of the urn. David said he had contacted the cemetery to see if a space was available in the plot. I said, "Mother really should be buried there." She has a plot already next to Ken, it has a dual gravestone that already has her name and birth date on it, it's pretty creepy; but I had been thinking that she should be buried in the Lakewood Cemetery with her family. It's so beautiful and peaceful there. David said, "I was checking for myself." That really surprised me. I never thought he'd be thinking about his own burial spot, nor did I think he would be so particular. Really, I shouldn't be surprised. Tom and I have had our burial plots for about twenty years. They are all nicely paid for in a beautiful cemetery although not as good as Lakewood; although it should have been. When the cemetery first opened we were told that a small lake was going to be made and there would be shade trees, etc. We chose our plots because they were going to be overlooking the lake. We were even going to donate some ducks for the lake because we love ducks so much. Unfortunately that didn't happen. Soon after, the cemetery started changing hands and things changed. But we will still be buried there—because we already have the plots. They tried to sell us one headstone instead of two and I threw a fit. No way was my name going on a stone like Mother (assuming Tom went first) and they said oh, no, no you don't have to put your name on it. I said, no way, I want my own headstone. I don't know why that bothers me so much, but it just does. Kind of funny really, but that's how I feel.

It was at this point that I came across the actual contract for the Lakewood plot. It was for one family plot with four grave sites. The grand total was $195.00. The date was 1935. The terms of the contract was for a down payment and then monthly payments of at least $5 a month or more. There was the receipt for the final payment of $65.00. There was also the original handbook Grandpa received from the cemetery laying out all of the rules. I skimmed through it noting that one of the rules is that you cannot remove anything from the cemetery including rocks, etc. That was rule number 10. I can't even imagine how much a plot would cost there now.

After finishing with the papers Tom and I came back to the motel. We stopped in the lobby and got a couple cups of coffee to take to the room with us and arrived at 10:00, just in time to watch *Men in Black*, again. I'm feeling very calm. It was a really good visit with Mother. I still find it strange that at a certain time she will be done with me and just get up and leave. I won't try to figure out how her mind works, I'll just follow her lead. I'll take whatever time with her that I can get. And it has been so nice seeing her in a good mood.

May 22, 2010

Tom got up this morning about 9:00. He went outside for a few minutes and then went and got us coffee and orange juice. I asked him how the weather was and he said it was really nice; warm and sunny. Good. The free breakfast also had cups of fresh fruit and he got a couple of them. As I sipped my coffee he started in on the fruit. He said, "This is really good, nice and cold." A minute later he said, "This fruit is frozen," and he put it aside. We were in no hurry to leave before check-out because we weren't meeting David at the nursing home until 1:00. As we finally started moving around we were surprised to hear a rumble of thunder and soon after we could hear drops of rain falling. Oh no. When we checked out at 11 the rain was coming down pretty good. We weren't too worried though because we still had a couple of hours and it would probably pass over. We went down the road to a restaurant for breakfast. As we sat there the rain started coming down full force. There was thunder and lightning and angry looking black clouds. Crap. The rain started coming down in sheets, whipping in the wind. Tom said, "You can forget the cemetery." I said we still have a little time.

After finishing breakfast we drove down the road to a small strip mall and went in a tobacco shop. It was still raining hard, not only that, but the temperature had dropped to 60° and the wind was blowing something awful. By then I was agreeing with Tom, the cemetery was out. Not only would everything be soaking wet but it was now cold and windy. We would be able to do it, but not Mother. Still, I wanted to wait and see what David thought. We went down to the Home Depot to get the flowers. The plants I wanted were outside, of course. Tom waited inside with a cart as I ducked outside in the pouring rain, the hood on my jacket up for a little protection. After several trips in and out we had the flowers and continued on to the nursing home, arriving about 12:45. David was already there. The rain had stopped but not the wind and the temperature was still sitting on 60.

Tom and I both went up to Mother's unit. We had left Chelsey in the truck because Tom would be going back out. As we entered we spotted Mother right away sitting at a table in the back of the dining area. David was squatting beside her. As I approached I heard him say, "Look who's here?" He is so patient with her. His love for her is obvious. As I reached Mother she got a big smile on her face, and said, "Well, hi there," and put her arms up for a hug. I gave her a hug then asked if she wanted to move to a different area. She said okay. She was still wearing a bib from lunch and I removed it and then led her into the visiting area. I sat her down in a chair and then went to get another one to set next to her for me. She said, "Don't leave!" I said, "I'm not leaving, I'm just getting a chair." I pulled a chair over and didn't put it directly in front of her but kind of a ninety degree angle. Tom talked with David for a minute, both agreeing that the cemetery was out. Tom left and David sat down in another chair that was next to Mother with a small table separating them.

Mother looked really happy. She was wearing the blue and white top I had requested and she had her shoes on, all ready to go. We knew that Mother didn't remember our conversation yesterday on taking her out so we didn't even mention it. David said when he had first arrived Mother was asleep with her head down on the table. He woke her up and when she saw him she smiled and said, "Well, hi there!" He seemed really impressed by that greeting. After a minute David said Tom was having trouble getting out of the unit and had to ask for help. I had forgotten to give him the pass code for the alarm system on the door. Later Tom told me that as he was walking towards the door a woman in a wheelchair approached him and asked for his help. I think she needed help moving her chair; he helped her then started towards the door again. She said, "Are you leaving?" He said, "Yes." She said, "Can I go with you?" He said, "No, sorry you can't." She said, "Will you give me a ride?" He said, "Where are you going?" She said, "To Lake Street." He said, "I'm not going in that direction."

David and I talked about many things. Once again it was hard to keep Mother in the conversation. I told David that he could have all of the flowers we bought and tomorrow he and Dorothy could go plant the urn. They had already been planning that before I called David and said I wanted to do it, so they will go back to their original plan. I started talking about something and Mother kept laughing. I think I was talking about how one year I planted tulips in my backyard and when they came up our pet ducks got to them first. I was saying that they had been really pretty but the ducks wouldn't leave them alone. One autumn after moving here we planted tulip and other bulbs on our land across the street, which is all forest. In the spring we went over to check on them and we found the stalks, but no flowers. The deer had eaten them. Mother thought that was so funny that she was laughing almost hysterically with tears running down her face. Of course that made David and I start laughing. I said, "I remember one time when she got sent from the dinner table for the same reason." David smiled and said, "I remember." David had started the trouble in the first place. He and I sat next to each other at the dinner table and on this particular evening he was goofing off and pulled the headband out of my hair. Daddy got mad and for punishment made David wear it all though dinner. He did look funny wearing my pink cloth headband over his buzz cut. Mother started laughing and couldn't stop; and of course she caused a disruption so Daddy sent her out of the room. By then the rest of us were having trouble holding back our laugher but we managed it so we wouldn't be sent away also.

There were a lot of people in the dining and visiting areas, but only a couple of visitors. I mentioned the lack of visitors and how I rarely see any. David agreed and said, "These are the forgotten people." That's so sad. He also said, "You'd expect there to be more visitors today because it's Saturday, but there never is." The inside doors to the vestibule were open; it's actually an exit but is now kept locked. By then the sun was out again and people were going out there to look out the windows. A nurse wheeled an elderly lady past going in that direction and as they passed near David the woman reached out and tried to grab him. I noticed it was Evelyn, the woman Mother can't stand. I hadn't seen her at all my last trip. I said, "Oh, there's Evelyn, I haven't seen her in a while. I also haven't seen Judy, or Ray." We looked around and spotted Judy nearby, also in a wheelchair now. She looked like she was trying to get over to where we were sitting but couldn't get her chair to move. There was no sign of Ray. David, thinking, said he hadn't seen Ray in a while either. He said he had come one day and Mother and Ray were walking down the hall together holding hands. Maybe that's why she always seems to be in a good mood now. David said when the nurse went to get Mother she couldn't get them apart because Ray had such a tight grip on Mother's hand. It took some effort but she finally managed to get Mother free. I said, "Why was she trying to get them apart?" He said so she could come and visit with him.

A nurse came over and handed Mother a small glass with the mysterious liquid. She said, "Here's your milkshake." Ah, that's what it is. Mother took the glass eagerly and began drinking it. I said, "Is that her medicine," and the nurse said yes. I asked what kind of medicine Mother is taking but she said she didn't really know. I'm surprised the nurse doesn't know exactly what she gives Mother. She said she thinks they give her something for high blood pressure and recently they started giving her a mild sedative to help her sleep. She'd begun getting up in the middle of the night, wandering, and falling down. Surely they don't give her a sedative at that time of day though, it must be in the evening. Mother sure did like the milkshake, when she emptied the glass she actually tried to lick the rest out.

There was a man in a wheelchair near us. He was completely stretched out, his legs in front of him, and he was asleep. He started to stir, looked around and saw David then called out to him for help. David went over to him but they just couldn't communicate; David just couldn't understand what the man was saying. It ended with both of them frustrated. A male nurse came walking down the hall holding the arm of a white haired lady. When they got to the end, right in front of the nurse fixing medication, the lady kind of started a ruckus so the man left her there. The lady was really upset and said to the nurse (yelled it really), "You can tell him to go to hell!" and looked back at the fleeing man. The nurse looked up from her work and said, "You're not happy?" She said, "No, I'm not happy!" The lady stood there for a minute then said, "Are you going to help me?" Finally an assistant came and led her away. A few minutes later a black female nurse came down the hall leading a female resident. The lady's head was bent completely forward. How frustrating I thought. I wonder what was causing it, osteoporosis maybe? They walked around the area for a moment then the lady got angry about something and started hitting the nurse. She couldn't do it very well, though, because she couldn't lift her head to see. Her punches just kind of glanced off the nurse. Finally a young woman came and got her, I think she was an assistant of the activity director. This same young woman reappeared a few minutes later pushing a different woman in a wheelchair. They were going real fast like you would if giving a child a ride. The young assistant had her brown hair in pig tails and she really looked like she was having fun. I wonder if they get volunteers in that area. Come to think of it, I don't remember when I've last seen a candy striper, either in a nursing home or hospital. Do they even have them any more? Kelley would be really good at that.

At first Mother kept up a running commentary as we talked. She'd say things like, "Really? Oh I'm so glad you did that," or "That really happened?" After a while I noticed that she had become quiet. Every time I looked at her she'd kind of jump to attention and say something like, "I didn't do that," or "I didn't see that guy." I said to David,

"I always wonder what she's thinking about," and he said, "Mom?" I said, "Yes," then I turned to Mother and said, "What are you thinking about?" She said, "What am I thinking about...right now?" "Yes." "Well..." She said something but I swear it was complete gibberish, not one word made sense. I turned to David and said, "See?" Is that how her mind works, in complete gibberish? Does she try to think? Is that why she seems to want to keep moving, because she can't think clearly and rationally? How frustrating that would be, no wonder all of these people sleep so much; it's a good way to turn off the mind. I often wonder what she dreams about. Are her dreams also gibberish or are they clear? Is she able to float above the dementia while she's asleep?

I told David about the mystery of Mother's teddy bear blanket now being brown and how her roommate's bedspread was also brown. He was skeptical so I told him to go look at it. He got up and said he's go look and sign the calendar. He came back a minute later and said that he thought it was just turned over. Well, I had to check that out and got up. He told me to sign the calendar while I was in there. In the hallway near her room three Jamaican staff members (two men, one woman) were standing very close together talking. I wondered if they noticed we had both gone into Mother's room and I wondered what they thought. Going in I saw that the room was darkened and the roommate was in her bed asleep. I noticed her bedspread was actually a dark colored tan blanket. I quickly picked up the edge of Mother's cover and looked it over, finally seeing a manufacture's tag. Yup, David was right. I have never seen a blanket that has an underside like that. How strange. I signed the calendar and then quickly left. Back in my chair I told David about my visit yesterday with the Bible and photographs. I told him that I had stashed the Bible in the bottom of the tub in the closet for safety and that he could get it out and go through the pictures with Mother if he wanted to. He seemed impressed by her reactions and asked me how old the pictures were. I said I didn't have a lot of the really old pictures but the one of Emily that she was so engrossed in was her grade school picture. I said that I would go digging for some more of that time frame for my next visit. He seemed to be thinking about it so maybe he'll look through his own photographs and bring some to her.

Last night David said he and Dorothy are going on vacation the last week in July to the Black Hills. I know they have been there before and I wondered what the draw was. So, I asked him, "What's in the Black Hills?" He kind of looked at me like I was crazy and then said, "Mount Rushmore!" I thought, okay, but do you really need to see that more then once? So, I asked him, "What else is there?" He said, "Bears." "Bears?" "Yes, a lot of bears." I asked if you could actually see the bears and he said you can't help seeing them. It's a bear preserve that you drive through. They're in a huge fenced-in area and he said it's more like you're in a cage and they look at you as you drive through. I asked if there were signs all over saying 'please don't feed the bears.' He said, "No, there are signs that say don't get out of your vehicle." He said one time they were driving through and it was hot so he rolled his window part way down and then through a loudspeaker a man said, "Please roll up your window." I said, "They watch you through cameras;" which is why he said it felt like you were in a cage instead of the bears. I think that would be fun. We've been to a couple of drive-through safaris but the bears have never even gotten close. Not much fun really if you just spot them in the distance in the woods. I like interaction with animals.

The activity director came over pushing a cart. She asked Mother if she wanted some lime sherbet and Mother said no. She said, "Are you sure, you don't want any?" Mother said no again. David was amazed and said, "You don't want any ice cream?" Mother said, "Ice cream? Yes, I want ice cream." The woman handed Mother a small white Styrofoam bowl and a white plastic spoon. Mother dug right in, stirring it a bit first. I was eager to see her eat it because David had said that sometimes she couldn't remember how to feed herself. She started taking large spoonfuls of the sherbet and eating it. One time she dropped a small amount on the bottom of her shirt but it didn't slow her down. There were a couple of times when she got her spoon turned around and when she brought it up there was nothing on it, when she realized what was going on she was able to get the spoon turned back over. When the bowl was empty she started scraping it with the spoon, trying to get every drop in her mouth. Then she looked in it to see if there was any left. She held it out to me and said, "What is that?" I looked and saw a couple of drops she hadn't reached and scraped them up for her, handing her the spoon. She licked it up, put the spoon back in the bowl and then started looking for a place to put it. As she was reaching towards the table David said, "Here I'll take it," but Mother was already in mid aim and set it on the table, keeping the spoon in her hand. Once again David said, "Here I'll take it," again she was in mid aim trying to put the spoon in the bowl while David was trying to take it from her. This little interaction had both of them frustrated. David then picked up the bowl and spoon and went and threw them in the trash. When he returned he said, "You spilled some on your shirt," and she said, "Yes, I saw that," as she fiddled with the bottom of her shirt. I wonder how clearly she can see. She has always worn reading glasses, I know from my own experience how frustrating it is when something suddenly becomes blurry. It must be even more so for her because at least I know why it happens.

After a few more minutes David said, "How much longer are you going to stay?" I was actually waiting for him to make the first move. I was surprised he had lasted so long; we had been there for three hours and he looked really uncomfortable sitting in his chair a little sideways. I said, "Are you ready to go?" When he said yes I got up. I said to Mother, "Come and give me a hug." I helped her up and she wrapped her arms around my waist. I told her I loved her and she said I love you too. Then I said, "Are you going to give David a hug?" She said, "Yes," and they wrapped their arms around each other in a hug. While she still had her arms around his waist I said, "Tell David you love him." She looked up at his eyes and said, "I love you." I know that doesn't happen very often. I said, "I'll see you in two months," and she said, "Two months!" I said, "Well, it takes a long time to drive up here." David said, "Well, I'll be back in two days, I won't make you wait two months." We left her there and made our way back to the front entrance in silence.

Once outside we walked over to where our truck was parked. Tom was sitting in his chair reading, Chelsey at his feet in the grass. The same white stuff on the ground at the motel was here also. I pointed it out to David and he said, "That's from the dogwood trees." Hmm, I never would have figured that out. I don't remember ever seeing them before. Tom put his chair and Chelsey back in the truck and then showed David all the plants in the back. He asked if we could drive over to where his truck was parked so we could transfer them. We drove to the other side of the parking lot but there was nowhere to park so we just stopped in the drive-through and loaded everything in to the back of David's truck. He showed me the ivy plants he had bought and the special grass for the middle. The urn will look really good when he gets it planted. He had brought a plastic bag full of the helicopter seeds that he gathered up, which we forgot to get last night. We talked for a few minutes until a car pulled in the lot and we had to move.

Back out on the road headed for home I thought about the visit. I was disappointed we hadn't been able to take Mother out; I was really looking forward to it. But I still had a good visit. She has been in such a good mood these last two trips. Maybe on our next trip we'll be able to take her to the cemetery. Still, I really wanted her to help plant the urn. I wanted to see if it would bring up any memories and I wanted to see if she would get excited about having her hands in the dirt again. Maybe we'll have the chance to do it next year.

We stopped for gas and so I could smoke. Inside the little convenience store I saw a display of small bags of Old Dutch potato chips. I said, "Tom, look at these Old Dutch chips. You can only buy these in the north; we can't get them at home. I'm going to buy some for a special treat on Father's Day." I bought two small bags of regular chips, plus they had small bags of dill pickle so I got two of them. For our Father's Day cookout next month we'll split them up amongst everyone. I also still have the bottle of sarsaparilla that I was going to crack open at the cemetery but will portion out to everyone. I thought about the reaction I would get from the grandkids, "Sarsaparilla, what's that? I'm not drinking that!" It'll be funny.

We had a quiet drive out of the cities and through southern Minnesota. There wasn't any sign of the police cars from the other day, probably because the construction was stopped for the weekend. Tom was energized and planned on driving late into the night. The more we drive tonight the less we'll have to drive tomorrow. We were in Iowa when it started getting dark. The storms were gone and the sky was clear. I was dozing off and on feeling contented. Suddenly Tom was putting on the brakes. I looked up and saw a deer on the side of the road, wanting to cross. He said, "Deer are stupid, watch." The deer was looking at us (our lights anyway) and looked like it was going to dart out but then didn't. The thing with deer is that you never know when they're going to. You think they're going to wait for you to pass but then at the last minute dart out. Tom came to a complete stop; luckily there was no other traffic. We had to wait a couple of minutes and then the deer finally ran across the road. We waited another couple of minutes because deer are rarely alone. When no other deer appeared we continued on.

We are now at the motel in Chillicothe. It was the Best Western Inn, but now is just the Best Inn, soon to be the EconoLodge according to their sign. It was pretty late when we got here, going on midnight. The front entrance to the parking lot was blocked off because of repaving or something so we had to go around to the side. The parking lot was packed full; near the front were a few big utility trucks. Tom was able to find an empty spot next to one of them. He went into the office while I waited in the truck; and waited and waited. He was taking so long that I was beginning to get worried; I couldn't see the office due to being parked next to the utility truck. Finally, he came out. I said, what took so long? He said he had been having an argument with the clerks, about money. He told them that he always pays only $60 and they said they couldn't find him in the computer. The reason they couldn't find him in the computer is because we always pay cash when we stay here (do we even want to be in their computer?). Anyway, Tom won the argument. The place was so full though that we had to get a room on the second floor. We hate that, hate carrying all of our stuff up the stairs.

I can't smoke in the room here; the rooms downstairs have a rocking chair in front of each unit, but not on the second floor. However, there was a bench a couple of rooms down, and since it was already midnight, I asked Tom to help me move the bench to the front of our room, then he went to get ice for the cooler. I started running Chelsey's bath and once again this tub stopper didn't work. Tom finally put a small Styrofoam cup over it and that slowed it down but that was it. Chelsey was not happy. Tom said we really need to get one of those rubber stoppers and carry it with us. It took me a moment to understand what he was talking about and then I remembered way back many years ago we had a flat rubber disk that we could place over the drain and it would seal it up. Good idea, that's exactly what we need, and sometimes the sink doesn't have a stopper at all, I hate that. I'll be looking for one. I hope someone still makes them. Time for bed, I'm exhausted.

May 23, 2010

We were back on the road about 11:00 this morning. After leaving Chillicothe I was saddened when we drove past several dead deer on the side of the road. When we got to Malta Bend we were going to stop at The Waggin' Wheel for lunch but they were closed on Sundays. I had been so intrigued about this town that I looked for it in the Atlas. It wasn't there. But we started watching and Waverly is eight miles to the north. The population is 249. We had just passed through Sedalia and I was dozing a bit when Tom exited the Interstate. I said, "Where are you going?" He said, "I'm going back to that entrance ramp we just passed." I said, "Why?" He said, "There's a turtle on the side of the road." I said, "A turtle? You're joking right?" "No, you'll see. It's upside down. I have to help it." I don't know how in hell he saw that thing but we went back to the entrance ramp and he pulled onto the side. Sure enough there was a turtle lying there upside down. I could clearly see all the legs, tail, and head sticking out of the bowl shaped shell. It was a bit bigger than Chelsey. Tom got out of the truck, picked up the turtle, and put it in the grass next to the road. Getting back in the truck he said, "Dead." Tom is such a softie. If he see a turtle crossing the road he will stop, if possible, and move the turtle to the other side.

It was nice to get back into Arkansas. Once getting on Hwy. 7 in Harrison we started looking for the rest area we had found on the last trip. It's really nice, on top of a mountain with a great view, in the woods so it's nice and cool. Once we get off the Interstate there are no more rest areas so we were glad to discover this place. We found it; it's actually outside of Russellville. It even has a name, the Rotary Ann. The building is made out of stone and there are observation areas. There are probably trails leading off of them down the mountain. There are also a couple of picnic tables. We went over to one of the tables so I could smoke and Tom put his head down and went to sleep. I stayed quiet to give him some time to rest until he said, "Ready to go?" It's nice to be home. I miss Mother already.

May 24, 2010

During our trip I had been worried about a nest of baby birds we have. The nest is in a weird place. It is in the top of an iron motor-puller, in just a small square opening, exposed to the elements. With all of the rain I was afraid they'd get drenched. I've been watching the momma bird. I'm not sure what it is. It's a light blue with a red breast like a robin. The closest I can get to it in my books is a scrub jay. When I was growing up we had a huge tree in the front yard. In the summer it was so full of branches and leaves that you couldn't even see up in it. One day David and I were out there and I think he was throwing a ball up in the tree. All of a sudden a big blue jay came flying out and started dive bombing him. It was pretty funny although I made sure I stayed really close to the front door. David started screaming and running and waving his arms around. The blue jay must have had a nest of babies up there.

This evening when I went on my walk I checked on the baby birds, making sure momma wasn't around. They have grown so much, in just four days! They were completely naked when I left and now they're covered with gray fuzz and their eyes are open, actually looking at me looking at them. The very back corner of my walking area gets covered in water when we've had a lot of rain. Walking through it tonight I saw a ton of the teeniest tadpoles. I hope they hurry up and grow little legs before that water dries up. Finishing my walk I saw that the squash plants have yellow flowers blooming on them.

May 26, 2010

I guess I should feel good about Mother's nursing home. Arkansas' nursing homes have been rated as the worst in the nation. It's like you just can't find good people to work in nursing homes; nobody wants to take care of old people. I hear and read about so many horror stories: violence, missing (stolen) money, medication not being given (and being stolen), accidents not reported, recently in Arkansas a death wasn't even reported. I guess I should feel relieved that Mother only has missing flowers, vases, and stuffed animals. It's just all so frustrating. Looking in the news-paper at the classifieds I always see numerous ads wanting CNAs, training provided. And there's such a big turnover rate. There are times, around here at least, when the entire staff is replaced at one time. Why?

In Arkansas most deaths in nursing homes are due to choking on food. The staff is either not paying attention or not providing a proper diet (chicken instead of soft foods); coroners are often the ones who find the evidence. Mother is in a Masonic Home. I wonder if that makes a difference.

June 2, 2010

I was watching a medical program on TV this afternoon and they started talking about poison ivy. Mother used to get poison ivy really bad and would really suffer. It was kind of funny that I was not allergic to it at all. I was allergic to so many different things but not poison ivy. I would even prove it by sitting in a patch. I think Emily was also allergic to it. They would have to stay out of bushes, and pretty much all greenery and I could romp all I wanted. On the show a doctor was talking about how you should wash the rash with cold water. He said that hot water would open the pores and make it worse. You should wash it with soap and cold water. I wonder if Mother knew that. Today there are steroid creams and injections. Mother always covered herself with pink calamine lotion.

June 7, 2010

I was going through the photographs I had taken to Mother last month, just trying to form an idea on what I want to do for my next visit. I kept going back to the one of Mother just standing in her yard in Crosslake, the one in which she was wearing the white short sleeved cotton blouse and blue jeans. There is a big smile on her face. I finally took it out, put it in a frame, and set it on my office shelf where I can see it whenever I'm in there. This is how I remember Mother. This is how I want to remember Mother. This is how I <u>will</u> remember Mother.

June 9, 2010

Today I was looking through my flower reference books looking at the information on lady slippers and moccasins. It's pretty interesting. They are actually orchids. One of my books says that Native Americans used the powdered root as a sedative, tranquilizer, and pain reliever. Another book says that the lady slipper's genus name, *Cypridpedium*, can be broken into "*Cyprid*," the original name for the god Venus, and "*pedium*," Latin for "foot." Orchids are highly specialized plants needing their own special fungus growing on their roots to survive. This is why they are nearly impossible to transplant and should be enjoyed in the wild only. I want some.

June 11, 2010

There was a huge flash flood in Caddo Gap, on the Little Missouri River, and swept through a campground filled with people about 3:30 this morning. That's about 40 miles from here. It was so bad. The flood was measured at 10 feet higher than ever recorded. It just descended on the campground and swept all of the people out of their camp sites. There were so many people who died. It was like a Mother Nature massacre. It was on a small scale compared to all of the hurricanes and earthquakes, but still deadly and horrifying.

We had a close call one summer. We were camping in Crosslake. Daddy wanted to go to another town that had a huge campground and spend a few days there. Before we had a chance to pack up and leave a storm came up so we stayed put. The next morning we packed up and headed out. On the car radio we heard that there had been a big tornado that hit the campground during the night. Tents full of families had been buried. It was really scary. We drove through the town and could see all of the damage and we kept driving, going straight home in a state of shock. I don't remember the name of the town but it was one of those that when you get to the main intersection all traffic is at a standstill because a family of ducks is crossing the road.

June 15, 2010

We have a small turtle that's been coming into our feeding area each morning wanting to be fed when Tom's getting ready to leave for work. It's really funny because I hear him leave out the back door then he comes running back in the house and grabs some fruit out of the refrigerator and a knife then runs back out. Over the years we've had a lot of turtles coming around. Each year is different—from the type of turtle, to the size. But they all seem to like the same kind of fruit: strawberries, kiwis, and grapes. They have trouble biting into them so we cut everything up. This particular turtle always seems to know when Tom will be coming out and hangs around until he shows up.

One year, it must have been spring, Mother saw a turtle digging a hole and knew she was about to lay eggs. Mother watched really close and then when the turtle left she went out and put up a stick next to the hole to mark it. When she knew it was about time for the eggs to hatch she kept a watch on the spot. Sure enough, the baby turtles started digging themselves out. Mother was ready and picked up each small turtle and took them down to the lake. She really loved living in Crosslake. Her dream come true.

I got an email from David this evening. It actually started yesterday when he wrote and asked if we were under water, referring to the flood. He asked how close we were to it and I wrote and explained that we were about 40 miles away and how Scott, Ruth, and Trevor had been there just a few days earlier canoeing down one of the rivers that had flooded and that yesterday there was a big flood in Oklahoma City. David and Dorothy were going to plant the urn at Lakewood Cemetery over the weekend so I had asked how that went. In today's email he said that it had been a really nice day and that there was some construction going on at the cemetery, like they were building a new mausoleum, and there was a big crane set up. He said when they arrived at the urn it was already filled to the top with dirt and that the groundskeeper must have filled it.

June 16, 2010

I got a phone call this morning. When I answered a woman's voice said, "Hello, is this Lakewood?" That was creepy. I thought, that has to be a cemetery doesn't it? I've never heard of a Lakewood cemetery around here. I got out the phone book and looked it up. There is a Lakewood Convalescent Home and a Lakewood Residential Care Center. Neither has a phone number similar to mine. There is also a Lakewood Electric company whose first three numbers is the same as mine. I don't know who the woman was trying to reach but it was definitely creepy.

June 18, 2010

There was a tornado in Albert Lea today. I sent David an email asking how much damage there was. I also asked him if he knows what the tornado precautions are for Mother's nursing home. The nursing home I worked in during high school had a small basement where they would take the residents. Mother is on a higher level which scares me.

June 20, 2010

It's Father's Day. We had a big get together this evening with the kids. They had other plans during the day so everyone arrived around 6:15. We had a big cookout but since it was so hot and muggy we ate inside. Once everyone was settled with a plate of food I announced that we had brought some special treats home from Minnesota. First I brought out the Old Dutch potato chips explaining that you can only get them in the north. Tom had eaten one of the bags of the regular chips but no one seemed interested in them anyway. But they got excited about the Dill Pickle chips, although they didn't care where they came from. Next I got out the Sioux City Sarsaparilla. I said, "Whoever wants some of the sarsaparilla get a glass of ice and come get some." There was only one taker – Zakary. He'll try almost anything, he's sweet. He liked it but didn't ask for more. That was it. I guess Tom and I will get the rest.

After everyone had eaten I called all of the kids to come outside with me. Why, why, they asked. I said I have something new for you to play. What, what, they asked. I sat down in a chair with the bag of helicopter seeds in my lap. As everyone gathered around to see what was in it I opened it and…dam, they were wet! I had never opened the bag to check. David must have gathered them after the rain. Everyone shouted, what is it? I picked up a few of the seeds and threw them up in the air. Kelley yelled, "Helicopter seeds!" Everyone grabbed a handful and threw them in the air. Most fell to the ground in a lump but some free floated. I thought that we'll have to gather them back up and dry them and try again. So, my treats/surprises from Minnesota didn't turn out so well. That's the way it goes sometimes.

June 21, 2010

I received an email this evening form David in reply to the one I had sent him. He said that the storm had gone to the north of them, about 20 miles, and hit Wadena, that storm and the one that hit Albert Lea were both big and deadly. He said he had gone to see Mother but had forgotten to ask them about weather warnings.

July 5, 2010

Scott called Tom today and said that it is next week that Ben will be coming to stay with us while Trevor goes to band camp. I thought it was the following week but that's okay. I asked Tom if he had told Scott that we want to take Ben to Minnesota with us. He didn't so I told him to get back on the phone and make sure it's okay. He did and it is. So, it's set. We'll leave sometime next week.

July 6, 2010

This morning Tom said that he thinks we should go to Minnesota this week instead of next week. That caught me totally off guard. He said because he doesn't have any work this week and he does next week and it's supposed to rain anyway. I said but we'd have to leave tomorrow. I thought about it for a minute and couldn't think of any reason not to so I said okay. I said but you'll have to call Scott first and make sure it's okay to get Ben early. No problem with anyone. We ran into town and bought a bunch of fresh fruit and cookies for Mother and then I called the LaQuinta and made reservations. We had decided to stay an extra day because Ben is going with, makes it more like a vacation. I made the reservations for Thursday and Friday, a room with two beds. Thursday night is $64 but Friday night is $109. I said, "Wow! That's a big difference." And she said, "And we're almost full." So, the question is – why is the price so much higher? We have stayed there on a Friday before without a jack-up of the price. It'd better be a really nice room for that price. Then I called David and said we were coming. Boy was he surprised. He'll be out of town until Friday afternoon.

July 7, 2010

We left the house about 12:30 heading for Scott's to pick up Ben. It started raining really hard while we were on the Interstate. It was coming down so hard that we could hardly see the other vehicles around us. We started around a slight curve and Tom moved out of the left lane into the middle one. Just as we got around the curve we saw a small car in the left lane that was nose first into the retaining wall, the front of the car crumpled. I said, oh no, I hope that doesn't start something. It was raining so hard that no one would have even been able to stop and help the driver. I hope he had a cell phone. Awhile later Tom said he wondered how many vehicles had hit the car. He said that it wouldn't have been the first one that would have been bad but the next one. I said, and the one after that. He said the best thing he (the driver) could have done was to get out of the car and start walking. It doesn't matter how wet you get; you get as far away from the car as possible. I said but where would you walk. He said in the median. I said there is no median, just a concrete wall. He said then you walk next to the concrete wall and get as far away from the car as you can. I hope that I'm never in the position where I'll need to remember this information.

When I called David last night I explained why it was so last minute. He said that he had received several phone calls from the nursing home recently. The first call they said that Mother had gotten really angry about something and hit a staff member in the shoulder. They were then keeping a close eye on her, checking every 15 minutes to see where she was and what she was doing to make sure nothing else happened. They called him back later and said that after the initial outburst she had been fine. Another call said she'd been having extreme mood swings. One minute she'd be really happy, the next minute just the opposite. He said they had put her on some type of medication in the mornings but it hadn't helped any so they wanted to try giving her something at 5:00 in the evening. I said well they had put her on a mild sedative the last time I was there. He said they hadn't kept her on that for very long. Now they wanted to try something different. They'd actually already started it and when they started getting her ready for bed at 7:00 she went willingly. I asked him what the medication is and he didn't know but said we could find out while I'm there. I said surely they don't have her on anything strong. We don't want her groggy all the time (or drugged up). He said no.

We got to Scott's house a little after 2:00. Scott and Ruth were both at work of course. Tom and Trevor changed the tire on Scott's motorcycle for the race this weekend and we left there about 3:15 with Ben.

Chelsey rides in the front seat all of the time now. Today she stayed in the front of her travel bed so she could see everything until we got out of town then she went down, under the blanket. Once down she never comes back out. Ben has one suitcase, a large tote bag full of activities, and a fold-up chair which we told him to bring along. All of our stuff is piled up in the back seat leaving just enough room for one person to sit comfortably. I asked Ben if he wanted to ride in the front with Grandpa and Chelsey or in the back. He said, "In the front!" I said, okay, I'll ride in the back. I knew he would want that so I had already arranged the back seat for me with all of my stuff right where I want it. I even brought along a small pillow for napping. I didn't mind at all. I had my coffee, my camera, my work, and all the food. After leaving Tom got his phone out and called Scott and told him they'd gotten his tire on. He let Ben say good-bye to him then Tom called Ruth and let Ben say good-bye to her. He seemed really excited about the trip.

We took a back way out from Ben's house and didn't get on Hwy. 65 until we got to Mountain View. It was just a two lane but a nice change of scenery. There were lots of mountains and curvy roads. There were also a lot of goats, horses, and cows. We saw a real neat motorcycle that had what looked like an Amish buggy on the back. We stopped in Heber Springs so Tom could look at a map. He pulled into a convenience store and Ben asked if he could get something to eat. I said, tell me what you want and I'll tell you if I already have it. "Chicken." No, I don't have chicken. We went inside and got him a couple of pieces of chicken and looked through the drinks. There were some that looked like little plastic jugs and he said, "Those are cute, I want one of those." Kids are funny. I choose drinks according to what's inside but they choose drinks by what the bottle looks like. The stuff looked like colored sugar water. He got the blue stuff of course.

It doesn't matter which part of northern Arkansas you're in, it's always beautiful. The heavy rain had stopped and there were big fluffy white clouds everywhere. There was a little rain occasionally. Ben spent most of his time watching movies on his mini DVD player. What can you say, he's only 8. He did take one nap. Like I said, kids are funny, his head just flopped to the side and he was asleep. The seatbelt was the only thing that kept him from toppling over. We went through Searcy, Rosebud, and Romance— the town where everyone likes to get their Valentines postmarked. We went through Greer's Ferry where they have big fishing tournaments and big tornados. We went past a lot of signs advertising different types of cows; on the top they say BEEF, and underneath the brand of the cows. Up past Marshall was a big church. It looked like a plain cream colored hall except that it had a huge wooden cross on the end. We saw a lot of old barns, some falling down, some still in use. And why does it seem like all the newer barns are sitting right next to the road? We went past numerous small creeks that looked really low on water. Yesterday the weather man said we were 5 inches below average in rainfall. You can always tell when you're getting close to the Ozarks because the sides of the roads become lined with jutting rock walls. And it seems like you're always traveling upward and hopefully you won't get behind a big truck. And when you start going back down you're hoping there's no big truck behind you.

We drove until we got to Sedalia, about 11:00. Tom pulled into a Super 7 Motel. The motel stretched horizontally, one story, with the office in the middle. As Tom went inside several young men at the far end of the parking lot started shooting off fireworks. I was hoping Tom had seen them; I sure didn't want to be near that. When he came back out he said he had told the clerk that he wanted a room away from the fireworks. The guy had muttered, "Those guys!" So now we're in the very last room on the other end, as far away from them as possible. After getting everything in here it started raining so the fireworks stopped, but does that mean they'll be quiet? If they are so inconsiderate as to shoot off fireworks at 11:00 in a motel parking lot it's not likely they'll be quiet guests; they had been going in and out of several different rooms. I'm glad we're down here where it's quiet.

July 8, 2010

Is there a difference between a Super 8 Motel and a Super 7? Isn't there also a Super 6, or is that a Motel 6? Is the 8 supposed to be the better motel? That Super 8 we stopped at last year was definitely worse than the place last night. The Super 7 was older but it was comfortable, clean, and everything worked. That's all we need, plus it was only $59 total for all three of us. However, we got tiny bars of soap, but no shampoo, and we didn't even get free coffee this morning. But that's okay. Besides, I still had some coffee left in the thermos.

We slept until around 9:30 this morning and were back on the road by 11:00. Ben decided he wanted to ride in the back seat today. He started watching his movies again and of course he had full access to the food. When we stopped for lunch he wasn't hungry. Missouri is a beautiful state. There are a lot of ranches and we passed signs advertising bulls for sale.

"Grandma, are we almost to Minnesota?" "No, but almost to Iowa." The fields in Iowa were beautiful. Corn and bean fields all looking lush. Even Ben watched them as we drove past. Several times we saw white windmills stretched out as far as we could see in both directions. Our future maybe? There was a lot of road construction going on. Northern Iowa looked like it had some recent flooding. When we crossed the rivers the trees on the banks had limbs touching the water. Many fields had standing water in them. The weather today was beautiful, sunny with just a few clouds.

"Look, what does that sign say? "Minnesota!" We stopped at the rest area right past the state line. It was really nice with a lot of picnic tables and even a sand covered play area for the kids. There were vending machines inside and Ben wanted a hot chocolate. It came out in a paper cup with 'Poker' written on it; advertising for the Diamond Jim Casino which is nearby. We decided to sit at a table in the shade for a few minutes to kind of stretch our legs. Tom got Chelsey out and set her on the stone table. We're wary about putting her on the ground at rest areas because we don't know if they use poisonous chemical weed killers. I was a few steps behind Tom and Ben and when I reached the table Tom said, "There are mosquitoes." My arm got bit immediately. I looked at Ben and said, "Welcome to Minnesota." Later Tom said that as he was walking to the area a family was sitting nearby and all of a sudden the man said, "Oh Lord." He didn't think much of it and soon the man said it again, "Oh Lord." After a third time the family suddenly got up and quickly moved away. Tom then sat down at the same table and the mosquitoes started swarming. We tried to sit there but it was really bad.

Ben went to play on a tire swing and Tom suggested we move to a table in the sun. For some reason mosquitoes like the shade. We moved but then Tom was sitting right next to a wooded area (also a favorite place for mosquitoes). I could see them start swarming around his head. He left with Chelsey and I sat on the other side of the table, in the sun, away from the woods, and didn't have any problem, except that it was hot. We did, however, have to pass back through the shade to get to the truck. At the truck we each had to do a funny maneuver of brushing any mosquitoes off of us then getting the door open, jumping in, and closing the door. If a mosquito got in with you, you had to quickly get out, with the mosquito, brush it away, then jump back in, which we all had to do. Once we were all in we waited a minute, watching to see if we missed any. Tom said, "Look at the windows. They're watching us." There were numerous mosquitoes on the outside of the windows and they did look like they were watching us.

We didn't get to Minneapolis until after 7:00. Minneapolis looks so neat from a distance. The skyscrapers standing up real tall like in a circle makes it look like a floating city, almost like the Land of Oz beckoning us, always seeming to be surrounded by haze at that distance. Ben was surprised to see so many airplanes flying overhead. The airport is nearby. It was too late to go see Mother so we went straight to the LaQuinta, arriving about 8:00. As we checked in I asked the clerk about the different bed options. Well, she had said, "Two full beds?" She said they have rollaways and cots, plus queen size, and king size. We each had walked in with a suitcase and when we got the keys we took the cases to the room before going out to get another load. I stood in the room a minute; it just didn't look right. I said, "Wait a minute." I looked around, "There's no bath-tub. We have to have a bathtub. Go back and try to get another room. Try to get that room we had before." Tom left and came back and said we couldn't get that room but one just like it and she'd bring a rollaway. She had said that the only rooms that had bathtubs were the wheelchair accessible rooms. How strange. We carried everything back down the hallway to the new room. Tom and Ben finished unloading the truck while I waited for the rollaway. She finally arrived and then we all jumped into our swimming suits and headed for the pool.

We got to the pool at 8:30. We could not believe it but it was empty! We stuck a toe in the water and it was cold. We gingerly made our way in knowing it would be better once we got used to it. Tom's not much of a water person but I love it. Tom can't swim but he can dog paddle across the pool, of course the water didn't get over our heads. We had meant to get a ball but forgot so finally we got one of my flip flops and played catch with that. Ben loves doing cannon balls off the side. We tried out the hot tub and boy did that feel good. Tom turned on the jacuzzi for a few minutes, and then we went back in the pool which seemed even colder after the hot water. Tom was done by 9:30 and got out of the pool and started reading his book. But Ben wasn't about to leave until the pool closed at 10:00. We were standing in the shallow end and he said, "I never dreamed I could have so much fun in the pool with you and Grandpa." I said, "Really, you didn't think you'd have fun with us?" "No." "Did you think you'd be in the pool by yourself?" "Yes." We just kind of messed around, seeing how long we could stay under water, etc. until 10:00.

Back in our room we put the rollaway down, there wasn't much room for it but we got it into a space almost next to our bed and where he could watch TV. There was an indentation down the middle of the mattress. I laid down on it and it was comfortable; the indentation, like the mattress, was cradling me. We hadn't eaten any dinner so we sent Tom out on a run to Wendy's. After eating we took turns in the shower and bathtub and then went to bed. We were all pleasantly exhausted.

July 9, 2010
Our new room isn't as good as the other room we stayed in. The toilet paper holder was gone, just a piece of metal sticking out of the wall. Plus, the bathtub plug didn't work. What is it with all these plugs not working. I finally put a washcloth over the drain and that seemed to work. Tom got up early and went outside. The weather was beautiful. He brought back some muffins so that we could feed the ducks and geese out back. He then woke up Ben and asked him if he wanted to go to breakfast, they only serve it until 9:00. I told him to bring me a waffle right at 9:00 and I would try to eat it. I'm definitely not a morning person; it's hard for me to eat. I slept until they got back. He also brought back fresh fruit, orange juice, and coffee. I was able to eat a little. We weren't in any hurry to leave because we didn't want to get to the nursing home until after Mother ate lunch. When we did go out there was no wildlife to be seen. The hotel is sitting in a business district and the surrounding parking lots were crowded with vehicles. Usually we were there only on weekends so the lots had been empty. Today is Friday. We looked at the pond area but the greenery had grown up so much we couldn't see

anything. We left and drove to Target. I wanted to get some bug spray because we were planning on taking Mother to the cemetery and didn't know what to expect. I also got a disposable waterproof camera and a blowup beach ball for the pool.

We got to the nursing home a little after noon. The front parking lot was full so Tom just let me out in front and then went and parked around the side. I said I would call him when we were ready and he could drive around and get us. When I got to Mother's unit there were still a lot of people in the dining area. As I walked through I saw Mother leaving the area arm and arm with a nurse. It was the same nurse that I had been watching the one day when all the chair alarms were going off and she was running around sitting everyone back down. I walked up to them and the nurse said, "Oh, are you here to visit Sally?" I nodded and she turned to Mother and said, "You have a visitor." She looked up at me and I said, "Hello Mother." She let go of the nurse and put her arms around my waist. I told the nurse that I wanted to take Mother out for a while. She said, "Are you sure you want to take her? We've been having some behavior problems with her." I said, "Yes, I know, but she'll be fine with me." The nurse looked skeptical and I said I know she's been having extreme mood swings. I explained that I only get there every two months and that I wanted to take her out for a while. She said, "Oh, that's why I haven't seen you before."

She said, "Well, I gave her a bath this morning at 6:00." I was happy to know that she had been the one to bathe her. I asked her how Mother had liked that and she said that Mother had enjoyed the bath itself until she started to get out and she started shivering. I said, "And that's why she's wearing that sweatshirt, but we'll need to change it because it's hot outside. We'll also need to get her shoes on." Mother was standing there the entire time not saying a word. Then I made a mistake and accidently stepped on her toe, not hard, but she let out a howl. The nurse said, "Would you like to go out with your daughter?" Mother was pissed and said, "No!" She pulled away from us and took off. The nurse said, "We just let her walk it off." As Mother began walking down her hallway the nurse continued, "We'll catch her as she comes back around and see if she has changed her mind." We walked down the hall and met up with Mother as she was coming back down. The nurse went over to her and said, "Would you like to go with your daughter?" Mother said, "Okay."

We led Mother to her room and sat her down on the bed. All of her bedding was gone, to the laundry I guess—bath and laundry day. The mattress was covered with a dark blue vinyl fitted sheet. I thought, that looks good, it would be great for little kids. The nurse went over to the closet and started looking for a short sleeved shirt appropriate for 'going out.' I said there was a blue and white shirt that would look good. She started pulling shirts out but not the one I wanted so she just selected one. She sat down on the bed next to Mother and started to remove her sweatshirt, slowly pulling out her arm. I said, "Let me help," and I sat down on the other side of her and started pulling out her other arm. I saw that she wasn't wearing anything underneath. I said, "Does she have a bra you can put on her? We don't want her to look a little obscene when we get out." The nurse said she had tried to put a bra on her this morning but Mother had said it was too tight. She said we'd try it again. Before pulling the sweatshirt all the way off the nurse went back to the closet and looked for a bra.

All this time Mother had not said a word, just sat there quietly not looking at either one of us. Detached. I know I would have felt somewhat uncomfortable in such an intimate situation. The nurse came back with a bra and placed it on Mother then slipped off the sweatshirt and slipped on the new shirt. Mother let out a groan and I asked her if she was in pain. She said, "Yes," and the nurse, sounding a little alarmed said, "Where?" Mother said, "All over." I said, "I hurt all over too." (motel bed) The nurse quickly put on Mother's shoes. I wondered how she did that so easily because the day I did it I was really having trouble getting them on. One of Mother's toes was sticking out of her sock (toenail too long?) but the nurse didn't mention it. I asked if she thought Mother should use the bathroom first and she said she would try. She got Mother off the bed and into the bathroom explaining what she was doing. She sat Mother on the toilet, scooting her back on the seat, still explaining what she was doing. As she was doing this I pulled out my cell phone and called Tom telling him we'd be down in a few minutes. Mother sat on the toilet looking straight ahead at nothing until the nurse went back in and finished her up. The nurse got Mother off the toilet, got her pants back up, then handed her over to me. She told Mother that her bed would be all made up again by the time she got back. Mother said okay and then the nurse left the room. That nurse is so nice, she's gentle and caring; I really like her.

For the first time Mother looked directly at me and smiled. I said, "Would you like to get out of here for a while?" She said, "Oh yes." I said, "Then let's go sign you out." She said, "Okay." We entwined our arms together and started down the hallway. When we got to the visiting area one of the Jamaican men hurried up to us; Manoa, I think his name tag said. I said I was going to take her out and asked him where I was supposed to sign her out. I already knew but it was easier to just ask him. He led us to the nurse's station and pulled out a sign-out book. As I started to write a black nurse in the station came over and eyed me suspiciously. She said, "Where are you taking her?" I didn't want to say I was taking her to a cemetery so I said out for a ride. She asked when we would be back and I said we'd be back by 5. She said, "Five?" Like she couldn't believe I would take her for so long. I said, "We'll be back by 5:00, in time for dinner." She said, "Are you sure? We've been having some behavior problems with her." I said, "She'll be fine with me." She said that was the wrong book and she got a different one out. There were only five entries in the book and David's name caught my eye at the top. He had checked her out last December and took her to his house. It was sad that in over six months only five people from that unit had gotten out. The nurse asked me who I was and I told her and I said that my brother, David, will probably meet up with us. As I was signing the book she was over at her desk quickly looking through a binder. I'm sure she was looking to see if my name was in there and that it was okay to take Mother.

As we walked away form the nurse's station I looked at Mother and said, "Let's skip this joint." She smiled and said, "Yes." When we got close to the door I told her to wait as I punched in the code so she wouldn't set off the alarm with her bracelet. I opened the door and said, "Let's go." As we passed through the door the alarm went off anyway but we kept on going without a glance back. We walked through the first hallway quickly—I know Mother was going as fast as she could. When we got on the bridge I slowed down somewhat and I could see her relax. And her nose started dripping. I said, "Your nose is dripping." She said, "I know," and laughed. I said, "Well, when we get outside I'll get you a tissue." She said okay. But then I saw drops actually falling to the floor. There is a bathroom at the end of the bridge so when we got there I told her we'd better get a tissue now. I turned on the light and stepped inside, Mother right behind me. I looked around but didn't see any tissue so I tore off a small piece of toilet paper and then wiped Mother's nose. She said, "That feels better." As we got on the elevator I told her that Tom was waiting for us downstairs. She said, "Tom?" She always says that. I don't know if the name is familiar to her or if she just wonders who the man Tom is. I said, "Ben is here also, my grandson, your great-grandson. You remember Ben don't you?" "Oh, yes." She doesn't of course, how could she, they'd only met once a few years ago and Ben doesn't even remember her. That just shows her pat answer whenever someone asks if she remembers something.

I signed out at the front desk saying that I had signed Mother out upstairs. We made our way through the front doors; they are so heavy, I had a little trouble getting it open then holding it open as I maneuvered Mother through them. But we finally got out. I thought Tom would be parked right in front of the entrance, but he wasn't. I saw him and Ben sitting in the grass nearby in their chairs. They jumped up as soon as I came out and we all walked over to the truck. I opened the back door just as Tom walked up. He said hello to Mother and they gave each other a big hug. I do think she remembers him. I said that I was going to get in first so that I could pull Mother in. She said laughing, "You're going to pull me in?" I said, "Yes, and Tom is going to push." And that's what we did. It wasn't easy. We got her on the seat but had some trouble getting her legs in. We finally got them in and I got her buckled up.

I said, "Before we leave I want to call David and tell him we're taking her and get directions to the cemetery." I pulled out my cell and called him. I said, "David, we're at the nursing home and we have Mother out in the truck with us." He said, "You do?" I said, "Yes, we want to take her to the cemetery." He said, "Do you know how to get there?" I said, "No, that's why I called you." He started giving me directions and I tried to remember everything—down Lake Street, past Lake Calhoun, past so many stop lights, and then at the big intersection (but I don't remember the name of the road he said) it's right there. I asked, "What time are you getting off work? Maybe you could meet us out there." He hesitated and then said no, he wouldn't do that but he was getting off about 2:00 and could be at the nursing home about 2:30. I said we wouldn't be there. He said, you won't? I said, no, we won't be back that soon. It was then just after 12:30. He said, "Then I'll just see you at the house later."

Mother looked so calm as we drove along. She looked out the window and dozed a little. As we made our way to Lake Street we could see Minneapolis ahead of us. There was a lot of traffic. We drove past Lake Calhoun and it brought up some childhood memories, the grassy areas next to the beach especially. I said, "This is where Mother would take us swimming," and I turned to her and said, "remember?" She smiled and said yes. We went past the lake and then couldn't make out David's directions. Tom said, "I remember this area now, are you sure David said to turn right? And which intersection?" At that point Tom let his internal compass take over. He turned left and we knew right away that was wrong. There were a lot of young people around there. The college was nearby. There was a girl jogging and Tom rolled down his window and she came over, removing her small headphones. Tom asked her if she had ever heard of Lakewood Cemetery. She said no, then after a moment she said there was a cemetery but she didn't know the name of it. She said we would have to go back to Lake Street then go down to Hennepin and turn right. We followed her directions and there it was.

Lakewood is a huge cemetery. Tom said, "Now where do we go?" I said, "David said it was on the west side of the lake." We found our way to the lake and determined which the west side was. After that it was just a matter of looking for the graves. David had said to look for a green urn that was off by itself. The graves have flat headstones so I got out and walked up to the green urns by themselves and read the names on the stones. It didn't take too long before I found them. The graves were right out in the sun but there was a big tree nearby right next to the road. I got Mother out of the truck. As she stood up it was like her knees were giving out and I had to give her a moment to steady herself and stand up straight. Tom got the chairs out and set them up in the shade. I walked Mother over and placed her in one of the chairs. She landed with a big sigh. She really does act like she's in pain. I still think it's the osteoporosis that they're not treating. But how can she walk so much when she's in pain? Maybe it feels better after walking.

I had brought along a small white teddy bear for Ben to give to Mother so I got that out and handed it to him explaining that he was to give it to her. I had my camera ready. He gave it to her without a word. The ever talkative boy was suddenly completely silent. I said, "Ben has brought a bear for you." Mother's face lit up as she took the bear and she started stroking it. I got the two of them together for my camera. It may be the last time they will be together. Ben placed his chair near Mother's but there was no talking from either of them. That's okay. I know that even though he doesn't remember his last visit with her he will remember this one.

I asked Mother if she would like to walk over and look at the flowers in the urn but she said no. I had wanted to show her the graves; I was hoping being there would stir up some kind of memories. I walked over to the urn David and Dorothy had planted. The flowers were really beautiful, but they were not the ones I had bought on the last trip. A few of the ones I had bought were there along the bottom edge but in the top were different ones. I was a little disappointed but had to agree that these looked better—and expensive. Unfortunately I'm not in a position right now to buy anything expensive. I went back and sat next to Mother. There was a nice breeze and it was blowing through Mother's hair. Her hair has gotten longer and is a little shaggy looking. I noticed she had a couple of dry flakey spots on her face. She looked so peaceful sitting there. Next to me Tom said, "She's really happy." I said I wanted to write down the dates on the headstones and went to the truck and got out some paper. Mother's parents and grandparents are buried there; two on either side of the urn. Her grandfather, Louis, was born in 1875 and died in 1933. I wondered how he had died, he was my age now. Mother's grandmother, Olive, was born in 1881 and died in 1958. I wondered if I had ever met her. I don't remember if I did. I also wondered what she had done after her husband had died; how she had survived daily life. Mother's daddy was born in 1898 and died in 1981. Her mother was born in 1901 and died in 1983. Mother is now older than all of them had been when they died.

I went to the truck and fixed a bowl of cookies and blueberries and gave them to Mother. She seemed pleased and touched them but didn't eat anything. I noticed that she was wearing bright red nail polish; her nails looked good, recently manicured. The rest of us ate some cookies. Mother looked kind of zoned out, just enjoying being there. The place had changed since we had been there last. At that time we were able to walk right down to the edge of the lake but now there is greenery growing all around it. I had wanted to take Mother to the edge but not when we'd have to wade through the plants. I asked Tom if he wanted to take Ben down to the lake and they left. There were several

Hispanic men working in the area, watering the plants, etc. They were speaking to each other in Spanish. At one point I saw a couple of them look at Mother then say something to each other and then start laughing, some comment about her being there soon herself. People can be cruel, and they don't realize that their voices carry in an open area, and that a lot of people can speak Spanish. But nothing was going to disturb Mother.

Chelsey was out of the truck of course. Tom had put her on the ground and she had walked over to Mother's chair and was watching the men from underneath. When the men left the area Chelsey took off. I was going to let her wander a little but she was going pretty fast so I had to go get her. I put her back and a minute later she took off again in the same direction. It looked like she was heading for a large standing headstone. I guess she was looking for a place to burrow. I brought her back again and put her on the chair with me. She wasn't going for that however, so I got a little blanket out of the truck and put her back under Mother's chair and placed the blanket over her. That settled her down. Mother and I didn't feel the need to talk. The weather was just right under the shade tree. Tom and Ben came back and said there had been a lot of mosquitos by the lake. Of course, mosquitos love lakes. There was a water spigot so I got a cup out of the truck and watered the flowers in the urn. Pretty soon Tom said we needed to leave so we could beat rush hour. I asked Mother if she was ready to go and she said no. Tom and I looked at each other thinking, oh oh. We packed up everything else then went back to her and said it was time to go. She said okay.

As I led Mother over to the truck I told Tom that it would be easier for her to ride in the front seat instead of the back. It was, so much easier, she just slid onto the seat then I pushed her legs in. I tried to hold the bowl of cookies and blueberries (which she had not touched) while she got in but she wouldn't let go of it. She had placed the teddy bear in the bowl also so that she would have at least one hand free. Once in she set the bowl on her lap then started straightening her pants. They were a dark blue stretchy material. She started tugging them into place although they already looked all right to me. She finally stopped and I strapped her in and got into the back seat with Ben. It was about 3:00. It was such a successful outing. It didn't go exactly as I had planned (but what ever does?) but it was good. It was so nice to see her out of the nursing home, so nice to see her enjoying herself, so nice to see her smiling. We'll have to do this again; maybe not the cemetery but somewhere just as nice. Maybe even Lake Calhoun. The parking lot is really close to the lake that it wouldn't take much of a walk. Tom had suggested going to Minnehaha Falls (for Ben) but I said Mother wouldn't be able to walk very far; still, it's something to think about.

Driving back to the nursing home Tom kept a conversation going with Mother, and, she was keeping up her end. It was like she was completely normal! How does she do that? Tom pulled up to the front entrance and I started getting Mother out. She finally let me hold the bowl. Once out it was like her legs gave out again and I gave her a moment to steady herself. We entered the building and I signed back in and we headed for the elevator. I pointed to the railing and told her to hold on. She laughed then turned to face the wall and held onto the railing with both hands. We made our way through the other unit and around the corner to the bridge. We walked hand in hand; I was still holding the bowl. She was walking pretty slowly down the bridge and I asked her if she was tired and she said yes.

We went down her hallway and when we got to the door of her unit I let go of her hand so I could push the unlock button on the wall. The button is very large, red, and flat. I pushed then tried to open the door but it wouldn't open. That was strange; I'd never had a problem before. I pushed it again, it still wouldn't open, I pushed it again, harder, and it still wouldn't open. I said to Mother, "I need you to push this button while I try to open the door." She said okay but I could see her looking at the wall but not seeing the button. I walked over to the wall and pointed out the button, "Here, do you see it?" She said yes. I walked over to the door and said, "Now." Mother leaned on that button with both hands as hard as she could. It was funny. The door opened and I held it as I took Mother's hand again.

Inside the unit I could see two young women rushing towards us. They had seen me struggling with the door. When they reached us I said I couldn't get the door open. One of them said that it was the teleresponder on Mother's arm, if she gets too close to the door it won't unlock. I didn't know that. I guess when Mother walked over to the wall she was a safe distance away from it. The woman greeted Mother looking really surprised that she had been out. She said, "Where did you go?" I said, "We went to a cemetery." I knew she would think this was really strange so I continued, "We sat in the shade in chairs in the grass and looked at the lake." She looked at Mother and said, "Did you have a good time?" In a very serious voice Mother said, "A really good time. A really good time." We kept on moving through the area and made our way to Mother's room. I set her bowl on the nightstand and helped her sit down on the bed. I said, "Lets' slip off your shoes," and when I got them off she said, "That feels better." I said, "Would you like to lie down for a while?" She said yes and I laid her back on the bed. I kissed her and said I love you. She said, "I love you too." I said I'll see you tomorrow and she said okay. I left her room and went to the nurse's desk. There was now different people working so I told another black woman that I needed to sign Mother back in and she gave me the book. I finished then made my way out of the unit and back downstairs, stopping to sign myself back out again. Tom and Ben were sitting in their chairs again and I said, "Let's go."

We went back to the motel for a few minutes to freshen up. Ben was about to get reacquainted with his cousins who were all over at David's. On Ben's last trip to Minnesota the twins were still newborns. But then Ben said he doesn't remember that trip at all. It was 4 ½ years ago. When I was at David's last summer he had a huge blow-up pool for the kids to play in so I told Ben to bring along his swimming trunks in case they were playing in it. I called and let them know we were on our way and off we went. We stopped at the Holiday store in Osseo so Tom and I could get coffee. I was in dire need of immediate caffeine having only one cup earlier. When we got to David's house we could see Vincent in the backyard wearing his swimming suit and all wet. Ben got a little excited. I got out of the truck and just happened to be next to the living room window, which was open. I heard a small voice and looked up to see one of the twins standing there. He said he was watching a movie and then held up the DVD case for me to see. I think it was *He Man*. I was so surprised because neither of the twins had ever said a word to me before. They are extremely shy. I don't know which twin he was because I can't tell them apart. Tom told me later that when he got in the backyard one of the boys ran up to him and said hi and gave him a hug. It had to have been Vincent; he's not shy at all. It sure took a long time to break the ice with those boys. As I walked past the flower garden I saw that the lady slippers were now just brown plants.

When we got into the backyard Vincent was standing in the middle of a tiny blow-up pool. I said that I thought they might still have that big pool but David said it hadn't survived. I asked Ben if he wanted to play in the small pool and he said no. We all sat down and started talking. Ben and Alexsis were both sitting with us but neither one of them would say a word. It was kind of funny. We asked Ben if now that he was here he remembered his last time but he said no. After a while David said he had a slip-and-slide and he went and set it up. All of the kids put on their swimming gear and began playing together in the water. They may not really have been talking to each other but they were having fun.

I asked David if he was surprised when I called him and said I had Mother out in the truck with us. He said yes he was, but that the nurse had called him a few minutes earlier and said that I had taken her; wanting to make sure it was okay. He said that he remembered me saying last time that I wanted to take her to the cemetery and he figured that's where we were going. He asked if we found it okay and I said yes, but not by his directions. He said, really? I said well, at a certain point Tom said he could find it on his own. He asked if the flowers looked good and I said yes. I told him I had watered them. I asked him about his lady slippers and he said they just bloom for a couple of weeks and that's it. I told him about my conversations with the nurses, how they had questioned my taking Mother because they had been having behavior problems with her, but that I didn't have any trouble at all. When I said the nurse had given her a bath this morning David said, yes, Friday morning. I wondered about that because I know she used to get a bath on Sunday evenings. I wonder how often they change up her routines.

Ben hadn't talked to his parents since leaving Arkansas so Tom gave them a call so he could talk to them. When Ben got on the phone with Ruth he didn't say much except that he had gone swimming. Then he just sat quietly saying yes or no. When he hung up he was sitting at the table with a glum look on his face. I said, "Are you in trouble for something?" He said no. I said, "Well, you look like you're in trouble." He shook his head. Tom said, "It isn't that; he misses his mommy." I said, "Are you homesick already?" He nodded yes. He'd only been gone two days. He's so sweet.

David said a nurse had recently called and said they wanted to schedule Mother for a haircut and they would just put the charge on her monthly bill. David told her that there was already an account for that. The nurse hadn't known that and said, "She does?" Why hadn't she known? Was she a new employee? And I'm surprised that they were going to set it up themselves since the family had always done that. Her hair didn't look that bad. David also talked about how he had gone up to see her one afternoon and she had been sitting in the vestibule, asleep in the chair. He had started tapping the leg of the chair with his foot and she had woken saying, "Stop that!" He had said, "What? I didn't do anything." She had said, "Yes you did." He laughed as he was telling me. Dorothy fixed everyone dinner and after talking for awhile longer we headed back to the motel.

Ben and I wanted to go back to the pool of course so we, along with Tom, got into our suits and got to the pool about 9:00. We were the only ones there again, but just for a couple of minutes when two teenage boys came in and headed for the hot tub. A few other people had arrived but the pool wasn't too crowded. After a few minutes, Tom, who was standing a short distance from me said, "That little girl just threw up in the pool." I turned to look and at the same time Ben, who was standing on the pool edge yelled out, "Gross! She just puked in the water!" And he jumped in. I said, "Come on, let's go." He was pretty upset, "I don't want to go!" I said, "We have to. We can't stay in the pool now." He looked over at the girl and her Mother had gotten a towel and was trying to scoop the puke out. Ben said, "It's okay she's cleaning it up." I said, "No, she can't clean it up, we have to leave." It was disappointing and the little girl was really embarrassed and of course she got a scolding from her mother. You couldn't really blame her, though, she was only about 5 or 6 years old; I'm sure she hadn't yet received the advice on how to puke politely. When you're a kid you just puke wherever you happen to be. We went back to the room and watched TV the rest of the night.

July 10, 2010

Happy birthday TJ! We checked out of the motel about 11:30 and went back to Target so I could get Ben a Minnesota T-shirt. We had kind of looked them over yesterday but all we could find were sports related shirts; the Gophers, the Twins, the Vikings. I just wanted a Minnesota shirt, but I needed to get something. Tom said we would stop at Cabela's, in southern Minnesota, but I didn't want to risk not finding one. Tom waited in the truck and Ben and I went in. He also had a toy picked out he wanted to get. We settled on a Minnesota Twins shirt and I also got him a large activity book for on the way home.

We arrived at the nursing home about 12:30 or so. Tom and Ben stayed outside and I went up alone. I crossed through the front areas of Mother's unit and didn't see her. There are occasional smells of urine in this unit. I walked over to the vestibule and there she was. The vestibule looked smaller than I remembered. Mother was on one side, the chair up against the wall and there was a man in a wheelchair in the middle; he was asleep but Mother wasn't. She was just sitting quietly, looking out the window. I walked up to her, squatted down to her level and said, "Hi Mother." She looked at me, smiled, and said hi. It's always a relief when she greets me in that way. I gave her a hug. I glanced down at her feet and both socks had holes in them. Her left foot had four toes sticking out, and her right foot had one toe sticking out. I couldn't believe they'd put those socks on her. I said, "Look at your toes sticking out." She said, "They're not." I said, "Yes they are, look," and I ran my fingers over her bare toes. She looked down but just smiled, it didn't bother her a bit. I asked her if she'd like to walk down to her room with me and she said yes. I got her out of the chair and off we went.

I sat Mother down on the edge of her bed, noting that her roommate was in hers in what sounded like a deep sleep. The teddy bear and bowl of cookies were sitting on the nightstand. I said, "Oh, here's your teddy bear from yesterday," and she looked and said, "Isn't it cute." I said, "Do you remember getting it? Do you remember going out with me yesterday?" She said, "Oh, yes." I said, "Here's your bowl of cookies and blueberries. Would you like to eat one?" She said, "Do you want me to eat one?" I held the bowl out to her and said, "Do you want one? See the blueberries, do you want some?" She ran her fingertips over the berries like yesterday but didn't pick one up, just let her hand drop. I handed her a cookie and put the bowl back on the nightstand as she started to eat it. I took down the calendar and signed it as she was eating. When she finished it I handed her another cookie and she took that one also and started to eat it.

It was really dark in her room and I looked for a light. The only one in there was the long florescent up on the wall behind her bed. I thought it was turned off so I pulled the string and it went even darker. I pulled the string again then realized that half the tube was burned out and the other half was headed in that direction. I wondered why they had let it go so bad without replacing it and wondered how they managed without a light. Then realized they probably didn't need it—it was light out when she got up and still light out when she went to bed. A nice little payback from when she made me and Emily go to bed at 8:00 all summer long. But I wanted more light. I finally went over to the window to open some of the curtains. The roommate's wheelchair was sitting there with pieces of it all over the floor. I had to step among all the pieces to get to the window. I managed to get through it all without stepping on anything and pulled back the end of the curtain a short way. It let in only a small amount of light but it was better than nothing.

By then Mother was finished with her cookie so I headed for the closet so I could get out the Bible and photographs from my last visit. At first I couldn't get the door open and eventually I had to open the roommate's door slightly in order to get Mother's open. Looking inside I was horrified to see that the tub containing all of the cards was gone. I thought, "Oh no! Someone has stolen the tub and probably the Bible." The cards were all piled up on the shelf so I grabbed them and hurried over to the bed and started flipping through the stack and then found the Bible. I thought how strange that just the tub was gone. I was sitting next to Mother and I quickly removed all of the photos then handed the Bible to her. Once again she was very pleased with the Bible. And, once again she opened the cover and stared at the two front pages, which were black. I wasn't paying much attention, however, and said, "Can you read it?" Then I noticed she was running her fingers over the black pages. I said, "Should we get your glasses?" I opened the top drawer and got out the reading glasses and put them on her then opened the Bible to actual writing. I said, "Does that help?" She said, "Not really." I'm sure she doesn't remember how to read. I started handing her the photographs one by one. When we got to the one of her mother she ran her fingertips over her face and softly said, "She's so pretty." And that was it. None of the other photos interested her at all.

I left her for a moment to look at the pictures by herself and walked back over to the closet. I wanted to look over her socks. All of the white socks had holes in them. They were only four months old, how come they already had holes in them? On my last visit there were three pairs of colored socks in the drawer. Today there was just a pair of light blue ones. I'm assuming the others are in the laundry. The blue pair had no holes in them, so why didn't they put those on her this morning? I'm going to start bringing socks whenever I come. I just didn't think they would wear out that fast. Probably because she rarely wears her shoes, and maybe she shuffles her feet when she walks. As I turned back from the closet Mother had looked over to where I had been sitting next to her and then said, "Where did you go?" I said, "I'm right here." How strange that she didn't see me get up.

I sat back down next to Mother and asked if she'd like to look at the pictures on the calendars. She said yes, so we started going through them. "Here's David." "Yes." "He's standing in front of your house." "Yes." We went through all three calendars; the only interest I saw was when her dog was in the picture. She went back to looking at the photographs in the Bible and I went through the drawers in the nightstand. In the middle drawer was the missing tub. Her denture stuff was in it. The bottom drawer which wouldn't open before now opened. The stuff in the bottom drawer had been in the middle drawer and that stuff had been in the top drawer but now everything was back to the way it had been. Mother was being very quiet today. We started looking through all the greeting cards one by one. After a while I saw that she really wasn't interested and stopped and just sat next to her. A nurse came in and went to the closet, explaining she was getting a chart out. She retrieved some papers from both closets and then said, "Are you looking at pictures?" I smiled and said yes and then she was gone. Mother had glanced up at her but didn't say anything.

There was a radio playing next to the roommate. When I had first noticed it hip hop music was playing but now as I tuned in to it I realized that it was all types of music that was playing. Mother started tapping her fingers to the tune. She was holding a few of the photographs and she started tapping them against the Bible; tap, tap, tap. Her eyes closed and she was gone—tap, tap, tap. She wasn't asleep but in that strange state I've seen before—in a world all her own. She was smiling like she was listening to some inner dialogue. Tap, tap, tap. She chuckled and said, "Oh, Johnny Foot." I said, "Johnny Foot?" She said yes and I asked, "Who is that?" She didn't answer just kept tapping and smiling. I sat quietly next to her until she started swaying back and forth in sleep. She eventually jerked herself awake and I asked her if she wanted to lie down and take a nap. She said yes so I put all the cards in the nightstand drawer and I stuck the Bible back on the closet shelf, pushing it out of sight. I helped Mother to lie down on the bed, got her legs on, and put the pillow under her head. She smiled tiredly. I kissed her forehead and said, "I love you," she said, "I love you too." I told her I'd see her soon, she said okay. Again I said, "I love you," and she said, "Okay, bye." She was done with me. I left. I'd only been there about an hour. I made my way downstairs and outside where Tom, Ben, and Chelsey were waiting for me. I said, "Let's go."

We all climbed in, Ben in front, and quietly began our drive back towards Minneapolis and southern Minnesota. I don't think we were even out of the city before Ben fell asleep. I rested also while we drove thinking about Mother. We drove to the Cabela store in Owatonna. I don't know why Tom wanted to stop here; it's a huge sporting goods store. I was there a few years ago with Tommy and the kids and we spent a bunch of money on winter gear; but this isn't the type of store Tom and I shop in very often. Still, there's some neat stuff. As we walked through the store we saw a big display in the back that was a huge artificial mountain with various stuffed wildlife positioned around it. We went upstairs to use the bathrooms and saw a restaurant. Tom wanted to eat so we got some lunch. In the dining area the back wall was a giant fish aquarium filled with local fish. We sat next to it and Ben enjoyed watching the fish swimming back and forth. On our way out we asked a sales clerk if they had any Minnesota shirts but all they had was some University of Owatonna shirts; not what we were looking for. Good thing we got the shirt at Target. Right down the street from Cabela is a small military airport. There is a display right in front of three jets that look like they are zooming straight up in the air. We stopped and got out so we could take some pictures of Ben standing in front of the jets. It was extremely windy so we didn't stay long.

Back on the road Ben promptly went back to sleep. It was a quiet drive until we were approaching Indianola in Iowa. In the distance we could see three colorful hot air balloons floating over the road. Tom woke Ben up and I pulled out the camera. As we got nearer to them they seemed to be splitting in slightly different directions. One of them came very near us and started coming down. It looked like it was about to land in a Walgreen's parking lot that was right next to the highway. I said, "I doubt that's where they were planning on landing." Right down the road the second one was also coming down but it was a little ways from the highway, from where we were it looked as though it was about to hit the wall of a large building. We were driving through town at that point with a lot of traffic so we just watched what we could see as we passed. Continuing on down the road the third balloon was still pretty high up and was clipping along. If it was a race, that one was winning.

Tonight we are back in the Super 7 Motel in Sedalia. When Tom was checking us in he just asked for room 25, which is the same room as before. So here we are, nice and comfortable. After sleeping most of the way it still didn't take Ben very long to go to sleep. It didn't take Tom very long, and I don't think it will take me very long either. We should get home tomorrow early evening. I already miss Mother.

July 17, 2010

We had a yard sale today. I think it's been around 25 years since my last one. There's so much work involved. However, things have been piling up and we thought it would be a good way to make a little extra money. Tom got up early and got all of the stuff set up and the signs put out. It was set to start at 8:00 but I noticed he got his first customer at 7:30. I went out at 8 and of course I didn't like how he had set it up and had to rearrange everything.

Tom and I took turns going in the house because it was so hot and had so few customers that both of us didn't need to be out there. About 3:00 dark clouds moved in and it started thundering. We were ready to move at the first drop. However, with our luck, there were no warning drops and when the rain hit, it hit hard. We jumped and started rushing everything into the storage trailer. The boxes were getting soaked so we had to throw them inside and then carry everything by armloads. Chelsey was outside with us sitting on the lounge chair, snoozing under a towel. When the rain started she came out from under the towel and watched us like she couldn't believe we were making her sit in the rain. When we finally got everything under cover Tom and I were drenched. We looked like we had just taken a shower with our clothes on. I grabbed Chelsey and ran for the house. What a bust!

Mother loved yard sales. She had them all of the time. My first yard sale memory was when I was still in grade school. All of the neighbors got together and had a huge garage sale. I remember walking through it and seeing long tables all lined up loaded with stuff. Seeing it through my child eyes it was a lot bigger than my neighbor's garage actually was. Mother had asked me if I wanted to put anything in the sale. I put my baby doll in it. I don't remember what my thinking process had been but I'm sure I had decided that I was just finished with it, that I was past the point of needing it any longer. After the sale Mother came up to me and said, "Your baby doll was sold." Then she put her arms around me and held me close. It was so strange for her to do that and I thought, "She must think I'm going to cry, that I'm sorry I did that." But I didn't cry, I wasn't sad at all. That's all I remember about those garage sales, I'm sure they had one every year. I don't think Mother had one after we moved into Ken's house until after I left home. I don't know when they started, but once she started she kept having them. When we were at Rebecca's wedding reception Judy asked me about a big round coffee table that had been in her father's house, asked if I had seen it. It took me awhile just to remember the table and I told her I hadn't seen it. She said, "Sally probably sold it in one of her yard sales." She made it sound like Mother had sold off all of Ken's stuff after he died; she didn't. But when she sold the house and moved to Crosslake I'm sure she sold a lot of the furniture and stuff.

Once Mother was living in Crosslake she had a lot of yard sales. David would often help her. While cleaning out her house we came across some of her yard sale stuff, still with price tags on. Mother also loved going to yard sales. She enjoyed buying handmade items and she loved buying straight-back chairs. She bought every one that she found. It wasn't like she needed those chairs but she loved restoring them. One time she showed me a chair that was completely restored. She had sanded it, painted it, and rewoven the seat. Most of the chairs were just solid wood but that one had a cane seat. I don't know where she learned how to do it; she took numerous art classes over the years. She was definitely talented.

July 19, 2010

There was a special on TV tonight about Shirley Temple. We watched her movies a lot when we were kids. Mother once told me that when she was young a lot of people thought she was named after her, but Mother was actually older then Shirley Temple. Maybe it was the other way around. Ha!

August 1, 2010

There was an article in the paper today about the Boeing plant in Seattle (reprinted from *The Seattle Times*) that is going to be demolished. There was a ceremony last week honoring the history of Plant 2. Plant 2 was big enough to hold eight football fields. They made bomber planes during WWII. There was a fake neighborhood on the roof of the plant during the war. Houses, streets, and plants were assembled out of plywood, clapboard, chicken wire, and burlap. The theory was that if any Japanese bombers made it that far east hopefully their pilots would mistake the plant for a quiet residential neighborhood. At the ceremony was an 89-year-old woman who was one of the "Rosie the Riveter" workers. The woman said she got paid 65 cents an hour for drilling holes in B-17 wing panels. There were also two B-17 WWII bomber pilots who spoke.

Mother was a senior in high school when WWII was declared. She worked in a war plant as a draftsman, which she had learned to do at one of her other jobs during high school. She had always had a job after school. I bet she loved that kind of work. After the war Mother worked at the telephone company as a draftsman tracer (not that I know what that is).

August 7, 2010

Ben and TJ are spending a week with us. Today we took them, along with Kelley and Zakary, to Mid America Science Museum. This year's theme is dinosaurs. They have things like a giant dinosaur skeleton. There were also numerous video games. To play you sit in a seat facing a large screen. You "become" the dinosaur and use the controls to traverse through the environment. The goal is to stay alive. To keep the game (and yourself) powered you have to do certain things like eat, drink, and poop. Along the way you learn different facts about your particular dinosaur. Zakary and Ben really liked the games; especially Ben, I had trouble getting him off.

We all had a lot of fun at the museum. I took Mother there one time. I don't remember how long ago it was but I know the boys were still pretty young. I'm not sure who was on the trip with her; but I think maybe it was Amy and Patrick. I don't remember what the theme was that year but I do remember there was a huge cast iron pig. I loved getting Mother to do different things so I said, "Mother, climb on that pig and I'll take your picture." She climbed right on that pig's back. It was so funny. The museum also has a Tesla machine. It's a huge metal ball; you stand next to it and put your hand on it. A man then touches the ball with some type of metal rod and the person with their hand on the ball gets some kind of energy that makes their hair stand straight up. "Mother, go up there." She did. I still have the photographs someplace; she had a big smile on her face. I always had a lot of fun with her.

August 12, 2010

I keep thinking about Lake Calhoun, probably because it's 100° here. Funny, when David was giving me the directions to the cemetery it didn't stir one memory. It wasn't until we were driving past the lake that it dawned on me that Mother used to bring us there. I remembered the big parking lot very close to the lake and the big sandy beach. But on either side of the beach, stretching around the lake was grass and in some places trees. It was the grassy areas where we always went. I even remember the water; it was very shallow at the shoreline, very clear, and numerous small pebbles. The memories are very relaxing.

I think this would be a good place to take Mother. We could set up our chairs in the grass and even bring an umbrella if we needed it. Mother would love to sit and watch the lake. I wonder if it would bring up memories of Crosslake for her. We'd have to check it out first, especially if there would be too much walking for her. And of course it would depend on the weather. It's something to think about anyway.

August 19, 2010

I was watching a program on the weather channel about storm disasters. They were showing a previous ice storm in Oklahoma, how trees were being split apart, and how icicles were turning into missiles. We had a huge ice storm the winter Mother was here. It was awful; extremely cold and windy. The power went off in the evening. I had just given Tom a round battery operated heater for his garage for Christmas. He set it up in the living room and we huddled around it. You don't really do very much when your power goes off because you expect it to come back on at any minute. But it didn't come back on and we just sat there in the dark. Mother finally went to bed. Our problem was keeping the iguanas warm, so Tom slept in his recliner with Buddy on his chest under a blanket, and I slept on the couch with Ruffles under the blanket. In the morning there was still no power. Tom then dragged out his generator and hooked up the refrigerator and the coffeemaker. We still had water and natural gas. Our kitchen was gas and so was the furnace, but it had an electric blower. We were able to cook but had to heat water for the dishes. We lit up a lantern in the kitchen and dug out all of the flashlights we could find. Note to self: always keep fresh batteries on hand.

It was really beautiful outside, everything encased in ice. In the backyard we had a huge pear tree and one of the branches had split from the trunk and was lying on the ground. It was so sad to see the tree like that; we had gotten it when it was just a sapling when we first bought the house. The sun came out and I have pictures of Ruffles lying on the downed limb, soaking up the warm rays. The house warmed up pretty good during the day. The iguanas took turns on top of the stove, lying across the pilot lights; one of their favorite spots. That evening Tom unplugged the refrigerator from the generator and plugged in the TV and a lamp. We were pretty bored by that time. The power didn't come back on that day but we were all able to sleep in our beds. The next day we still didn't have power. Tom took his backhoe out in the county and started clearing fallen trees that were blocking the roads. I was able to work in my office all day although no computer use. I don't know what Mother did, same as every other day I guess. In the evening, after dinner, Tom said, "Should we plug in the refrigerator or the TV?" Mother spoke right up, "The TV!" I said, "No, we have to keep the refrigerator plugged in." Another dark, boring night, and the next day the power finally came back on.

August 25, 2010

David had made copies of some of Mother's papers and sent them to me. Looking through them I found a chart she had made. She had told me about this chart the last time I visited her in Crosslake before she went down. She said that Linda was working on a college project and asked for her help. She wanted her to make up a chart on the highs and lows of her life. I asked Mother if I could see the chart, thinking that I may need to defend myself in some way. Mother said no, no one could see it until after she died. That made me think even more that I might need to defend myself in some way, but what could I do? Granted, she's not dead yet, but I looked at the chart anyway. Not to worry, none of my bad behavior was included.

The chart is really interesting. It starts by saying she had a very happy childhood, and then goes all the way through her life until she was 66 years old in 1992. She wrote about how in Junior High her father went to Alaska as the purchasing agent for the work on the Alaskan Highway. She had been talking about that during that last visit and was showing me the photographs of him in the deep snow, wearing a heavy, fur-lined parka. There were also photos of bears in the distance. It had been a difficult time for the family he had left behind to fend for themselves. Grandma had been horrified to discover that her husband had left a stack of unpaid bills behind without telling her. She went to business school and then got a job.

While in the 12th grade Mother noted a low point saying, the war is on. That was the same year she met Daddy, at work she said. The next year she said that her mother moved to Chicago, leaving her with no home. There was a high point when the war ended. The next high points were when she and Daddy got married and the children started being born. The chart goes up and down from there. One amusing point started out as a high point when she married her third husband, Bob, then she went back and added a notation saying that had been a false high point.

After the chart it looks like she just started writing about her life, everything she could remember; and she had an incredible memory at that time. I have to assume this was in 1992 because that's where the chart ended. She wrote about every house she had lived in while growing up, describing her bedrooms, and even the complete addresses. She even remembered the names of their neighbors. She wrote about every school she had attended (they moved around a lot), including the full names of her classmates. She wrote about how she loved taking dance lessons. She remembered the teacher's name, the address of the dance studio, and her classmates' names. She even wrote about the recitals and the dresses they wore. There are old black-and-white photographs somewhere of a dance recital; she was wearing leotards and was holding big balloons. She described this recital saying they had silver balloons fastened around the waist.

August 31, 2010

I keep thinking about a photograph I found of Mother sitting in the canoe. She had the biggest smile on her face. We all spent so much time in that canoe, as a family and as individuals. It was good for getting a little time alone. Even I could take it out by myself. I remember the entire family climbing in, taking along a picnic basket, paddling across the lake(s), and finding a neat spot to have lunch.

One year Emily and I were in the canoe with Grandpa. They didn't spend much time in Crosslake so it was always a treat to be with Grandma and Grandpa. This particular day the three of us were in the canoe and we had paddled out to the island. The water was very calm that day and we were just kind of floating very close to the shoreline. I looked out at the lake and was surprised to see a small airplane skimming across the water. It was the first time I'd seen a water plane and it was coming directly at us. Grandpa hadn't said a word and I quickly looked at him. He was watching the plane with a calm, happy look on his face. I knew then that we weren't in any danger and I turned back to watch the plane. It skimmed across the water a ways then lifted up into the air. It was exciting.

Another time Grandma and Grandpa took us kids to the nearby town of Emily. When we arrived at the town sign Grandpa pulled over and made Emily stand in front of the sign so he could take her picture. She and I were still in grade school at the time. We went on into the town and there was a large black bear in a huge cage. Back then we often saw wild animals in cages on public view. Sometime before that we saw a bear that would drink bottles of soda pop. I don't think it was in Crosslake but somewhere nearby. I remember it standing (chained?) in front of a store and when there was a crowd of people someone would hand the bear a bottle and he would drink it. Being a small child at the time I was amazed. So, back in the town of Emily, Grandpa parked the car and told us kids to go stand in front of the cage. We lined up in front and looked at Grandpa's camera. Suddenly that big black bear reached his paw out through the bars and scratched the back of my leg with his long claws. It scared the hell out of me, of course, and I started screaming. Grandpa said, "Stop crying so I can take the picture." I sucked it up and afterwards Grandma wiped the blood off my leg with a tissue. I was able to bury that memory for many years until I got interested in Native American studies then the memory came flooding back in. And, of course, I was kind of wishing those claws had left a scar—that would be pretty neat. "How'd you get that scar?" "I was attacked by a bear; how'd you get your scar?" I began looking for that photograph but still haven't found it, although I did find one of the soda pop drinking bear.

One more Grandpa in Crosslake story. Emily and I sunburned very easily, usually the first day. I have had some nasty burns during my life. So, this particular summer Emily and I were past the sunburn and on to the peeling. We were peeling badly, all over. We were in the cabin, in the spare bedroom, each of us laying on one of the beds. We started pulling our dead skin off and naturally it turned into a competition to see who could pull off the most. We each had a growing pile of dead skin on the floor between the beds. We were laughing and having a good time. Then

Grandpa came in and freaked. He thundered at us, "What are you doing?" We were startled to say the least, then he yelled, "Get outside!" We jumped up, grabbed our pile of dead skin and took off running. We never did figure out why he was so mad. Did he think we were going to leave the mess on the floor? We weren't. He was mad at us quite often now that I think about it. It was like he just didn't want to see us during the day. Too bad. He never really got to know any of us. Their visits to us from Florida weren't very often.

September 1, 2010
I fixed fish for dinner tonight. I hate cooking fish; I'm a bad fish eater. I know that it's really healthy, but I just have trouble eating it. It's strange because I grew up eating fish and didn't have any trouble with it. Maybe it's different when you catch the fish yourself. We did a lot of fishing of course. I was actually pretty good at it. We kids had bamboo poles. I had no problem putting a worm on the hook. I couldn't catch anything big with that pole but I pulled in my share of perch and sunfish. I could take the fish off the hook myself also. Daddy taught me the technique of not getting my hands sliced up by the gills or teeth.

Mother and Daddy were always big on fishing. I remember one year they loaded up the canoe and went all the way up to Canada. It was supposed to be a fishing trip but there was a photograph of Mother sitting on a huge rock in her swimming suit so maybe it was a 'get away from the kids' trip. That's the only trip I remember Mother taking away from us. Daddy went on trips often with his friends; fishing and hunting. However, Mother fished in Crosslake all of the time. She had a fishing license every year until she went down. In winter men would come and put their fishing houses out on the ice. She'd let them park their trucks in her driveway and they'd give her fish in return.

One summer, while Mother was married to Bob(2), Tom and I went up for a visit. Bob was all excited and wanted to have a fish fry with his fresh catch. He said, "I'll clean the fish." He had a table outside to prepare the fish and he started giving Mother orders—get me this, get me that. After Mother did all of the work, except the actual cutting of the fish, she was so mad and said to us, "He wants to clean the fish but I do all the work! It would have been easier if I just did everything." When we started eating I didn't like it at all. It was overcooked, dry and crisp, and still had bones in it. As a child we always ate around the bones but by then it was just too much work. I was constantly pulling bones out of my mouth. There's nothing worse than getting a fish bone stuck in your gums or between your teeth.

September 10, 2010

I came across an article today, written by Emily Main for Rodale, on a possible cancer link detected for popular osteoporosis medications. The article says that osteoporosis can hit a third of women between the ages of 45 and 60, when menopause and a drop in hormones lead to a rapid loss of bone mass. But the drugs being used to treat the condition are coming under increasing scrutiny for possibly triggering esophageal cancer.

The medications in question belong to a class called bisphosphonates, which includes brand names like Fosamax, Actonel, Reclast, and Boniva. As far back as 1994, these medications were suspected of causing cancers in the esophagus, and a study published in the *New England Journal of Medicine* in January 2009 added to the evidence. This month, a study in the *British Medical Journal* has found that the cancer risk could be particularly high among women who take the drugs for three years or longer.

Of course doctors don't want people who are taking these medications to panic. One doctor was quoted as saying, "Esophageal cancer is uncommon, and overall, relatively few people would be expected to develop the cancer as a result of using bisphosphonates, even if the risk we found is confirmed." That said, there is mounting evidence that the drugs can cause long-term harm. They don't know why bisphosphonates trigger esophageal cancer, they do know that these drugs are liable to irritate the esophagus, and that chronic irritation/inflammation has been linked to esophageal cancer. And all forms of the drug seem equally at fault.

The article stated that the study didn't look at whether patients are taking the drugs properly, which could influence the likelihood that someone could develop cancer. The medicine has to be taken first thing in the morning with a full glass of water, at least 30 minutes to one hour before eating or drinking anything. They can't lie down for at least 30 minutes to one hour after taking them, and not until after they eat something. The doctor here put Mother on Fosamax. She hated taking it and I really felt for her. To have to drink a large glass of water first thing in the morning would be hard enough, then have to sit straight up for at least half an hour. At first she had to take a pill every morning but as time went on she was able to get some that she only had to take once a month.

Prevention, of course, is always better. After Mother retired to Crosslake her doctor there told her she needed to increase her calcium intake. He told her to just take Tums every day, "That's all my wife does." I thought that was strange, how much calcium could be in Tums. Mother developed osteoporosis, I wonder if the doctor's wife did also. For years we were all told to take calcium supplements, the more the better. Now there's some evidence that calcium supplements may increase the risk of heart attacks. Just eat healthy they say, lots of leafy greens, low-fat dairy, and fatty fish.

September 16, 2010

David called me tonight. I said, "Are you wondering when we're coming, because it's September?" He said, "Yeah." That's something that's been on my mind a lot also. I didn't tell David that business has been so bad this year that I've been out looking for a job and if I get the one I'm hoping for I'll be working weekends through October. Jobs have been far between all year until the heat of August hit and then Tom finally started working steadily. But we're now so far in debt that I need something else. I told David, "Well, Tom's finally been working and there's a motorcycle race this weekend." (It's kind of funny how Tom can always find the money for motorcycle racing.) David said, "And it'll be a last minute trip." "Yes, always the last minute." I explained there are two races this month and last weekend was Trevor's birthday and then the month is almost over but I'm hoping to come in the next few weeks. Of course I was thinking, "Where is that money going to come from?"

David said the nursing home is putting together memory books for all of the residents and asked him to provide photographs and names, etc. And then every so often they'll sit down with the resident and the book and see if there are any memories. My first thought was that they had stolen my idea after seeing me showing Mother pictures. But, that's selfish of me. The truth is that any interaction with the residents would be good. However, there's still the thought that if they do that too often then Mother won't want to look at pictures with me. I told David how outside of the other wing they had big displays of those resident's photographs doing fun stuff but nothing like that for Mother's wing. David has seen the displays of course. I asked him if he thought they'd leave the memory books in the resident's room and he said no, they probably wouldn't because then they'd have people all over walking off with them. I'd like to see it when it's finished. David said he had about 25 photographs and he had to write all the names on the backs and then take them up there tomorrow after work.

He also said the nursing home had called him recently and said they had taken some pictures of Mother and they wanted to use one in the monthly newsletter. They needed his permission. The next time he's there he'll have to sign a release. I said he'd have to get a bunch of copies. I didn't even know they have a monthly newsletter. I wonder if they mail them to the families. I'll have to ask him.

We talked about the weather. David said he thought it got up to 67° today. Wow. We've been having record high heat this year. It's been in the high 90s here and has been for quite a while. I'm not complaining though, I'm afraid if it stops being hot we'll instantly be in winter. I don't want that yet. David said they've had a lot of rain this year. We've had hardly any. He said the nursing home had put in a small patio outside the far door of Mother's unit. I'm not sure where that is; I'm only familiar with one door. He said the area is all fenced in and has chairs. I said that's good, now they can go outside when they want to. He said no, you have to put in a code first to open the door. He took Mother outside one day when it was about 75 degrees. There was a man out there at the same time and after about 30 minutes he got up and went back inside and Mother got up also and said, "It's time to go in." David asked if she was sure she didn't want to stay out longer but she said, "No, it's time to go inside." That's surprising; you'd think it would be just the opposite, maybe there wasn't anything to look at out there and she got bored or itchy feet and needed to walk. I wonder how often she does get to go out.

September 19, 2010

There was an article in the paper (*USA Weekend*) today, written by Jean Carper, entitled "Stay Sharp." It started with, "Did you know that 25% of us have the Alzheimer's gene?" The article says that millions of Americans without a genetic susceptibility develop Alzheimer's, and many with the genes do not. Gary Small, M.D., director of the UCLA Center on Aging said that the idea that Alzheimer's is entirely genetic and unpreventable is perhaps the greatest misconception about the disease. Researchers now know that Alzheimer's, like heart disease and cancer, develops over decades and can be easily influenced by lifestyle factors including cholesterol, blood pressure, obesity, depression, education, nutrition, sleep and mental, physical and social activity. There is a huge amount of research which reveals that simple things you do every day might cut your odds of losing your mind to Alzheimer's. In search of scientific ways to delay and outlive Alzheimer's and other dementias, the author, Jean Carper, tracked down thousands of studies and interviewed dozens of experts. She wrote the book, *100 Simple Things You Can Do to*

Prevent Alzheimer's and Age-Related Memory Loss. Here are 10 strategies she found the most surprising:

Coffee. Coffee is the new brain tonic. A large European study showed that drinking three to five cups of coffee a day in midlife cut Alzheimer's risk 65% in late life. Caffeine reduces dementia-causing amyloid in animal brains. Coffee also contains antioxidants.

Floss. The health of your teeth and gums help predict dementia. Research has found that having periodontal disease before 35 quadrupled the odds of dementia years later. Older people with tooth and gum disease score lower on memory and cognition tests, studies show, experts speculate that inflammation in diseased mouths migrates to the brain.

Google. Doing an online search can stimulate your aging brain even more than reading a book, MRIs prove it. Novice internet surfers, ages 55 to 78, activated key memory and learning centers in the brain after only a week of web surfing for an hour a day.

Grow new brain cells. Scientists used to think this was impossible. Now it's believed that thousands of brain cells are born daily. The trick is to keep them alive. There are several ways to do that. Aerobic exercise (such as a brisk 30-minute walk every day), strenuous mental activity, eating salmon and other fatty fish, and avoiding obesity, chronic stress, sleep deprivation, heavy drinking, and vitamin B deficiency.

Apple juice. Apple juice can push production of the "memory chemical" acetylcholine. Researchers were surprised that old mice given apple juice did better on learning and memory tests than mice that received water. The recommended amount is 16 ounces, or two to three apples a day.

Protect your head. Blows to the head, even mild ones early in life, increase the odds of dementia years later. Pro football players have 19 times the typical rate of memory-related diseases. Alzheimer's is four times more common in elderly who suffer a head injury. Accidental falls doubled an older person's odds of dementia five years later in another study.

Meditate. Brain scans show that people who meditate regularly have less cognitive decline and brain shrinkage—a classic sign of Alzheimer's—as they age. A study showed that a yoga meditation of 12 minutes a day for two months improved blood flow and cognitive functioning in seniors with memory problems.

Take vitamin D. An alarming study showed that a severe deficiency of vitamin D boosts older people's risk of cognitive impairment 394%. Most people lack vitamin D. Experts recommend a daily dose of 800 IU to 2,000 IU of vitamin D3.

Fill your brain. It's called "cognitive reserve." A rich accumulation of life experiences—education, marriage, socializing, a stimulating job, language skills, having a purpose in life, physical activity, and mentally demanding leisure activities—makes your brain better able to tolerate plaques and tangles. You can even have significant Alzheimer's pathology and no symptoms of dementia if you have high cognitive reserve.

Avoid infection. Astonishing new evidence ties Alzheimer's to cold sores, gastric ulcers, Lyme disease, pneumonia, and the flu. One researcher estimates the cold-sore herpes simplex virus is incriminated in 60% of Alzheimer's cases. The theory is that infections trigger excessive beta amyloid "gunk" that kills brain cells. Proof is still lacking but it's still best to avoid common infections.

September 28, 2010

Yesterday I sent an email to David asking how Mother was doing. I also told him that we're so broke that I had to go out and get a job and that I'll be working weekends until November. I saw they had some flooding up there and asked about that. I told him we still haven't had much rain but in the last couple of days it dropped from the 90s to the 60s. We froze our butts off yesterday because it was really windy. Today I received an email from him. He said that Mother is doing about the same. She fell down again but she didn't get hurt. They put together the memory book for everyone at the nursing home and he had brought in his pictures and filled out a questionnaire about her life. Nancy brought in some pictures also and added more information.

He said the book turned out really good. He didn't hear about any flooding in the Cities, just in southern Minnesota. He said it was too bad that I have to wait until November before we can get up there and hopefully it will be above freezing. He also said he would be hunting the first and second weekend, unless they get two deer the first weekend. He said to let him know when we'll be coming and to have a safe trip. I hate waiting, and I hate working.

October 3, 2010

Ruth's mother died this morning. It's very sad; such a loss, she was only 59. She'd been battling cancer for years. She'd gone into remission but it came back earlier this year. I wish I could give Ruth a big hug right now. It's during times like this that I find myself thinking about all of the other deaths I've experienced.

I had a strange experience when Grandma died. It was back in 1983. I had been in town and after arriving home I sat down in the kitchen. Suddenly I got so cold that I started shivering. I put on a sweater but it didn't help. No matter what I did I could not stop that shivering. I knew something bad had happened. So I sat and shivered, waiting for the phone call.

Grandma's journey with dementia wasn't nearly as long as Mother's has been. Grandma had had a history of small strokes but she seemed fine otherwise. They were living in a small apartment near Mother. One day Grandpa fell and broke his hip. He ended up in a nursing home and never walked again. Grandma was so angry about it. She was mad at the nursing home saying it was their fault for not getting him out of the chair and making him walk. He died after a couple of years.

When Grandpa first went into the nursing home Grandma had stayed in their little apartment by herself. One day (according to her) one of her stove burners stopped working. She said 'the guy' told her to turn the stove on at high power and the problem would fix itself. It didn't, of course; instead it burned out the entire stove and she was evicted. You can't blame the apartment people though; obviously she didn't need to be living alone.

I believe Grandpa in the nursing home and his death accelerated her decline into dementia. Her whole world had revolved around him. Grandma had been a writer. She wrote magazine articles on various subjects. I remember one article was on secretary etiquette. It instructed secretaries on the proper way to sit—back straight, knees together, ankles crossed, skirt pulled over the knees. That was back in the 1960s. When Grandpa retired he told her she'd have to quit writing so she could spend all of her time taking care of him. And she did! If Tom said that to me I'd laugh in his face. But, Grandma was a different generation. I don't think Mother would have done it either. She was way too independent and enjoyed her way of life too much to give it up.

Once Grandma got evicted she moved in with David and Dorothy for a while. Her journey was already in motion though and she started doing strange things like dressing in reverse order; she'd put her underclothes on the outside. When her dementia had progressed to a certain point and David and Dorothy could no longer take care of her she had to move into a nursing home.

When the phone call came that day it had been from Nancy. She said Mother had received a call from the nursing home telling her to come immediately. Mother had sat by Grandma's side as she died, although she didn't know who Mother was. She died of infected bed sores. A completely inexcusable way to die. Grandma had been a tiny, tiny woman. In the nursing home she had become so frail that one day her hip broke just by her turning over in bed. She had to have been eaten up with osteoporosis. I hope I never get that way. Grandma Ruth wasn't small like that so I'll just trade in on her genes and keep my bones padded a little.

Nancy was mad at Mother when she called me. She said that when the nursing home called Mother she had in turn called Nancy. Nancy had told her to call her as soon as she got back home. I wonder why Nancy didn't go to the nursing home also. Why didn't she meet her there. Maybe that's why Mother had called her, hoping she would. Nancy could have given Mother some support and love, a shoulder to cry on, a hug, a ride home, or just so she wouldn't have to go through her mother's death alone. But she didn't. And Mother didn't call Nancy as soon as she got home. Instead she went out and shoveled the driveway. Nancy was dumbfounded. "Shoveled the driveway! I was waiting for the phone call!" But I understood. I understood completely why Mother would want just a little time alone; to let it all sink in. Sometimes you can hang onto your control a bit longer if you just don't have to speak those words.

October 10, 2010

It is still so hot here. It was 90° today. The leaves should be turning beautiful colors; instead they are just drying up and falling off the trees. The yard is dying. The hummingbirds are all but gone; just an occasional one that makes a pit stop on its flight further south. I can't stop thinking about Mother. When someone you know loses their mother, like Ruth just did, it makes you think much more about your own. I am really missing her and it'll be next month before we'll get to go up there.

October 14, 2010

There's been a lot of talk about the State Fair lately. One year while Mother was married to Ken they went to the State Fair to watch the tractor pull. Emily and I got to go with, although they didn't invite us to the tractor pull with them. At that fair every year there was a giant pair of blue jeans extended into the air. It was a good meeting spot for families. When we arrived Emily and I had no money, of course, so Ken handed us each a five dollar bill and said see you later and they walked off. Emily and I just looked at each other for a minute. An entire day at the State Fair with only five dollars? What should we do with it? Should we eat? Should we go on a ride? Should we play a game? I don't remember exactly what we did but I know we did a lot of walking and sitting around that day. Knowing us we probably still had some of that money in our pockets at the end of the day.

October 19, 2010

I got an email from David today that says, "Here is the picture of Mom they used in an ad for North Ridge." The photograph shows Mother sitting outside on a bench with some children. I'm surprised they used this photo because Mother was sitting right up against a girl holding a little boy on her lap. Mother was looking down at the boy with a strange little smile on her face and that little boy was really crying, looking totally scared of her, terrified actually.

October 22, 2010

I have found several creepy looking spiders trying to get into the house. They are black, fuzzy looking, with a white spot on the rear. They are about an inch in circumference. Our weather has finally cooled off into the 70s so I guess the spiders are trying to get inside for the winter. I don't kill them so I either just keep them from coming inside or take them back out.

At one time, as a child, I wanted to be an entomologist. I didn't actually know the word but I knew I wanted to work with the creepy crawlers. But then I had an unpleasant experience. In the summer Mother always hung the laundry outside on the clothesline. People often talk about how fresh your laundry feels and smells from drying outside. In my own experience, however, everything is stiff as a board and smells like dust. But Mother always hung everything out; I suspect to save money. On this particular day Mother had washed my bed sheets. As I climbed into bed that night I felt something go over my foot. I picked up the covers and looked and saw a spider run across the foot of my bed. I started screaming. Mother ran in, Daddy not far behind. "What's wrong?" "There's a spider in my bed!" Mother pulled off the covers and looked and looked but the spider was gone. Granted, it was a small spider, but it was enough. My parents were probably glad my fascination with insects had ended. It hasn't though, not at all. I take numerous photographs of unique looking insects. I just don't want them to touch me. I can't even guess how many times I've jumped out of lawn chairs.

October 25, 2010

I have been feeling very crafty lately. I kind of go in streaks with it. Sometimes I just like to work with my hands; I need to create. I tried selling my crafts at my yard sales in the past but that wasn't very successful. I never had enough stuff to actually rent a booth at a craft fair but tried putting things in consignment stores; however, I had a lot of items stolen so I stopped. When Mother started selling her items at a shop in Crosslake I began mailing some of my stuff to her and they went into the shop also. I still have the inventory list of what was sent and sold. Mother's and my creative talents have always been different. She was an expert with her sewing machine; I'm doing good if I can get mine to turn on. My specialty is needlepoint.

Mother was also an artist. Her canvas paintings could hang in galleries; ships, landscapes, lighthouses, covered bridges, etc. My artwork is miniscule in comparison. I can manage a childish looking snowman and Christmas trees.

For a while Mother was putting together model ships. She'd use kits, very elaborate ones, with numerous tiny pieces that had to be glued together. The ships, when finished, were huge. She had one that was very beautiful. She was extremely proud of it and placed it on top of the television set for all to see. One day we had all gone somewhere and it was dark when we returned home. There was a lamp also on top of the television set; I reached out to turn it on and my heavy coat sleeve accidently brushed against the ship and sent it crashing to the floor. Daddy yelled at me, "That's what happens when you swing your arms around!" I hadn't been swinging my arms around but I didn't say anything, it had been my fault. As I ran to my room in tears I saw Mother, also with tears in her eyes, pick up the ship. She never did repair it, just put it in the basement. She and I never mentioned it, but I carried that guilt for quite a while. She'd put a lot of work in that ship.

I can't help but wonder how Mother is doing it? How is she able to turn off her creativity? How did she make it stop, or did she? Is it still flitting around the edges of her mind? Is she sewing in her dreams? Mother had numerous books on sewing and designs and notebooks full of her ideas. I'm the same way. If I wasn't able to write down my ideas and thoughts I'd go nuts. I did get Mother to sew on a button while she was here, so I knew she could still do it, but I couldn't interest her in anything else. Does Mother's inability to create add to her frustration or is her mind just empty of it all? Does she feel the need to do something with her hands? Is that what causes her restlessness?

October 28, 2010

I was looking through a box of Mother's stuff. Most of it is sewing materials, but there are also some charts she made of her living expenses, probably when she first moved to Crosslake full time. Using large graph paper she recorded every expense and all incomes. It includes every month of the year and every day of the month. Every penny she spent, down to the stamp she purchased that day. There wasn't a lot of income, mostly government checks, money from sewing, and miniscule stock royalties. She even listed the coupons she used at the grocery store. It was a major undertaking. You'd have to have a lot of time on your hands. I know that once she retired she was on a very tight budget, so I guess that was her way of knowing every little detail of her finances.

Mother kept <u>everything</u> over the years. There are grade school report cards, school pictures, handmade cards from her grandchildren, and so many journals. I didn't even know she kept journals. I can track them back to her marriage with Ken, but they may go back even farther. She saved all the letters I wrote to her when I first left home. What a flashback they bring. We even had arguments through the mail. Funny.

Still going through the box I found something folded up in a paper bag. I opened it and found something from my childhood. It was a Christmas decoration I had made while in Blue Birds. Mother was our leader for a while. We did a lot of crafts. This one was made out of a can lid. In those days we used big metal cans for storage instead of cardboards boxes. The lid is about 12 inches across. There are dried petals glued in a circular flower design and then spray-painted gold. Small, colored glass Christmas balls had been glued all over the place. When I took it out of the bag the petals were still in place but the balls had all come loose. Amazing that she had kept it. I'm going to glue the balls back on and display it for Christmas.

After Blue Birds I went on to Camp Fire Girls. We didn't earn badges, like the Girl Scouts, but wooden beads. We had a felt vest that we then sewed the beads onto and then wore the vests to our meetings. Mother taught me how to sew the beads on in flower patterns. I still have the vest somewhere with a pile of the beads I never got around to sewing on. I'm glad Mother saved those things for me.

Once I was in Camp Fire Girls I got to go to camp in the summer. There were two sessions I got to choose from. I didn't really like any of the other girls in our group so I found out which session they were all going to and then picked the other. It was refreshing really, not knowing a single person, or I should say, not a single person who knew me. I could have any personality that I wanted. Daddy drove me to the departure designation where we were loaded onto buses and drove to the camp. It was way early in the morning, still dark when we left the house. I slept the entire way. The first year after arriving Daddy gave me a look of skepticism and a little worry, wondering if I was actually going to do it. I did. Did he wait to leave until I was on the bus, and made sure the bus left with me on it? There was such a freedom being away from the house and my family; like a little respite.

The camp was on a lake of course. During the day they split us into groups determined by our swimming level. One thing Mother did not teach me was how to swim. The first year they asked me if I could swim and I said, "Oh yes, I can swim." It was just a little fib; I could swim under water like a fish, I could float on my back all day, and I could tread water; that was good enough for me. They put me in diving lessons. We dived off the dock and there was always an instructor right there with a long pole to grab on to. I loved it.

The second year they asked me if I could swim and I said, "Oh yes, I can swim." They said prove it. I couldn't. They put me in shallow water and told me to swim. No one had ever taught me the strokes. And there's something about shallow water, the bottom just calls out to you, 'come on down.' If you're in deep water your body tells you to stay on the surface, and you swim. The entire two weeks and I never could pass their swimming test. They told me that if I came back the next year I'd have to go back into that beginner class. I thought not; that plus the ten mile hike they made us go on. Camp time was over. I wonder if Mother kept all of my letters. Letter writing was mandatory. I'd like to see them. She kept everything else.

November 13, 2010

Our temperature dropped 25 degrees overnight. All week it had been sunny and in the 70s. Chelsey and I sat outside every afternoon. About midnight it started raining. It wasn't a hard rain, just enough to bring winter to our door. At least we didn't get snow like Minnesota. Everyone's in the deer woods this weekend; including Kelley. She's been hunting for years, she loves it. She takes after her mama. Trisha has been hunting for a long time with her father and brother. When I was growing up women didn't deer hunt. Never once did I hear of a woman hunting. Daddy did teach us how to shoot. One time in Crosslake he set up some targets and then showed us how to use a rifle. I liked shooting but not enough to pursue it.

During the first hunting weekend, a few weeks ago, we were up at Tommy's for dinner when everyone came out of the woods. They were all so excited, especially Kelley, talking about their day and the deer they had seen. Zakary has also started going occasionally. It made me think of the deer Daddy had hanging in the garage one time when I was a kid. I was curious but a little horrified of the death.

All this talk about deer hunting reminded me about David's first deer hunting trip when he got lost in the woods. David and Daddy were having a really rocky relationship at the time. David was in his early teens. Years later Mother talked to me about how she had hoped the trip would improve their relationship. When they got back home Mother asked Daddy what he and David had talked about (on the trip) and he said, "Nothing." She said you mean the whole trip up there and back and you two didn't talk at all? He said that's how it was.

November 14, 2010

We were watching the weather channel this morning and David, in Maple Grove, received 12 inches of snow. Crystal, on the other side of Mother, received 8 inches. What a difference in amounts for the two cities so close together. In Crystal they were having a big bicycle race. The video was so funny, it was snowing so hard we could barely see the riders. I wonder how Mother is liking the snow. We're planning on going up there sometime in the next week, depending on how much work Tom has. Yesterday we had new tires put on the truck.

November 17, 2010

I thought we were leaving for Minnesota in the morning. I told Tom last night that I needed to make our motel reservation as soon as I could. But, he came home for lunch and said, "It won't be tomorrow." Maybe the next day— Friday. He had a bunch of excuses then ended it with, "…this way you'll be the only one mad at me." I love being at the bottom of his totem pole.

While Tom was eating lunch there was a program on TV and they were talking about how hard it is to be a parent nowadays. One woman was saying she had to make several trips to her children's school every day. I laughed and said, "When we were kids our parents just rushed us out the door in the morning and said see you after school. There were no trips to the school—no one drove us there in the morning or picked us up in the afternoon." The woman also talked about how they were so busy that they never had time to eat dinner together. I said, "We ate dinner together every night."

There's a winter "clipper" moving across the country today. There's a nice sleet storm in Kansas City. Tom said, "I hope that's not coming our way." I said, "Yup, it is." We'll see what happens with that.

November 18, 2010

Tom went off to work this morning then called me at 9:00 and said, "Let's go to Minnesota." I said, "Today?" He said the rain we had last night saturated his job site and it would have to dry out before he could do any more work. I didn't have even one thing packed because I was expecting to leave tomorrow. I called LaQuinta and made a reservation for tomorrow night then began packing. At least I had all the laundry done so I just had to get things in the suitcases and gather snacks and Chelsey's things. This is a strange time of year for traveling. It was in the 50s at home but got steadily colder as we moved north. So we started out in shirt sleeves, then we moved to light jackets, and tomorrow we'll switch to winter jackets. We had to stop in town at the bank and finally left town at 2:00.

We had an uneventful drive through Arkansas. There were hardly any colorful autumn trees because our warm weather lasted so long. When we stopped for gas I called David. I said, "Guess what, we're in your driveway!" He said, "You are? I'm in western Minnesota." I told him we were really in northern Arkansas and would get in tomorrow afternoon some time. He said he'd be getting back in town early tomorrow afternoon. He is going to stop and see Mother on his way home but I'm sure he'll get there way before us. I told him I'd call when we get to the motel.

It got dark about 5:00. That's so hard to get used to. There was so much traffic everywhere. Tom drove all the way to Chillicothe then stopped at the motel that used to be the

Best Western, then the Best Inn and now has the new EconoLodge sign up. I watched as he went in. The office has a big glass picture window on the side and you can see everything that goes on. A man had arrived the same time we did and he rushed inside. Tom held back and let the man check in (he had a reservation) and got himself a cup of coffee. When the man left Tom approached the woman working. She was young, in her 20s, and had really long blond hair. They seemed to be talking forever but he finally came out. Getting back in the truck he said, "Nope, too high." He said that he had been trying to negotiate the 60 dollars we'd been paying and she wouldn't go for it. She finally had said that they do have 60 dollar rooms but they were all full; all the other rooms were $71. The parking lot wasn't even half full. It was already about 11:00 but Tom said he was energized and unless I just needed to stop now that he wanted to keep driving. I said, "Go for it." I was wide awake also although my back was getting sore. But I knew that the longer we drove tonight the less we'll have to drive tomorrow.

So now we're in Indianola at the Apple Tree Inn. We haven't been here for awhile because I'd been having trouble with the excessive amounts of bleach and chlorine they use. But, it was going on 1:00 and I was very ready to stop. Surprisingly, it's not too bad in here; they've reduced the amounts. Either people were complaining or they're trying to save money. Whatever, it's a lot nicer. Since we were paying cash for the room we had to pay a $50 deposit. They've mentioned it before but never made us actually pay it. Their explanation has been because young people come in and party and do damage. Tonight we had to pay. Chelsey has been bathed and fed and she and Tom are cuddled together in bed asleep. Now I can take my shower and get to bed.

November 19, 2010
This morning after having coffee and loading the truck it was after 10:00. It was so cold out it was unbelievable. The wind was blowing extremely hard making it even worse. I said, "Let's hurry up and ger out of this state." We hit the

interstate in Des Moines and made really good time. I can't smoke at any of the rest stops in Iowa so we just bypassed all of them and then stopped at the first Minnesota rest area. Standing outside in the sun wasn't too bad. The wind had died down and even though there was about 6 inches of snow on the ground the sun felt good. Continuing on we stopped at a Wendy's for lunch before hitting the traffic in Minneapolis.

Driving so late last night really paid off and we got to the nursing home around 3:30. I left Tom and Chelsey to their own resources and made my way up to Mother's unit. As soon as I went through the door I saw her sitting there. She was sitting in the middle of the common area in a chair with her back to me. I was impressed that I recognized her from the back of her head; which was bowed, obviously asleep. Just to make sure I circled around the front of her and then sat down in a chair that was right next to her. I said, "Mother," and she instantly opened her eyes and smiled at me. She wasn't very talkative however, so we watched the activity around us. Mother was wearing a light blue, long sleeve, button up shirt that had little purple and yellow flowers on it. I don't remember seeing it before although it was old; the collar was frayed and it was coming apart at the seams.

She was also wearing her dark green stretch pants and white socks with a big hole in the toe. I said, "Where are your shoes?" She said, "On my feet." I said, "Really, show me." She lifted her legs straight out so she could see her feet. I said, "No shoes, just a big hole in your sock." There was a woman I'd never seen before walking around the area very rapidly, in a nervous like way. She kept pulling on her orange and white striped sweater. She had on gray stretch pants and like Mother she wasn't wearing shoes and had a big hole in her sock. She went over to a table and tried moving the chairs, then went over to the doors and looked out in the hallway. Suddenly she came over to me and said, "Hey, come on and let's go." I looked at her but didn't really say anything. She said, "Come on and let's go!" I mumbled something and she said, "We'll go tomorrow." I said, "Yes, we'll go tomorrow." She started stroking the top of my head and was looking at me with a puzzled look on her face, like maybe she was trying to recognize me.

I asked Mother the standard questions – how are you, are you eating, are you sleeping, etc. There was a young woman interacting with the residents. She pushed a woman in a wheelchair around the area a couple of times. She was wearing a blue knit top and khaki pants—one of the activity people. There was another young woman in the dining area wearing the same outfit. I had never seen either one of them before. Some of the same residents were doing the same things as always. The one woman was pushing around a walker that had two naked baby dolls. The one woman was chanting, "help me, help me." And the first young woman would reach out to them – "what are your babies' names?" "How can I help you?" Very caring. It makes me think of young social workers; they're so enthusiastic in the beginning, out to help people, to make a difference. Then they burn out quickly when they realize they've just been going around in circles, doing the same things over and over without changing anything. The activity girl pushed a woman in a wheelchair into the area very fast and went around the area, like she was giving her a ride. I said, "She's going for a ride." Mother smiled, nodded her head and said yes. I have seen her before. That time she was also pushing the woman across the entire unit and when she got it going fast she'd step up on the back of the chair and go gliding.

One by one the residents arrived, being pushed by a nurse and then placed at the edge of the room. The first was a woman in a high backed wheelchair. I've learned that these are called rolling bed chairs. Her legs were stretched out in front of her with a soft medical boot on her left leg. She was awake and very vocal. She kept yelling out a word. I thought she was saying "Live," but after a while I realized she was saying "Five." She would just yell it out. Her head shook slightly constantly. She had pure white hair and a tanned looking face. She looked very dignified and I could tell she had been very beautiful. I felt sorry for her family—having to visit their loved one in such a bad shape; at least I can sit and interact with my mother. Soon after another woman was wheeled out and placed next to the first. She was also in a high backed chair with her legs stretched out. After awhile the young activity girl (for lack of a better term) moved tables in front of the women. It's interesting how they do that. They don't move the resident to the table they move the table to the resident. They were getting set up for dinner. Once the second woman's table was set up the girl started asking her questions. I couldn't really hear them but Mother thought she was talking to her and Mother was answering. They were kind of behind Mother so she couldn't see them. But the girl would ask something and then Mother would say something like, "No." Then the girl would ask something else and Mother would say something like, "I don't know." I leaned over to Mother and said, "She's not talking to you." The girl asked another question and Mother started getting upset and said something like, "I don't know!" I leaned over to her again and said louder, "Mother, she's not talking to you." She said, "Oh," and got quiet. Mother had her eyes closed the entire time so even if she could have seen her she wouldn't have. The one woman came back over to me and said, "Come on let's go!" I said, "We'll go tomorrow." She said okay and then started stroking the back of my hair.

Mother's nose started dripping and she wiped it off with her shirt sleeve. I asked her if she wanted me to go get her a tissue and she said okay. I took off for her room hoping Mother wouldn't get up and leave because I left my purse sitting under the chair. But I knew that the activity girl would probably keep an eye on it. In Mother's room I was going to sign her calendar but it was gone. I opened her drawers but no calendar anywhere. The other two calendars were gone also. Her dentures were also gone although the empty case was there. I looked quickly in the closet and the things weren't in there either. Mother's roommate was gone. That side of the room was completely empty. I wonder what happened to her. I grabbed a tissue and headed back to Mother. She hadn't moved; she was probably too tired to move, she kept dozing off. I handed the tissue to Mother but instead of wiping her nose with it she laid it on her leg and started smoothing it out. She worked and worked on it trying to get it in a perfect square. She stopped at one point and started pulling at her pant leg. She pulled on the side all the way down the leg as far as she could reach. I watched her, amused, because her eyes were closed again, wondering what was going through her mind. When she finished with her pant leg she went back to straightening the tissue. She pulled and patted until she had it just the way she wanted it to be. I see some of this compulsiveness in me. Just recently Tom and I were working in Tommy's booster club concession stand and there was one deep fryer I couldn't use because it was sitting on the counter really crooked. When Tom straightened it out for me I was able to use it. Stupid, I know, but I can't stand things being out of place that bad. I would have had to stand sideways in order to use it. When Mother got the tissue just right she smiled and said, "There, now it's done." I said, "It's okay now?" and she said, "Yes." Her eyes were still closed.

The other activity woman was in the dining area, which was really full, there were women sitting at all of the tables. I didn't see any men. The activity woman had a television set in the middle of the area that had a computer program on it. She was actually trying to teach the women how to use a computer. That must be frustrating I thought. Some of the women had magazines. They were all off to my side so I wasn't paying much attention but I could hear snippets of conversation—like the chanting woman and one time the activity woman said, "Don't hit me. Remember the rules?" I was watching Mother as she dozed next to me and then I glanced up and one of the women residents was standing right next to me. I hadn't heard her come up and it really startled me to see her standing there. I jumped about a mile. The first activity girl saw it happen and she came towards me saying, "I'm sorry." I smiled at her and said, "She just startled me."

The woman was the one I had seen on a previous visit that can't lift up her head. The time I had seen her she was walking with a nurse and she had hit her. Since she can't lift up her head her hair hangs down, obscuring her face. The activity girl said to her, "Do you need to use the bathroom?" The woman started walking towards her and I saw that her hands were down in the back of her pants like maybe she was going to take them off. However, the woman said no and then walked off. The activity girl came over to me and asked if I had seen the memory book that they had made up for Mother. I said no, I hadn't seen it but that I wanted to. She said she would get it for me and walked over to a cart along the wall. I followed her over to it and she went all through the cart looking for the book. I noticed on top were some children's games, one being Ants in the Pants. After looking in the drawers and not finding the book the girl said it had been there but they have a new leader and she's changing things around. I said that was okay I'd be back tomorrow and would see it then.

Mother was still dozing and I touched her arm and said, "Are you going to sleep all day?" She smiled, opened her eyes and said no. But it wasn't long before her chin was resting on her chest again. I decided it was a good time to leave. I told Mother I'd be back tomorrow and she said okay without even opening her eyes. I got up and the activity girl said, "You're leaving?" I said, "Yes, I'll let her sleep but I'll be back tomorrow." The girl said, "She's so much fun." I said, "She is?" "Yes." I thought, wow, what's Mother been up to.

I was trying to remember the code number to get out of the unit but a woman pushing a food cart got to the door first. I held it open for her and then headed out. Downstairs I signed out and saw that I had been there nearly an hour and a half. Tom said he would probably be down in the vending area so I walked down the hall and got him and Chelsey. We drove down to the LaQuinta and checked in. After getting to our room I called David and said we were here. He asked if we were coming over and I said yes after we unload the truck and he said he was ordering pizza and it should get there the same time we do. We unloaded the truck and got Chelsey settled in amongst the pillows and blankets on the bed then headed his way. It was dark out and once again we couldn't find that simple route to David's house. I don't know what's wrong with us, we just can't find it. However, we at least head in the right direction and eventually find our way.

The pizza beat us by about 10 minutes so we all started eating right away and talked. David had been to visit Mother and actually left about 20 minutes before we got there. He said that when he arrived they were all watching a movie and when that ended they started another one. David always sits and watches the movie with her. Mother of course went to sleep and after about 10 minutes he had left. I said when I got there she was sitting all alone in the middle of the room asleep in her chair. I asked if that's where she had been when he left and he said yes, except all the other people had been there also watching the movie. Afterwards everyone had left the area and just left her sitting there asleep. I said there was an empty chair next to Mother and asked if that's where he had been sitting and he said yes.

Funny, when she went to sleep David was next to her and when she woke up I was next to her. David said he had gone into Mother's room to sign the calendar and it was gone, along with the pen that hangs with it. He had looked in the drawers but it wasn't there. I said I had done the same thing. He went to the nurse's desk and said that it was gone and wondered if the nurse knew what had happened to it, saying she couldn't miss it, he'd been signing his name on it all year. She didn't know but said she would look for it. I told David the other two calendars were gone also and her dentures, although the container was still there. He said who would want her dentures? I said I didn't know. It makes me a little queasy thinking about someone putting them in their mouth. I told him that tomorrow I would go through everything thoroughly. I asked if he knew what had happened to her roommate and he didn't but said he had received a letter saying she was going to get a new roommate December 11. Too bad, she'd probably be better off alone. We talked for a while longer then started to leave, making plans to meet up for breakfast in the morning. As we were getting in the truck David said, "Have a good night don't let the bed bugs bite." I said, "Yeah, I'm glad we're not in New York." He said, "They're here too."

Back at the motel we stopped in the dining area and got coffee then headed for the room. We watched television for a while, drinking our coffee then I said I was ready to go to the pool. By this time it was hot in the room. Motel rooms really heat up fast and I usually end up turning on the air for better sleeping. But I knew that I would be freezing when I got back from the pool and would welcome the heat so I left it alone. Tom didn't want to get in the pool so he just went along with me and his book. There was just one small family in the pool room when we entered; a couple and their two daughters. The females were all in the hot tub/jacuzzi and the father was in the pool. I stepped into the pool and the water was freezing cold of course. I just slowly walked the length of the pool to the deep end where the water was up to my shoulders, then dove. About this time one of the daughters jumped in. She was a teenager and she and her father started playing in the water. They were nice enough to leave me one edge of the pool so I could swim laps. Boy, I am so out of shape. I was breathing so hard in the beginning. After awhile a big group of people came in. I was surprised because it was already 9:30 and the pool closes at 10. Most of the group went to the hot tub but one couple started tiptoeing into the pool (it's cold!). Time to leave. I shivered and dripped all the way back to our room. Tom and Chelsey are now both asleep and I am feeling sleepy enough to go to bed.

November 20, 2010

What a night I had. I got in the bed and the room was so hot I couldn't go to sleep. I finally got up and turned the air on. Back in bed I was just about to go to sleep when my back started itching. I was squirming all over trying to scratch it and realized it felt like something was biting me. I thought, 'Oh no, surely there aren't any bed bugs in here.' I kept itching and finally got out of bed and quickly turned on the light. Assuring myself there were no bugs in the bed I turned off the light and got back in. The itching continued. Then I thought, 'Oh no, what if I picked up bugs last night at the other motel and now they are in my pajamas.' I got back out of bed and made my way into the bathroom, in the dark. I took off my pajama top and quickly turned on the light. No bed bugs. I went back to bed and finally went to sleep. Thanks David.

This morning after checking out of the motel we met David and Dorothy at the Lynde's Restaurant. The place was packed being Saturday morning. We had a leisurely breakfast with a lot of talking then we all left. Tom and I went to Target and did a little shopping. We don't have a Target at home but we get their sale paper and I saw that they had microwaves on sale and since ours had recently gone out I thought I would go get one. I got some pretty fresh-cut yellow flowers for Mother and then we went back to David's house because he was giving us a garden tractor to take home. After that was all loaded up we said our good-byes, see you in a couple of months. We headed for the nursing home. The parking lot was full but a man came out and motioned for us to follow him because he was leaving. That was nice and we were able to park right in the front.

Chelsey and I went in and left Tom to his own devices. We were later than usual so it was after 2:00 when I got upstairs. Entering the unit I saw everyone gathered around the television set in the large open visiting area. The activity woman from yesterday had that computer program on there again. Everyone was watching her with, what looked like, extreme attention, including Mother right in the front. I walked over and could hear the woman explaining the computer program and pointing to different graphics on the screen. She stopped talking when I approached and I said, "I'm going to steal Sally from you." Mother looked up with a smile and said, "Really?" I said,

"Yes," and held my hand out to her. "Come with me." Mother took my hand and stood up and started walking with me. The other young activity girl was right there and she said she had found Mother's memory book and she opened a cabinet and dug it out handing it to me. I took it and said we were going down to Mother's room and I would return the book when we were finished with it.

Boy, did I have an armful of stuff. I was holding Chelsey's tote bag plus the flowers, which I put in a glass soft drink bottle, and the book under my arm; my other hand was a hold of Mother's. As we walked to her room I was hoping I wouldn't drop anything. In Mother's hallway a man was standing in a spot right in the middle looking down at something on the floor. Then he walked forward a bit and bent down again looking at the floor. As we got closer I could see there was some type of circular metal plate on the floor—like a drain but surely couldn't have been a drain. I don't know what it was and I guess he didn't either but he sure was fascinated with it. He was right in the middle of the hall so when we got close I maneuvered Mother over to the wall so that we could pass. As I was doing this Mother said with a smile, "There he is." I didn't know what she was talking about of course so I just kept her moving towards her room.

Once we got into Mother's room I sat her down on the edge of her bed, then I set down Chelsey's tote bag, the flowers, and the memory book. Today Mother was wearing the blue and white top I had given her. I was surprised because it was short sleeved and it was really cold out. She was also wearing dark blue stretch pants and her shoes! I got out my camera and then handed the flowers to her saying, "Look at the flowers I brought you." She took them and said, "How pretty." She was holding them in front of her and I said, "Why don't you smell them." She said, "I did." I said, "Hold them up to your face and smell them." I moved the flowers closer to her face. Of course I was trying to get a good photo op but she was getting a little irritated so I took a couple of shots then put the camera away and put the flowers on her night stand. I took Chelsey out of her bag and held her out in front of Mother saying, "Look who came to see you. It's Chelsey." Mother made oohing sounds and I placed Chelsey on the back of the bed. Mother turned slightly so that she could see her then reached out and touched Chelsey's front leg. I watched to see what they would do and Mother kept touching the leg and finally I could see that she was pulling on it. Chelsey can be stubborn however and she was keeping a tight hold on the leg; it didn't move at all. I said, "What are you doing?" and I gently removed her hand. She said, "Well, I didn't know where he would go." I said, "She's not going anywhere. I'm going to put this blanket over her and she's going to hunker down and go to sleep." I put the baby blanket over Chelsey but instead of hunkering down she stayed at the very edge where she could look out and watch us. She stayed that way the entire time.

I grabbed the memory book and sat down next to Mother. The book wasn't what I had been expecting. I thought it would be one of those small hard-cover books that the photo stores are printing up now. But this was a loose leaf binder with a soft red vinyl cover. The pages were just computer paper with the photos scanned onto them and typed words on the bottom. Mother looked eager to start. I opened the book and the first page was a picture of Mother. On the bottom it said something like, "This is a picture of you Sally." I said, "Who is this?" Mother said with a smile, "It's me!" I said, "That's right." The next page was a picture of Ken and it said, "This is your second husband, Ken." I asked who that was but she didn't answer even though she was really looking hard at it. I said it was Ken, her husband. The next page was an old small black-and-white print of David, very young, and Daddy. I had never seen that picture before. On the bottom it said, "This is your son, David, and his father, your first husband Bob." I explained that photo then went on. There were really a lot of pictures in the book. There was one of Tom and me that is a really bad picture. We were sitting very close together on Mother's couch, still teenagers, looking at each other and smiling. It would have been a good picture except that my long hair was real thin looking and I had a really bad rash on my face. I wondered who had supplied that awful picture—David or Nancy? I said to Mother, "Here's a picture of me and Tom. I hate this picture." She said, "Why?" I said, "Well, I have that bad rash on my face. It's an ugly picture." She said, "You were never ugly." That really surprised me. She actually sounded like she remembered me and our life together. Could it be, or was she just being polite? The picture was dated December 1972, which means I was pregnant with Scott at the time.

There were a lot of pictures. Mother wearing a two piece swimming suit standing next to a lake and smiling. I had never seen her wearing a two piece—well, not that I remember. The suit was turquoise, not a bikini of course, the bottom had a pleated skirt. There were pictures of her parents and one of Mother and Aunt Laurie sitting together in front of the fireplace in Mother's cabin. There was one of David and me sitting with Mother in her apartment at the assisted living place. That was actually a good picture of me. There were a couple of Nancy, and Caroline. There were several pictures of when Scott and his family came up with me to visit Mother. The pictures were taken at David's house. The pictures were of Mother holding the twins; one at a time. They were just little babies. Mother was really smiling. Trevor and Ben were included in some of these pictures, and Alexsis. And Mother was wearing the same shirt that she was wearing yesterday! The one that I said I had never seen before. Obviously I have.

I didn't read any of the writing on the bottom except the first couple of pages. I wanted to go through the pictures my way. In the front there was also a small history of Mother's life and her family tree. I'll read all of that the next time. I was just really interested in the pictures. After we finished the memory book I pulled out the pictures I carry with me and we went through them. I had a new one that I came across since my last visit. It's an old black-and-white snapshot of us four kids standing on the backyard patio. Mother had written 1963 on the back, making me around 11, depending on the month. We were all dressed up, David even wearing a tie, so it had to be an Easter photograph. I handed the photo to Mother and said, "Do you know who these people are?" She looked real closely then she put her finger on Nancy and said, "Oh, that's..." I said, "Nancy." I knew she had recognized her but couldn't put an identity to her.

After we finished with the photos I got up and went through the drawers in Mother's nightstand and then went through the entire closet. No calendars. But I did find a large plastic bag that had all of the greeting cards. I sat back down on the bed and pulled everything out of the bag. I grabbed the Bible and handed it to Mother then we went through all of the photos I had stashed in there. The first Bible I had given her was there also. Funny how things disappear and then mysteriously reappear. I had written her name in the front of it. We started going through the greeting cards. Mother didn't seem very interested today; I had trouble keeping her attention. She kept looking out into the hallway. A black man in a wheelchair had gone past and a short time later he came back. Two men in this hallway. I wondered if they had rooms here. I forgot; the new outdoor area is at the end of that hallway.

The help me, help me, woman was in the room across the hall. The rooms are scattered so they aren't exactly across from each other. But we could hear her calling out. She kept saying a woman's name. It's always the same name that she calls out, but I can't remember what it is. After going through all of the cards I rearranged the ones on display around her bed. There's a metal strip all along the wall about mid-level and the cards are easily tucked into the top. I picked out the cards I thought were her favorites then spaced them out all around her bed. I realized that the teddy bear that had been sitting on her bed for quite awhile was now gone. When I was done I sat next to Mother again and didn't know what to do next. She usually would be dozing by now but she seemed wide awake. I said, "What would you like to do now?" She said, "I don't know, what do you want to do?" I said, "I don't know. Do you want to lie down and take a nap?" She said, "No." We sat there for a minute or so then she got up and left the room. Okay, I thought, visit's over. I packed up Chelsey and left also.

As I got into the hallway I could see Mother at the far end walking. I knew she had already forgotten me so I went the other way towards the exit. There were a lot of people sitting around. They'd be setting up for supper soon. I stopped the activity girl and gave her the memory book. She took it and walked me to the door. She's very friendly. She asked if I had read it to her as we went along and I said yes. She said that she reads it to her once or twice a day. I wondered why she did it so often, do they think she'll actually remember anything? She said she wished there were more pictures of her kids in there and I explained that I have all of Mother's photos at my house and I didn't find out in time that they were putting the memory book together and that since I live in Arkansas I only get up there every couple of months. While we were talking the girl opened the door for me and I was edging out. The woman from yesterday who kept saying, "Come on, let's go," was really watching us and finally she came closer and the alarm went off. She backed up really quick and it stopped. I finally left and told the girl I'd be back in a couple of months.

I walked down the bridge and crossed through the other unit heading for the elevator. Something was going on. The part of the unit I cross is the dining room. In the back is the food serving station. There was a line of women standing in front of it. They were all wearing their winter coats. The rest of the area was empty. That's odd, I thought. Focusing in, I could see that the one woman at the end of the line (or the front of the line) had some kind of object on her head, like a tiara maybe? I realized it was some kind of Masonic ceremony. I was in front of the elevator and I really wanted to watch this; doesn't everyone want to watch a Masonic ceremony? A nurse came by, looked at the women very briefly and then went on. I thought I'd better do the same. If the nurse had stopped and watched I would have been right by her side.

I made my way downstairs and signed out. Tom was sitting in the lobby reading his book. He had my jacket. I don't like wearing it in because then I have to carry it around. We left and were on our way. We drove a short distance to a service station where we always stop and got gas and coffee, then headed south. There was still a lot of snow on the ground and cold, but at least the wind wasn't blowing. We had a quiet ride as I filled Tom in on my visit. It got dark soon. We drove through Malta Bend. For some reason this little town really intrigues us. Tom looked down at the speedometer and said, "We are exactly half way home." That explains it, it's our halfway point and we didn't even realize it.

We got to Chillicothe and Tom just had to stop at the Best Western, Best Inn, now EconoLodge. It's like an obsession with him. He parked in the check-in spot and went inside. The spot is right in front of the first room and there was a man standing on the porch area right in front of the door. Tom had left the truck running and the headlights were on so I could see the man clearly although the lights were probably blinding him. I wondered what he was doing standing there; there were no lights on in the room or outside. At first I thought he was just smoking but he wasn't. He was probably around thirty with short dark hair. He was wearing a big olive green parka with a hood up around his neck. It was really cold out and I kept wondering what he was doing standing there. I could see Tom in the office talking with the same girl that was there the other night. She was young and pretty with long blond hair. And she was alone.

I kept watching the man and he seemed to be watching me although I'm sure he couldn't actually see me with the headlights on. Finally it looked like he was going to leave; he started forward a bit but then Tom came out of the office and the man moved back into the corner. I had my eyes on him when Tom opened the truck door, illuminating me with the dome light. The man suddenly darted out of the corner and took off really fast towards the rest of the motel, away from the office. When Tom got in the truck he said that he had gotten the girl to admit that they had recently raised all of the prices. We wouldn't be staying there any more. Back out on the road, we drove on to Carrollton and stopped at a Super 8 and got a room. And here we are. The room isn't as bad as the one we had stopped at before. But, the towels are still stained and the sheets don't fit the bed. It's like they use single bed flat sheets instead of full bed fitted sheets. Tom's side of the sheet is already off the bed. I'm going to try and keep mine on, and I'm not letting the blanket and comforter anywhere near my face.

November 21, 2010

Well, we survived the night. Tom went down to the office this morning and got us some coffee. We didn't dawdle and were soon on our way. Home was beckoning. Last night and even this morning we saw a lot of deer lying dead on the side of the road. Tom drives so careful at night. One time last night he came to a complete stop because a deer was standing next to the road. He waited until the deer crossed before starting up again. Luckily there was no other traffic. Today was clear but still cold. It was so nice to get back to Arkansas. As soon as we got in the mountains we started looking for the Rotary Ann rest area. It's always farther than we think. We're always excited to get there because it's usually our last stop before getting home. We got out and it was extremely cold and windy. But we always have to walk around a little bit. There is a big observation area looking out over a valley. We didn't stay long and continued our drive south. There was snow there in the higher elevation but as we passed through the mountains the temperature started warming up. We pulled into our driveway at 6:10 pm. It was just getting dark. As we drove towards the house we saw two deer standing in our field. They just stood there looking at us, their eyes reflected by our headlights. Welcome home.

November 30, 2010

I had been explaining to David and Dorothy my dilemma about having to buy Mother the same cards over and over because I couldn't find any new designs. They said they had a bunch of extra cards they'd never use and I could have some. They had brought out a big box and started going through it. They were the cards you get free from charities. I used to receive them also until the charities realized I wasn't going to send them any money. They gave me a big stack of cards. A lot of them are blank on the inside so I'll have to write something myself. Today a little message popped into my mind so I sent off a card to Mother that said, "This little bird has come to say, seeing you has made my day." I'll have to get my creativity flowing. I'm really missing her.

December 9, 2010

I was browsing around on the internet today - Christmas coming and all that - and I came across a really neat Scrabble board. It was an anniversary board or something in a wooden box. I'd really like to have it. I haven't played Scrabble in years. Matter of fact, the last time I played was with Mother. It was during my trip to see her just as she was beginning this journey, in 1999. I was surprised one evening when she pulled it out. I thought that I could easily win. She was already having memory problems. David had to write out her checks and show her where to sign her name. I'm a writer, words are my life. There was no way I could lose. Mother whipped my butt. I even checked the dictionary a couple of times. I made her play again of course. I won the second game. Then we had to play again—the tie breaker. She won. I was suitably humbled.

December 13, 2010

Minnesota had a major snowstorm over the weekend, nearly 2 feet of snow in some parts of the state. The roof of the Metrodome even collapsed; right before a big football game, which had to be moved to Detroit. I sent David an email saying, "Yes, David, all of us in the south are laughing at all of you in the north." Today I received this email from him. "You shouldn't laugh too loud. When you get a little snow or freezing rain you shut the whole town down until it's gone." He said they ended up with about a foot and a half of snow, the 5th biggest snowfall on record, and winter isn't even there yet. He said it is really cold now. He said he's not working on Mondays and Fridays any more, burning up some vacation time because March 1st is his last day at work. Then it's retirement time. He also said he made it to the nursing home on Friday just in time for the Christmas party. I wrote back asking, "Did you get your picture taken with Santa?"

December 15, 2010

I got an email back from David today saying, "We got our picture taken, but not with Santa this time."

December 17, 2010

Today I wrapped up Mother's Christmas presents and got everything ready to mail. I'm giving her socks. What else could she possibly need anyway? There is a pair of thick black socks and a pair of white ones. Then I included two pairs of those real fuzzy ones that are really too thick to wear with shoes. One pair is a bright orange and the other is neon green. I actually took them out of my own drawer because I never wear them. Maybe they'll have some of my energy on them that will make her feel good.

December 26, 2010

A few months ago someone gave Tom a large shop. All he had to do was get it moved here. We got up the money and paid a house-mover to get it here and set it up all nice and level on blocks. Tom has been so busy that he hasn't done anything with it except for some clearing out and cleaning. He actually destroyed my vacuum cleaner by accidently throwing away the filter. He got a new shop vac which is what we're using in the house now. He spent a lot of time out there today and got the electricity working (he'd been running an extension cord). This evening he asked me to come out and see all of his lights. It was so cold out but I stumbled my way through the dark yard to his brightly lit shop. He proudly showed me around, pointing out the lights; so and so gave me this one, so and so gave me this one…it's going to be a really nice shop for him. Sitting on the floor, leaning against the wall was a piece of pegboard. I said, "Didn't my mother give you one of those peg-boards?" He said, yes. I remember when she showed up one year with the huge board for his garage. She had hooks and everything. It was really nice. Tom said that when he tried to remove it while we were moving here the board fell apart. It was that old and worn out.

January 7, 2011

There are record snowfalls going on right now, especially on the east coast. People are getting stranded in their vehicles as traffic comes to a complete standstill. I can't imagine going through that. I would have to pee right away. People are also getting stuck in airports as flights are being cancelled. Tom and I were watching all of this on the news and then Tom started flicking through the channels. One of Tom Hanks' movies was on, "Terminal," I think is its name. It's the true story of where the man gets stranded in the airport because he doesn't have the proper paperwork. I said, "You know, that's the biggest fear of anyone who travels alone. I know it's always been my biggest fear." Then I told him about what happened at the Chicago airport when Aunt Laurie died. I went up for the funeral and I was meeting Mother at the airport. My plane got in an hour earlier than hers so I had to wait for her. At the appointed time I went to her gate and when the plane landed I was eagerly awaiting her. Only Mother didn't get off the plane. I went to the service counter and told the lady my mother was supposed to be on that plane. She got on her computer and then said her plane had been delayed an hour. What a relief. An hour later Mother arrived and I told her about my anxiety when she didn't get off that plane. I said, "I don't know what I would have done if you hadn't showed up." She smiled and said, "You would have figured it out." I don't think so. Linda was waiting for us in the baggage area but I didn't know about that; Mother made all of those arrangements. There were no cell phones in those days. I didn't even have Linda's home phone number with me, not that she would have been at home to answer it.

As I was telling all of this to Tom I said, "To this day I don't know what I would have done. I guess I would have called you." And he smiled and said, "And I would have told you what to do." Since that trip I have made sure I'm better prepared. I travel loaded down with phone numbers.

January 15, 2011

I had mixed feelings about the snow when I was young. I liked playing in it but I hated being cold. Our neighborhood park was just a few houses down from us. In the summer it was the baseball field; in the winter it was flooded for a skating rink. Mother taught all of us how to skate. There is a photograph somewhere of Mother holding my and Emily's hand. We were all bundled up. Even though the photo is in black and white you can still see that our cheeks were ruddy from the cold. It was quite a job putting those skates on, getting them all laced up. Once on they weren't coming off. There was a warming house where we'd change from boots to skates. Mother was probably glad when we were old enough to go it alone. David played hockey quite often. I'd skate round and round. A lot of the time the ice was rough and that made it difficult to skate and we fell a lot. Ice is very hard. Our mittens were knit and when they got wet they were soggy and cold. I didn't like being cold so I spent a lot of time in the warming house. They sold hot chocolate in there, but, of course, I couldn't have any.

One winter a woman started giving figure skating lessons – not plain skating lessons but fancy moves on skates lessons. The lessons were on Saturday mornings, very early, like at 8:00. I told Mother and Daddy I wanted to go. I wanted to do it. They didn't really believe me because I didn't like getting up early in the morning, and I didn't like being cold. I worked on them. They were afraid I'd start the lessons but then quit, because I didn't like getting up early in the morning and I didn't like getting cold. I finally convinced (promised) them that I would get up early every Saturday morning and that I would go to every lesson.

And I did. There weren't too many other students luckily so it was very individualized. It was very cold but I had fun. I learned a lot—how to hold my leg up behind me, bent forward, arms outstretched, how to pirouette, etc. Think ice skating at the Winter Olympics and then a grade school girl just starting out.

I only attended one year though, because...I don't like being cold. The year we went up to Crosslake to help pack up Mother's house it was cold. It was October so the days weren't too bad, but the nights...One evening we all went into town for dinner. When we got back to the house I was standing at the door with Mother and David. He was digging the key out and there was a bitterly cold wind blowing. They were both hunched forward and shivering. I said, "How do you two do it?" They looked at me and David said, "Do what?" I said, "How do you stand this cold?" He said, "You get used to it." I didn't. I was out of there at 18, heading south.

January 23, 2011

I saw this article in the newspaper today, written by Malcolm Ritter for *The Associated Press*: "Love Music? Thank a substance in your brain, study says." Music makes the brain release a chemical that gives pleasure, a new study says. Researchers say the brain substance is involved both in anticipating a particularly thrilling musical moment and in feeling the rush from it. It had already been discovered that dopamine is a substance that brain cells release to communicate with each other. While dopamine usually helps us feel the pleasure of eating or having sex, it also helps produce euphoria from illegal drugs. The new study scanned people's brains as they listened to music and it showed the dopamine happening directly. Dopamine is active in particular circuits of the brain.

The study used only instrumental music, showing that voices aren't necessary to produce the dopamine response. The study used eight volunteers for the brain-scanning experiments. The volunteers were chosen because they reliably felt chills from particular moments in some favorite pieces of music. That characteristic let the experimenters study how the brain handles both anticipation and arrival of a musical rush. Results showed that even if people aren't feeling chills they are still experiencing dopamine's effects. PET scans showed the participants' brains pumped out more dopamine in a region called the striatum when listening to favorite pieces of music than hearing other pieces. MRI scans showed where and when those releases happen. Dopamine surged in one part of the striatum during the 15 seconds leading up to a thrilling moment, and a different part when that musical highlight finally arrived. The researcher said that makes sense because the area linked to anticipation connects with parts of the brain involved with making predictions and responding to the environment, while the area reacting to the peak moment itself is linked to the brain's limbic system, which is involved in emotion.

And there's your new medical trivia for today. Seriously, I'm remembering Mother, with her eyes closed, tapping her fingers and swaying from side to side. She definitely remembers that old music and is reacting when she hears it. This article is going to make me watch her more closely while this is going on. I want to see if her emotions change as the music goes along. Will I be able to see her euphoria build, will I see chills? Will I be able to determine the climax of the musical piece? I want to watch her with new eyes.

January 26, 2011

On the news today they are still talking about all of the record snowfalls people are getting this month—especially on the east coast, like New York City and Boston. Schools have even been closed. Many have lost their electricity. They also said that Minneapolis has received 55 inches of snow so far this winter. I told Tom that it will probably be March before we go up there. I said that I would love to go up there tomorrow, but realistically that's not possible. Tom is working steady but we're so behind on bills that we need to get caught up, and I really don't want to go in 55 inches of snow; not to mention the record cold temperatures. We got 6 inches of snow here; big for us, and it shut down the job for a week.

January 27, 2011

I had sent David an email yesterday asking him if Mother is liking her new roommate and he replied today saying that the last two times he has been to see her he didn't see anyone in the room, and the bed wasn't made up; which means there is no new roommate yet. He said he's going over there tomorrow.

February 9, 2011

Today is Mother's birthday. 85! I had found her a card saying Happy 85th. It wasn't very pretty, but oh well. I sure miss her. I wish we could hurry up and go visit her. But this has been one crazy winter. If we have snow it's usually very light in January. But we are expecting our 3rd snowstorm tomorrow. They're predicting anywhere from 3 to 10 inches. Tom has been working steady all winter except when everything has to shut down because of snow and freezing temperatures. Yes, we've been having record lows also.

February 14, 2011

I had sent David an email a few days ago asking him how Mother's birthday went, if he had been able to go see her and if she has a new calendar for this year yet. I also asked him if his coworkers are planning on throwing him a big retirement party. I got an email from him today. He said he hadn't gone to see Mother on her birthday but went a couple of days later and brought her a chocolate cupcake with chocolate frosting. While she was eating it she said, "Oh, that was good," after every bite. He said she is doing good. She has a new calendar and the old calendar was back also. Nancy probably took it home to look at the pictures and get this year's calendar made up. He's not getting a retirement party but his boss and a few other people will be taking him out to lunch. He said he and Dorothy are planning a trip to Tennessee for the end of summer. This afternoon David was going to the nursing home for a Valentine party.

February 15, 2011

I came across an article today by Rich Laliberte for Rodale entitled, "Walking Reduces Alzheimer's Symptoms." The article says that adults with Alzheimer's disease, or with mild cognitive impairment, have healthier brains when they walk five to six miles a week. The effect not only preserves brain matter in areas that handle memory and learning, but actually slows the progression of Alzheimer's symptoms by 50%, according to a study made. One researcher said that the speed of walking didn't matter; slow or fast—it all had the same effect. Although that much walking is not always possible, any amount of walking is better than none. I wonder how many miles Mother walks in a week. I'd love to put a pedometer on her and find out. But I don't think all that walking is improving her memory any.

February 20, 2011

Today was Ben's 9th birthday party. His birthday was a few days ago but the party was today at a roller skating rink. He was wearing the Minnesota Twins shirt that we got him during his visit to Minnesota with us last year. Being at a roller skating rink brought back so many memories from when I used to skate when I was a teenager. The rink was pretty far away but one of the local schools had a bus that would take all of us down there and pick us back up. We had a lot of fun skating but we also had fun on the bus; mostly because we smoked up a storm.

One time I was lighting up a cigarette and someone was holding a lighter for me. I bent forward, forgetting my long hair and it swung down and 'poof,' it went up in flames. I put the fire out quickly and easily but what a smell. It just so happened that Grandma and Grandpa were in town. And of course it was Grandpa and Mother who came to get us at the school, in Grandpa's car. Well, there was a bunch of us kids and with my luck I had to sit in the front between Mother and Grandpa. I knew we all reeked of cigarette smoke and I was sure they could smell my burnt hair. But neither one of them said one word about it. However, it wasn't long before the bus driver said that smoking would no longer be allowed on the bus.

Sometime later Emily and I went bowling. Of course Mother had to drive us and pick us back up. This particular night I was smoking as usual. I don't think Emily ever smoked. I actually picked it up from David. It was my turn to bowl so I put my burning cigarette in the ashtray on the scoring table. When I turned back around there was Mother! Early! I thought, oh crap, I'm in trouble. Mother saw my unease and asked what was wrong. I just looked down at the ashtray and she said, "Oh I know you smoke." I put it out immediately of course; I wasn't going to smoke in front her.

March 1, 2011

We had an alarm system installed today. It's sad that we even feel the need, but we do. There's been some crime in the area and with us out of town a lot and me spending nights alone when Tom is off to his motorcycle races I've been feeling a need for more protection. When I was growing up we didn't even lock our doors. We rarely even closed the inside door if we were just running into town somewhere. We used to always have a big glass candy dish sitting on top of the TV. It was always full of lemon drops. One day one of Emily's friends from down the street told her that while we were gone she had snuck into the house and helped herself to some candy. I know I felt pretty betrayed and I'm sure Emily did also but we never told on her. We didn't want to start any trouble.

March 3, 2011

I sent David an email the other day asking him how he liked being a man of leisure. He sent me an email today saying he was getting used to taking it easy. He said, "We are expecting another big storm next week sometime. It's been a long winter and we still have over a month to go. Early this week Mom fell down in the middle of the night and she had a bruise on her hip and some pain, and pain in her shoulder too so they had both X-rayed for breaks, luckily both came back good. I stopped over there after work and the nurse said she had been walking around like nothing happened, she just had some swelling and black and blue on her hip but no pain."

I came across an article today on the Rodale website entitled, "Are You Eating the Saltiest Foods in America?" The article is about how americans are consuming way too much salt. The author wrote: It's well known that eating too much salt is linked to heart disease, stroke, and high blood pressure. But more and more research is finding that a high-salt diet causes other serious and life-threatening diseases, including these three: Cancer, Osteoporosis, and Dementia. Other studies have found a link between high blood pressure and dementia. Since too much salt can send blood pressure skyrocketing, cutting out excess sodium could help save your brain too. Researchers have shown that treating hypertension can reduce dementia due to Alzheimer's disease by half.

March 4, 2011

Last night I wore one of the nightgowns that Mother made me many years ago. It's made out of the softest flannel—turquoise with a small print design, trimmed in white lace. On the inside of the collar is a small label with a line drawing of three ducks in a basket, and it says, "From Mom with Love." The label is hand stitched on. I don't wear the nightgown very often because I don't want to wear it out. But I have been really missing her and wearing it makes me feel closer to her.

March 8, 2011

I came across an article today by Jeffrey Rossman, PhD, for Rodale entitled, "Is Sugar Sapping Your Memory?" The article says that it has long been known that problems with short-term memory are related to age-related decreases in blood flow in a part of the brain called the hippocampus. Recently, researchers discovered that decreased blood flow to the hippocampus is related to elevated blood sugar levels. The effects can be seen even when levels of blood sugar, or glucose, are only moderately elevated. This finding may help explain normal age-related cognitive decline, since our body's ability to regulate blood glucose levels worsen with age.

Our brain's primary fuel is glucose. If our blood sugar level drops too low, we'll have trouble paying attention, learning, and remembering information. But if our sugar level is consistently too high, the body pumps out excess insulin, which causes inflammation and oxidative stress that prematurely age our brain. So, a cup of coffee with sugar and a muffin can be just the thing to get us going in the morning; it quickly gets glucose into our brain and enhances our cognitive functioning. But over the long term, consuming a large volume of sugar—foods that are quickly converted by our body into sugar—will prematurely age our brain.

Like so many other things, it's about balance. A key to healthy cognitive function as we age is maintaining good blood sugar regulation, preserving the body's ability to keep the blood sugar neither too high not too low. The primary ways to do this are through exercise and diet. A healthy diet keeps us from overdosing on sugar, and regular aerobic exercise increases insulin sensitivity, enabling the cells of our body to efficiently utilize glucose for energy. This is a big part of why we feel more energetic when we exercise regularly, plus, it means our body doesn't have to produce as much insulin to get the job done. Here are some ways we can keep our blood sugar levels balanced, overcome sugar addiction and cravings, and keep our cognition in good working order:

- Minimize intake of sugar, and of the refined carbohydrates that our body quickly converts into sugar. When it comes to carbs, stick with fruits, vegetables, and whole grains. The fiber in these foods helps our body maintain consistent blood sugar levels and reduces cravings for more carbs. Avoid highly processed carbs, found in many cakes, cookies, breads, cereals, and pasta products.
- Eat healthy carbs with protein, which further enables our body to maintain consistent blood sugar levels. Eating protein stimulates our liver to produce glucagons, which slows down the absorption of glucose and makes it available longer.
- Eat healthy fats like omega-3 fatty acids. These also help to balance our blood sugar.
- Get regular aerobic exercise. This is the main way to increase insulin sensitivity and healthy glucose metabolism. Exercise also stimulates production of

brain-derived neurotrophic factor (BDNF), a substance that promotes the growth and connectivity of new brain cells.

- Be aware of our blood glucose level. If it's creeping up as we age, we should talk with our doctor about strategies for keeping it lower. With healthy lifestyle modifications, we can prevent type 2 diabetes, and stave off its precursor, insulin resistance, while keeping our brain sharp.
- Manage stress well. Prolonged, excessive stress can damage and impair functioning of the hippocampus. Slow, rhythmic breathing exercises and meditation can help to quiet the mind, relax the body, and reduce the effects of stress.

March 17, 2011

Spring is here. Today it was sunny and in the high 70s. Chelsey and I sat outside for a few hours. The yard is full of clover. Most of the grass is green. I saw the first bright yellow dandelion a couple of days ago. There are even several patches of beautiful purple wild violets blooming. Violets always makes me think of Mother. They were her favorite plant. There was always at least one violet plant in her house.

I got an email from David today. He said they are finally getting some warm weather, in the 50s, with a little rain. He also said that Mother is still doing good, some days she's crabby but he gets her to cheer up before he leaves. David has always been good at cheering her up. It doesn't take very long before he has her smiling and laughing. He has a certain way of teasing her that just melts her heart, even when she doesn't know who he is. This has got to be so hard for him, they always had such a close relationship. My heart hurts for him.

March 26, 2011

I was hoping to be in Minnesota this weekend, but that didn't happen. Tom is on a job he can't leave. April will be very tough; there are three birthdays and Easter. Plus, Tom has to work. It's hard to get him out of town when he has work. I suppose I should tell David. Not that we have money for a trip. Everything that comes in goes directly to the bills. Our weather this week has been beautiful. Sunny and warm. I was able to take Chelsey out twice. But now the temperature is suppose to be dropping into the 50s. That's how spring is around here; warm one week, cold the next.

I sure miss Mother. Today is really cloudy and windy. There was a huge flock of grackles in the yard. They'd cover the entire yard then something would spook them and they'd all go swoosh enmasse into the air. Then they'd fly like a black cloud to a different section of land covering the ground again. Then, swoosh, up they'd go, sometimes landing in the trees. A few times some of them would gather around the feeding area and get busy eating. It was quite entertaining and Tom and I watched them for quite a while, going from window to window. I love that part of spring.

April 7, 2011

In the newspaper today was an article by a doctor who does a question and answer section. The question was about Alzheimer's disease. I quote the doctor: the only true means of diagnosing Alzheimer's is through brain tissue samples after death, which will likely reveal twisted protein fragments within nerve cells that clog those cells, areas of dying nerve cells around protein and abnormal clusters of dead and dying nerve cells. Prior to death, a physician will base his thoughts on the results of a physical and mental examination to include testing of coordination, balance, muscle strength and tone, in-depth memory testing, asking the date, the name of the president, remembering three key words presented and more.

Now I'm confused. I thought there were actual tests that could determine Alzheimer's, like blood tests, etc. Mother never could have answered those questions such as in-depth memory testing, asking the date... How many elderly people can answer those questions? Yet, Mother was tested and found not to have Alzheimer's.

Reminds me of when the doctor here diagnosed Mother with lupus. He just asked her a bunch of questions about her health and aches and pains and then said, "She's got lupus." I asked why he thought that and he said she met 5 out of 8 criteria. I asked him what lupus is and he couldn't tell me. He just stuttered and stammered and said something about no one really knows for sure. Then he said, "You'll get it too." I wanted to say, "Excuse me? How can you just put that on me?" The doctor gave us a prescription for the aches and pains. I took Mother home and then went online and looked up lupus. Lupus is an autoimmune disease characterized by acute and chronic inflammation of various tissues of the body. Now how could I find out about it so easy and the doctor either didn't really know or wouldn't tell me. Mother's new doctor in Minnesota not only knew what it was but how to test for it and Mother doesn't have it.

The official definition from MedicineNet.com as of today is: a chronic inflammatory condition caused by an autoimmune disease. An autoimmune disease occurs when the body's tissues are attacked by its own immune system. Patients with lupus have unusual antibodies in their blood that are targeted against their own body tissues. Eleven criteria have been established for the diagnosis:

- Malar (over the cheeks of the face) "butterfly" rash
- Discoid skin rash: patchy redness that can cause scarring
- Photosensitivity: skin rash in reaction to sunlight exposure
- Mucus membrane ulcers: ulceration of the lining of the mouth, nose, or throat
- Arthritis: 2 or more swollen, tender joints of the extremities
- Pleuritis/pericarditis: inflammation of the lining tissue around the heart or lungs, usually associated with chest pain with breathing
- Kidney abnormalities: abnormal amounts of urine protein or cellular elements
- Brain irritation: manifested by seizures (convulsions) and/or psychosis

- Blood count abnormalities: low counts of white or red blood cells, or platelets
- Immunologic disorder: abnormal immune tests include anti-DNA or anti-SM (Smith) antibodies, falsely positive blood test for syphilis, anticardiolipin antibodies, lupus anticoagulant, or positive LE prep test
- Antinuclear antibody: positive ANA antibody testing

Looking at this list Mother had one of the criteria: arthritis

That's probably how they diagnosed fibromyalgia in the beginning also; what I would call a blanket label for women who are in a lot of pain and the doctors don't want to have to mess with them. Years ago I had a friend, Carolyn, whose health started going down. One of her main symptoms was a worsening overall weakness. She had a friend who was an EMT and finally called her. The woman came over and checked Carolyn's blood pressure and it was so low that the woman was surprised that Carolyn was even conscious. She took her to the hospital. The first doctor that examined her said that she had the "Menopausal Blues" and told her to go home and live with it. Carolyn refused to leave. A different doctor then took over and started running tests. Carolyn was dying of radiation poisoning from working in a poorly vented X-ray room at a veterinary clinic the year before in Arizona. The first doctor did apologize to her—small comfort.

April 19, 2011

I was watching the news on TV today and a doctor started talking about Alzheimer's disease. He said there is blood and spinal fluid tests to diagnose the disease, although there are no tests for the early stage. He said there are 3 stages.

Stage 1 – a chemical disturbance in the brain, but no outward symptoms
Stage 2 – some memory loss
Stage 3 – full blown Alzheimer's symptoms

Seems like there should be a stage in between 2 and 3 – that's when most people start seeking medical help. The doctor also said that 1 in 8 people have Alzheimer's, and that it takes decades to evolve. He said that the use of MRIs and other types of testing will lead to new and improved medication.

April 25, 2011

Imagine my surprise today when I opened the newspaper and saw an article entitled "New guidelines define pre-Alzheimer's disease." The article, written by Marilynn Marchione for *The Associated Press*, says that the first new guidelines for diagnosing Alzheimer's disease in nearly 30 years establish earlier stages of the disease, paving the way for spotting and possibly treating these conditions much sooner than they are now. The change reflects a modern view that Alzheimer's is a spectrum of mental decline, with damage that can start many years before symptoms appear. The new guidance describes three phases: early brain changes, mild cognitive impairment, and full-blown Alzheimer's.

Yet the guidelines do not advise doctors to change how they evaluate and treat patients now. Despite the hoopla about new brain scans and blood and spinal fluid tests that claim to show early signs of Alzheimer's they are not ready for prime time and should remain just tools for research. It's too soon right now to say these experimental biomarker tests will prove valid enough to be used in ordinary patient care, says Creighton Phelps, the Alzheimer's program chief at the National Institute on Aging. The article states that about 5.4 million americans and more than 26 million people worldwide have Alzheimer's, the most common form of dementia. Even before the mild cognitive impairment shows up, brain changes such as a buildup of sticky plaque or protein tangles inside nerves can suggest trouble ahead.

How can doctors tell what's going on? According to the guidelines, first, the doctors try to determine how fast symptoms are progressing and do tests to rule out an obvious cause such as a stroke or a new medication. If symptoms are gradual and progressive, doctors would likely diagnose mild cognitive impairment due to Alzheimer's. But they wouldn't know for sure without additional tests like the experimental biomarker and imaging scans rapidly being developed and researched.

One company has asked for government approval of a new type of brain scan it claims shows early signs of Alzheimer's. Other companies are working on tests for substances in blood and spinal fluid. The guidelines say these are helpful for sorting people into clinical trials or monitoring the effects of experimental drugs, but not for routine use in clinics and doctor's offices. One specialist involved in the guidelines, explained why. Unlike blood pressure tests that give fairly consistent readings regardless of what type of machine is used, the new biomarker tests are not yet standardized from one lab or location to the next. There are no agreed-upon cutoffs or levels for how much of a substance indicates impairment or Alzheimer's. There's not even enough research to validate that a particular substance or biomarker truly predicts progression of disease.

A bigger problem is what to do after impairment or dementia has been diagnosed. Current treatments do not alter the course of Alzheimer's, they just ease the symptoms. Many doctors believe drugs are being given too late, after symptoms are severe, so researchers more recently have started testing some in people with mild cognitive impairment. If you're only going to try them in people with advanced dementia, the chance of them working is not going to be that great, said one researcher. Early diagnosis is a first step, and something the Alzheimer's Association has long advocated. It allows people to anticipate what's going to happen in the future and plan their lives in ways to minimize the impact. People with the disease and their families cope better with their disease if they know what to expect.

April 27, 2011

Another birthday without Mother. I am so bummed out about not being able to see her. But Emily called this evening and that was very nice. She wished me happy birthday and asked me about the tornados that went through here two days ago. It was quite amazing. There were several tornados in our area and we watched the weatherman on TV as the tornados were tracked, watched how they hit an area, and then moved away from us. If you took a map and marked where each tornado hit it would form a near perfect circle, with us sitting right in the middle safe and sound. Like I said, amazing, although Tommy lost his electricity. He's just three miles from us. We did get heavy rain and wind but we didn't lose even a birdfeeder or birdhouse. I was telling Emily about this and told her that the storms were now hitting Mississippi and Alabama and it looks like it's going to be bad.

May 1, 2011

I'm about to go to bed but first I put on my boots and went outside. Sure enough, our entire yard is under about 5 inches of water. It's been raining almost nonstop since last night. It stopped for awhile this afternoon and Tom and I went out to the walking paths, but we couldn't go through it all because in a lot of places the water was higher than our boots. Tom has missed so much work. And it's still storming; lightning, thunder, and that incessant rain.

I was right when I told Emily the other night that the tornados heading for Mississippi and Alabama were going to be bad. They were bad all right; they were deadly bad, especially in Alabama. They were so much worse than around here. In our area a couple of communities were flattened. In Alabama entire towns were flattened! We had about five tornados, they had about ten. Our tornados were small, their tornados were huge, some a mile wide. Right now twelve people have died in Arkansas. Right now over 200 people are dead in Alabama. Over 500 people are missing. A lot of damage is in Tuscaloosa, the location where a lot of the missing people are. There's a big college there and the authorities think a lot of parents went and got their kids but didn't tell the college officials. Also, there are no cell phone towers still standing so no one can contact anyone. No electricity anywhere of course. The authorities also explained that a lot of the bodies can't be identified at the moment so they're still a part of the missing. This is supposed to be the deadliest outbreak of tornados since 1937. The pictures on TV are heartbreaking. And now all of the people (including the ones around here) are going through this new round of storms, even though there's no tornados this time.

What else happened today? Oh yeah, Osama bin Laden is dead. Amazing; everything that has occurred in the last ten years and Mother has been oblivious to all of it.

May 4, 2011

There was an article in the paper today entitled, "Sundowner's, Alzheimer's linked." The article says that Sundowner's, or sundowning, is confusion that generally occurs late in the day, although it has been known to occur during early-morning hours as well. The cause appears to be elusive and is often misunderstood.

The disorder is commonly seen in hospital or nursing-home settings where an older individual may be forced to adjust to a different setting. Or, in some cases, it can manifest following illness or surgery. Sundowner's may be temporary for some but prolonged in other instances. It is seen primarily in Alzheimer's patients, in those with Parkinson's, and with other forms of dementia. As a matter of fact, up to 25 percent of all diagnosed Alzheimer's patients have been found to exhibit sundowner's as well.

As the day progresses, a patient becomes fatigued and less able to deal with stress. In the case of hospital or nursing-home placement, it is likely all visitors have gone home for the day and there is less to occupy a person's mind. Perhaps medications have been administered prior to sleep. The patient who was stimulated earlier in the day has nothing to occupy his or her mind and appears increasingly forgetful and agitated. Memory loss seems greater. Blood-pressure readings may be lower. Patients may see things that aren't there or perceive things to be other than what they actually are. These visions can be extremely frightening.

Treatment might include establishing a repetitive routine that a patient can rely on. Continuity is good. Noise from the radio and television during evening hours may exacerbate agitation in some but help others. Allow the patient's sleeping area to remain lit during the night such as a nightlight. Review all medications to be assured they don't have insomnia or disrupted sleep patterns as a side effect. Anyone with sundowner's is unaware of the havoc that he or she may impose on family members and caregivers. The condition is not fatal but can be extremely difficult to deal with.

This sure sounds like Mother. The nursing home staff must be aware of sundowner's syndrome, but I wonder if they ever do anything about it, or do they just say she sure is crabby right now. Would they be able to do anything about it? It's very frustrating but think how frustrating it must be for Mother.

May 8, 2011

It's Mother's Day. Earlier last week I sent Mother a package with some new socks. The card was really funny. It was large with a picture of a monkey on the front; inside, the monkey's long arms come out of the card asking for a hug. What I wish I was doing today is bringing Mother a big bouquet of bright yellow flowers. Hopefully I'll be doing that very soon.

May 13, 2011

Today in the mail I received a cinnamon angel. I actually won it from a website called Pine Hollow Handcrafts. She gives away one every month. I wasn't really sure what to expect, but it's really cute. The angel has a round wooden head with some type of straw-like material for hair. She's wearing a flowered print dress. Her arms and legs are made out of thick cinnamon sticks. Wide red ribbon make her wings. I'm going to take her to Mother (hopefully next week). I just need to figure out how to put Mother's name on it someplace.

May 16, 2011

I came across an article today that says ruby red citrus compounds preserve brainpower. The article states that red grapefruit contains the citrus compound nobiletin as well as lycopene, the latter imbuing the fruit with its distinctive ruby hue. Studies tout the potential brain benefits of these phytochemicals, making red grapefruit a smart choice for overall health.

In one Japanese study, mice that had nobiletin mixed into their feed for four months had 56% less brain plaques (thought to be neurons). The nobiletin-fed mice were also 35% less likely to exhibit memory paralysis—the kind of brain freeze we've all experienced when we can't remember a name on the tip of our tongues. Lycopene – that other red grapefruit compound – was found to improve viability of brain cells by 38%, in one Petri dish experiment. While regular grapefruit has plenty of health perks, the red variety boasts 3,500% more vitamin A, 50% more fiber, and 60% more alpha linolenic acid (omega 3)!

Shopping list: one large bag of ruby red grapefruit.

May 19, 2011

I sent David an email last night telling him we'll probably be coming this weekend and asked him how the weather is. He replied today saying, "The weather will be in the low 70s and a small chance of rain, we'll be here."

May20, 2011

I woke up this morning to heavy rain. I thought, "Maybe we can go today instead of tomorrow. Surely Tom will be home soon." I jumped out of bed, had my coffee, and then started packing. Tom, however, didn't get home until 1:30 and he said we'll leave in the morning; as planned. Grumble, Grumble. We ran into town to the bank and did a little shopping. It's been raining off and on all day and is supposed to continue for several days. I called the LaQuinta and made a reservation. Our favorite room is no longer a smoking room. I told her we have to have a bathtub and she said she'd have to juggle things around then said okay, we're all set. The people there are really nice. I sent David an email saying we'd be getting in sometime Sunday afternoon. I'm excited. We haven't been up there since last November.

May 21, 2011

We left the house this morning a little after 10:00. I had most of the packing finished last night so I just had to get Chelsey's food together and last minute stuff. We drove through McDonalds for breakfast and headed out. They were predicting stormy weather all weekend but as we drove through Arkansas there were blue skies and big white fluffy clouds. I know that it's a bad time to travel because they're predicting really bad weather for the next few days along our entire route. But it's now or we'll have to wait quite a while, and I really need to see Mother.

We made good time all day. As we drove through Missouri we passed a lot of fields that had standing water in them. All bodies of water we passed were very high. We crossed into Iowa in the early evening. We could see dark clouds building in the distance and occasionally the flash of lightning. We were truckin' along and as Tom topped a hill there was a County Police car coming towards us. Tom said, "We just got a speeding ticket." We watched in the mirrors as the trooper turned around and came up behind us, finally turning on the red lights. Tom pulled over. He grabbed his wallet and started getting out. I said, "Don't get out! Don't you watch Cops?" He said, "It'll be alright." As soon as he got out we heard a voice from the car saying, "Get back in your vehicle sir." He climbed back in and I said, "Told ya."

It was actually a woman trooper that came up to the window. She had a smile on her face and said, "I know that you just passed through that other state where you can get out of your vehicle, but here in I. o. wa. you have to remain in your vehicle." Tom had removed his driver's license from his wallet and she said, "I'll take that now." Then she went back to her car. We sat there for a very long time before she finally came back. "Do you know why I stopped you sir?" "Absolutely, I sure do." She really was very nice, but very serious. She was probably in her 30s, with wire rimmed glasses, layered blondish hair, medium height, and somewhat stocky. I'd feel safe with her around. "In I. o. wa. all of the state highways are 55 miles per hour. You were doing 73." Crap, we're in trouble, I thought. But she said, "I'm giving you a written warning. Sign here. It's not an admission of guilt; it's just a written warning. The points on a CDL are pretty bad." Tom signed it and she gave him a copy and we were on our way—at 55 mph. It sure seemed slow. We were lucky. Tom has the squeakiest clean record ever.

We got to Indianola at 9:00 and Tom pulled into the Apple Tree Inn. The parking lot was pretty full. There were people standing inside and there was a small group of people standing outside. I was hoping if he couldn't get a smoking room that he'd at least get one on the ground floor because of the weather. As I waited it started raining a bit. When Tom finally came back he said there was a wedding and there were only two rooms left. He said he had to put it on the credit card. It was $75—higher than usual. He had tried to negotiate but wasn't successful. To pay cash he would have had to put down a $100 deposit. He said it was an elderly lady who could barely hear. We moved the truck into the parking lot then each of us grabbed an armful of stuff, including Chelsey in her tote bag. We hauled everything through all the people standing outside and in the lobby to our room. Luckily our room is a smoking room. It's also secluded from the other rooms so it's nice and quiet.

Tom told me to wait in the room and he'd get the rest of the stuff. When he came back with more stuff he was soaking wet. I looked out the window and it was really storming. That rain was coming down sideways. Tom was going to walk to the McDonalds right next door for our dinner but there was no way I was going to let him do that. He came back in with the last load and asked what I wanted. I said you can't walk over there in this rain. He said that he had moved the truck back to the front to unload it. I said okay. He left and I got Chelsey in the bath. As we ate Tom told me that a couple had entered the lobby after him and as he was unloading the woman came up to him and said they were glad they had called ahead and booked a room (they got the last one). She also said they watched him try to negotiate the price and knew he was familiar with the place. They were also but seeing that Tom was unsuccessful they didn't even try, they were just glad to get the room.

May 22, 2011

When Tom got up this morning he went outside for awhile then brought coffee from the lobby. I pulled Chelsey into bed with us as we sipped. When we finished the small cups of bad coffee Tom went to take a shower and I got out my Folgers and headed for the coffeemaker in the room. The Apple Tree Inn is the only motel we ever come across with a regular coffeemaker. I made two pots and filled our thermos and travel mugs. We packed up the truck and checked out about 10:00.

There's now a bypass around Des Moines and we got on that and it was really nice. We didn't stop at any of the Iowa nonsmoking rest areas (Tom doing the speed limit) and instead stopped at a convenience store and filled up with gas and got some lunch. The rain from last night was gone and the skies were clear.

It's always nice seeing that Minnesota sign. We stopped at a rest area just as it began to rain. Ugh. There was a big area right in front of the building that contains picnic tables and a big roof over them. The maintenance man was sitting on a table looking glum. We stood under the roof so I could smoke. It was a little chilly and the wind was really strong. When we left the rain was slacking off. All of the rest area entrances have a sign stating how far the next one is. They're all approximately 30 miles apart. I always make Tom stop at the last rest area before Minneapolis so I can smoke there and not at the nursing home. We can tell it's the last one because the sign says the next one is 60 something miles. The rest areas are really pretty and both were completely covered in bright yellow dandelions. I was pleased to see that other people were discovering the beauty of dandelions. Of course they won't look so good when they go to seed, but that's probably when they start mowing.

After leaving the last rest area we were almost immediately in Minneapolis. The traffic was horrific. Tom said, "It's 2:30 on a Sunday afternoon, what's all this traffic doing here?" Vehicles were just creeping along. After a short distance we could see four vehicles on the right shoulder with a police car right behind them—a fender bender. It was raining lightly and the roads were wet. We came to a dip in the road and it was flooded. Once we passed through the downtown area the traffic started moving normally.

We finally made it to the nursing home. There was a bus parked in front but we could see that the lot was full. Tom said he'd park around the corner. I got out and went inside. It was 3:00. A woman was in front of me signing in and arranging to have dinner with her mother. As I was signing in I could hear a radio playing. It was talking about a tornado. I asked the lady behind the desk if there had been a tornado. She was 60ish, grayish hair, wearing glasses. She didn't seem very interested and said, "Yeah, somewhere around Fridley." I didn't know where that was. As I was finishing up the radio said the tornado's activity was northwest of the metro area. I wasn't sure where we were in relation to that. I thought about going back out and telling Tom but figured he was smart enough that if it started looking bad out there he'd come inside.

I went down the hall to the bathroom but someone was in there; as I started back down the hall Tom came walking towards me. He just wanted to tell me he was now parked in front. I went up the elevator to the second floor and passed through the other area. People were playing bingo. I made my way to the other bathroom. I got in and settled and the door knob started rattling. I said, "Just a minute." It rattled again. Again I said, "Just a minute," only a little louder. I heard a woman's voice say, "Okay." I finished up and went out. There was an elderly woman facing the wall, grasping the hand rail with both hands. She said, "Sorry dear, I didn't mean to disturb you." I said that was okay and went on my way to Mother's unit.

I crossed through the front area and didn't see Mother so I headed for her room. Partway down the hall was a chair in front of the wall with Mother sitting in it asleep. I went up to her chair and squatted on the right side and said, "Mother." She didn't respond so I said it again and her head came up and she looked at me. I said, "Hi Mother." She smiled and said hello. I said, "What are you doing?" She said, "Oh...just sitting here." I said, "Just sitting there sleeping?" She said, "Yeah." I said, "Why are you sitting here?" She got kind of a puzzled look on her face and kind of said something that didn't make sense. I said, "You just saw a chair and thought you'd just sit down and take a nap?" "Yup." "Are you going to sleep all day?" "Maybe." I said, "Might as well, it's raining. I know there are days when I just feel like sleeping all day, but I'd rather do it lying in the bed, not sitting in a chair." She was still smiling at this point. She was wearing a purple sweatshirt with some silver embroidery on the top, black jeans, and the navy blue socks I had sent her, no shoes. I said, "Where's your room?" She started to point to the room right next to her but it was on the wrong side of the hallway, then pointed across from her but there was no room there, then she said, "It's around here somewhere." I said, "No it isn't, it's down there," and I pointed down the hall. I could tell that she was starting to get a little irritated.

Her mood always seems to change when I start asking her questions. But I don't know what else to do to start a conversation. And I kept on asking, "Did David come to see you today?" "David! Why would he come here?" She said it very loudly and sounded angry. I said, "To visit you." "No, he doesn't come around here." "Has Nancy been to see you?" "No." "Just me? I'm the only one who's come to visit?" "Yes." Her smiles had turned to anger—that fast. Yet I kept going. "It's been six months since I've seen you." Silence. "I couldn't come because there was about 50 inches of snow." Silence. "It was winter." Silence. "Now it's raining." Silence. "I drove all the way from Arkansas to see you." In an angry tone she said, "Arkansue?" I said, "Arkansas." "Arkansay?" "Arkansas." Silence. She definitely didn't recognize me. That's what I get for not coming for so long. "Do you know who I am?" Angrily, she said, "Of course I know who you are!"

There was a man walking up and down the hallway. He had beautiful white hair and stood ramrod straight. The first time he came by I said hello and he returned my greeting; Mother didn't even look up. David had said that they created an outdoor area where family can take the residents and I wondered if it was down this hallway. "Can you go outside down there?" I asked Mother. "Yes." "Do you like going outside?" "Oh yes, I go outside all of the time, whenever I want." "Do you want to go outside now?" "No." "I'm going to your room a minute then see if you can go out down there. I'll be right back." "Okay."

I walked down to her room and saw another name on the wall so I know she has a new roommate. The door was closed but not tight so I pushed it open a bit and peeked in. It was empty. I went inside and was surprised to see a small TV on a stand. It was on. I turned on the light next to Mother's bed and was happy to see that it finally works right. Mother's memory book was sitting open on her night-stand and the Easter card I sent her was lying on top. I signed her calendar then turned the light back off and left the room. I walked to the end of the hall but that's just an emergency exit. There are long windows along the sides but they are made out of colorful stained glass. I went back out the other way, through the sitting area, and to the other outside doors. There was the new little patio area, but only part of it had a roof over it and it was raining. I turned around and watched the birds in the enclosure for a minute then went back to Mother.

She had her head bowed again. "Are you asleep again?" She looked up but didn't say anything. She probably wished I would just go away. I wonder if this is sundowner syndrome I had just been reading about. Two aides came walking up. They looked just alike. Jamaican, early 20s, with their black hair pulled back in a curly ponytail. They were both wearing a purple flowered top and purple pants. The three of us greeted each other, smiling and saying hello. One of the girls went into the room next to where Mother was sitting and the other went down the hall. Then the girl came back out of the room slightly and said, "Shirlee Thomas? Are you Shirlee Thomas?" Mother said yes. "How are you today?" I said, "She's crabby." Mother started talking, kind of angrily, but she wasn't making any sense. It was like the gibberish of a toddler. We were both listening to her but couldn't make anything out. She seemed to be kind of struggling to make coherent words. I could feel her frustration and that was so sad. Then she said something that sounded like duck and I jumped on it. "Duck? Do you have a duck?" First she said yes then very precisely and with effort she slowly said, "No, I have a picture of a duck." "I know you do, I sent you that duck picture for Easter. I just saw it in your room. It's sitting on your memory book. Would you like to go look at your memory book?" "No." Then with some difficulty she said something like, "I always walk down there and look at that. Then I walk back. Then I walk down there and look at it again. Then I walk back. Then I walk down there again…" She added some other words that didn't make sense but I got her message that she looks at that book all the time and didn't want to look at it again right now.

Her fingernails were a pretty pink. I said, "I see you had your nails done." She said, "Yup." I said, "They're very pretty, very fancy." "I just walked down there and they do it." The girl had an amused look on her face and went back in the room. Mother was still angry and still talking, well, kind of muttering by then, when the second girl walked back up and started into the room. She said, "Are you Shirlee Thomas?" Mother just gave her a look of disgust and turned away. Like I said, the girls looked just alike and didn't she just get done asking if she was Shirlee Thomas?

Down the hall a ways three women came out of a room. One was a physical therapist and she was helping an older woman and she put a walker in front of her. The woman was wearing a light rose colored robe. There was a younger woman behind her pushing a wheelchair. They started walking our way. The therapist was telling the woman that she needs to walk up and down the hallway every day. They were walking on our side of the hallway and they were nearly upon us when the younger one said, "You'll have to go around Mother." The older woman said, "Really?" I guess she expected us to jump out of her way, but Mother hadn't moved, or even looked in their direction. The daughter said, "If you don't you'll run right into them." I smiled and said, "That might wake her up." She said, with a smile, "Nothing bothers her, huh?" They went on around us then continued down the hall.

A few minutes later Mother put her hands on the arms of her chair and raised herself up. I said, "Where are you going?" She just muttered something, went across the hall, took a hold of the rail on the wall, and started walking. I stood up also and turning around I almost bumped into the man that was walking up and down the hallway. It really startled me. I said, "Oh! I'm sorry, I almost ran over you." He was nice and kept going in the opposite direction. I quickly went to Mother and started walking next to her. When we got to her room I said, "Here's your room, are you sure you don't want to go in?" She muttered something and kept walking. I said, "Okay, I'll see you tomorrow. Bye." Without even slowing down or turning around she said, "Okay. Bye." The three women had reached the end of the hallway and were coming back, the one woman now in the wheelchair. I left the unit and made my way back to the front door. I signed out at 3:30. Tom sure was surprised to see me walking up. I said, "She is really crabby. Bad crabby. Let's go."

We drove down to the motel and as we began checking in I saw a TV. The sound was muted but I could see there was a weather report on. I asked the guy, "Was there a tornado?" He said, with obvious relief, "It's past us now." He gave us a paper to sign and as I scanned it I noticed our member number wasn't on it. Then I noticed our street name was spelled wrong again. It was the same spelling the woman had used the first time we stayed there. I asked the man if he had our member number since it wasn't on the paper. He said no, so I dug it out and handed it to him and said the address was spelled wrong. He said when he puts in the number the address would be correct. You'd think that after all of the times we've been here they'd have our address correct by now. Tom signed the paper and the man handed us the keys. Then he said that they had been booked solid last night so our room wasn't ready yet. He said he'd go check and he took off. He came right back and said she was working on it right now. Tom asked if the mosquitos were bad and he said not yet. He said sometimes they get really bad because of the pond out back, especially at night, and there are times when he actually has to put on a jacket.

Tom grabbed a luggage cart and quickly unloaded the truck. We went into the dining area to wait. I called David and told him we were at the motel and would be over in a while. I mentioned the tornado and he said it had started last night and he'd been really surprised because they had been predicting a slight chance of rain. It just took a couple of minutes and our room was ready. I was still talking to David so Tom took the cart in and unloaded it, brought it back, then picked up Chelsey in her tote bag, and took my arm and led us to our room. Room 134, the same room they told me on the phone had been converted to a nonsmoking room.

As soon as we got inside I said turn on the TV and find that weather channel. When it came on we saw that a tornado had hit north Minneapolis at 2:15, damaging six houses. If we hadn't stopped for that last cigarette break we would have been sitting on the interstate with everyone else while that tornado went over our heads. No wonder traffic was barely moving. A scary thought. I said, "Call the boys." Tom got on his phone and called Scott and said that he knew he hadn't heard about the tornado yet but he just wanted to let him know that we're safe. Then he called Tommy but he didn't answer. His phone has been messed up. He can make and receive calls but the screen is completely blank so he can't tell if he misses any calls or retrieve messages. I said we'd call him later.

We went outside for a tobacco break and walked down to the pond behind the motel. The neighborhood is a business section but all of the nearby parking lots were empty. We walked near the pond for awhile but didn't see any wildlife.

As we were heading back it started raining again; we ended up jogging the last few yards. We had entered in through the front door and instantly smelled fresh popcorn. We spotted an old-fashioned popcorn popper that looked like a glass enclosed trailer on wheels. We went over and filled two small bags, started munching immediately, and came back to the room. We scarfed down the popcorn pretty fast then loaded up Chelsey and headed for David's house.

Tom finally remembers the quick way now. Getting out of the truck I could see David's yellow lady slipper plants in full bloom. They're so pretty. The weather had cleared up nicely and the sun was out so Chelsey and I sat outside for a while. Dorothy made another delicious dinner; fried chicken and potato salad, baked potato wedges and corn on the cob. She had also made an Italian dessert which was like a cream pie (I can't remember what she called it) that had the liqueur amoretto in it. It was really good. We were just finishing when Tom's phone started ringing. It was Tommy and he was really upset. Tom handed the phone to me and I took it in the other room. He said he had just heard about the tornado and had been really worried about us and was a little mad that we hadn't called him. He said he hadn't known anything was going on until Trisha's mother had said, "You got out of Minnesota just in time." Tommy had said, why, what's going on, mom and dad are there. Trisha had just been here for a conference. I told Tommy that we had called but he didn't answer. I asked if he had gotten his phone fixed yet and he said no. I said, well, we called at 4:00. He said, 4:00? Yes. 4:00—I was out on the lake. I said that we would have called you this evening, but right now we are having dinner. He said he knew we would have called him. I guess he had panicked. I was able to calm him down. We're all just pretty wary of tornados right now.

I asked David how Mother is liking her new roommate. He said he didn't know how she liked her but that he had met her several times and that she was really nice. He had also met her daughter, and one day a man was visiting who he assumed was her son. We didn't really talk about Mother too much. I told him about my brief visit this afternoon and how

I had sent Mother socks for her birthday, that I always send socks now because she wears them out so fast. He said he and Dorothy were going through Mother's clothes the other day and her gray sweatpants had two holes in them, near the knee. He said she still has plenty of clothes, however.

About 8:00 Tom started yawning and said it was time to go. We made plans to meet for breakfast at Perkins. Back here at the motel we picked up coffee in the dining area and headed for the room. Tom climbed into bed and promptly fell asleep. I turned on the TV. There was a new Jesse Stone movie with Tom Selleck on that I wanted to watch. Tom was looking forward to it also, but he was out. I would have liked to go to the pool but I wanted to watch the movie more. I put Chelsey in bed with Tom then settled in with my coffee, and Tom's.

The movie is now long over, Chelsey has been bathed (although all of the water drained out of the tub before she was finished) and fed and back cuddled up with Tom. I'm finally getting sleepy, and of course my thoughts are on Mother, hoping our visit will be better tomorrow. I recently read a small article about how a phone call from your mom is like a good hug, the article said that when moms hug their kids it releases the "love hormone," oxytocin. A study suggested that a phone call from mom might have the same effect. (I guess that would depend on your mom, I know some moms...) While I won't be receiving any more phone calls from Mother I'm determined to get a hug from her tomorrow whether she wants to or not.

May 23, 2011

This morning Tom woke early and went outside for a walk around the pond. He came back to the room with coffee and orange juice, and then he went back for mini muffins and doughnuts. We turned on the TV and saw that a huge tornado hit Joplin, Missouri last evening. The video footage was heartbreaking. We packed up, checked out, and met up with David and Dorothy.

I checked in at the nursing home a little before noon and made my way to Mother's unit. There were still a lot of people in the dining area eating lunch. One of the male Jamaican aides came walking towards me and I said, "Hi, is Shirley Thomas still in here?" He said yes, turned slightly and pointed saying, "That's her there in the pink." I said, "Is she asleep?" He said no. I walked over. Mother was the only one sitting at the table. I squatted next to her and said, "Hi Mother." She looked at me, smiled, and said, "Well hi." She was just sitting there fingering the label on the bottom of her bib, her lunch sitting there partway eaten. I said, "Are you still eating lunch?" She said, "No." I said, "Do you want to eat some more?" "No." I looked over her food. I'd been curious about what they feed her. There was a plate of some kind of meat and bread, looking all smashed; a bowl of what looked like pureed peas; and a small plate that looked like some kind of smashed dessert. It looked like she had eaten a little of everything. On the back of the tray I could see a bowl of what looked like purple pudding. I picked it up saying, "I wonder what this is." I had Mother's interest and she said, "I don't know." I was looking it over and said, "There are little blueberries in there." "Oh, really?" I sniffed it and couldn't smell anything. I said, "I wonder what it is. Do you want some?" "Okay." I picked up a spoon and gave her a bite. Immediately two Jamaican ladies said, "No!" I looked up and they rushed to a table behind me, pulled out a chair and brought it over to me saying, "Sit here." I thanked them and sat down gratefully, getting out of that squat. I said to Mother, "Do you want some more?" She said yes eagerly. I gave her another small bite and she said, "Oh, that's so good."

A female Hispanic aide, probably late 30s, came up to the table pushing an elderly woman in a wheelchair and rolled her up to the table next to me. The woman was somewhat overweight, wearing a bright red knit hat. Someone placed a tray of food in front of her and the aide sat down in the chair on the other side of her. I kept feeding Mother the blueberry dessert and the aide tried feeding the new lady. She said, "Do you want some hotdog?" I looked at her plate and saw the same thing Mother had except it wasn't smashed, just kind of sliced throughout the length. They didn't look like the hotdogs I feed the grandkids; these were a lot bigger. The lady didn't say anything and wouldn't eat. I kept watching as the aide tried to feed her and the aide watched as I fed Mother. Then she asked me, "How old is she?" I said, "She's 85." She said, "She's small." I said, "Yes, she never passed five feet. All of us were bigger then her by the time we were teenagers." (I don't know why I said that, because Mother has always been 5'2) I asked her if Mother usually feeds herself. She said, "Yes she feeds herself. If we try to feed her something she won't let us. But if it's someone she knows she lets them. She must know you since she's letting you feed her." I smiled, looked at Mother and said, "She'd better know me, I'm her daughter!" Mother smiled and said, "I know who you are." I was glad to see that she was following the conversation.

The aide didn't have any luck getting a response from the lady. When the hotdog didn't work she said, "Do you want a peanut butter and jelly sandwich?" I looked over to see the sandwich cut in quarters. There was still no response. Mother, meanwhile, had eaten every bite of the purple stuff with blueberries. There were some drinks on the tray also; a small glass of milk, a smaller glass of apple juice, and a cup of either tea or coffee. I picked up the apple juice and handed it to Mother explaining what it was. She began drinking, holding it with both hands, and kept saying, "Oh, that's good." It was then that I saw there was a printed menu on the tray, under the drinks. I began reading. It said she was a Level 1. There was a hotdog – pureed. It actually looked like someone had finely chopped it. Also peas – pureed. And a sugar, cinnamon cookie – pureed, which looked like someone had tried to mash it up with a spoon. The purple stuff was actually yogurt! I hadn't even considered that; no wonder there wasn't any smell to it. I tried to get Mother to eat some of the other food but she said no. I asked her if she wanted some milk and she said no. I picked up the cup and sniffed it. I said, "This is either tea or coffee." She used to drink a lot of tea. She even had a collection of little, pretty, tin tea boxes. Over the years she had drank her way through them and in later years they just stood empty in a wooden rack. I think her favorite had been orange pekoe. I took a sip out of the cup and said, "It's coffee, do you want some?" She said, "No, you can have it." I took a big drink. It was actually good even though it was black. I was going to drink it all but then thought about that long walk back to the bathroom on the far side of the bridge.

All this time Mother was fingering the label sewn into the bottom of her bib. I asked if she wanted to walk down to her room and she said okay. I said let's take the bib off first. I took it from around her neck. She was really working on that label however and I had to actually pry her fingers off saying, "Let go." I finally got it away from her and put the bib on the table. I walked around her chair to help her up but she put her hands on the arms of the chair, stood up, then pretty much picked up the chair, moved it backward and stepped away from it. I took her hand and we were on our way. There were still a lot of people in the area and we had to maneuver around some of them. As we moved slowly I said, "Look out, we don't want to step on anyone." She said, "No, we don't want to do that." I couldn't tell if she was joking.

We finally got to her room and I helped her sit down on the edge of the bed. Once again she ran her fingers over the blanket and said, "Oh isn't that pretty? That's..." I said, "Teddy bears." I put Chelsey, in her tote bag, on the floor then squatted down and said, "I have something for you." I pulled out the plastic bag holding the cinnamon angel, then took it out and handed it to her. "It's an angel." Mother didn't look very impressed. "Isn't she pretty?" No comment. I took out my camera and said, "Hold up the angel and let me take your picture." She held it up a bit more and looked at it more closely. I wonder if it reminded her of her own work. I should bring some of her stuff with me next time and see if she recognized it. I said, "Isn't she pretty?" This time she said yes. I said, "Where shall we put her?" "I don't know." I looked around and saw that the only places to hang it were the calendar or the spot on the wall behind her bed; there were already a couple of things hanging from that nail but there was still some room left. I hung the angel there

then said, "Now she can watch over you while you sleep."
"Good."

I took Chelsey out of her bag and said, "Look who came to see you. It's Chelsey." Mother looked, but no comment. I put Chelsey on the back of the bed with her blanket covering her so that she could see out. She kept moving around though and I kept rearranging the blanket. She was finally still so I got Mother's memory book off the nightstand and sat down next to her. I said, "Do you want to look at this book of pictures?" "Yes." Just then I heard a thump behind me and sure enough, Chelsey had fallen off the bed. She landed on her side between the bed and the wall. I pulled her out, set her between Mother and me and covered her partway with the blanket. She settled right down. I guess she wanted to be where she could watch everything.

Last time I went through the memory book pretty fast because I wanted to see the pictures. Today I took my time reading everything out loud; except for the family tree which was large and would have been confusing for her. I changed things up a bit though as I read. They had it reading like, "I was born…I went to school…" That would only work if she was reading it herself, but I was reading it to her so I said, "You were born…you went to school…" She looked intently at every picture and listened to my every word, sometimes saying, "Oh really?" About half way through I remembered my packet of photos that I always show her was out in the truck. I learned something new. It said she attended college in Northfield. I didn't know where she had gone to college. It said her favorite subjects were math, science, history, geography, drafting, Latin, and art. But that's not true. She hated college. She told me about it one time. Her father made her attend, even though she fought him on it. At that time it was a status symbol for your children to attend college and Grandpa was big on that. He won though and off she went. She didn't get good grades, probably a C average. I bet she was tempted to flunk out but knew that would be bad in the long run. The only subject she liked was art. The other ones they had listed as her favorites were probably just all of the subjects she was taking; well, she probably liked drafting also. I waited for Mother to be finished with each picture before moving on. Her interest in the book seemed a lot more than last time. I wonder if it is stirring up some kind of memories.

I put the book back on the nightstand and took down the calendar hanging on the wall. There was a pen hanging on it so I signed my name on it then sat back down with it. I hadn't seen this particular calendar before because it was the new one Nancy had made up for Mother. I was anxious to see the pictures and we began going through them. Mother was looking at each picture intently. I explained where each picture had been taken and what everything was, trying to add a few details to each one. For example there were a couple of sunset pictures and I told her from where on her land they were each taken and then added, "Isn't that pretty?" "Yes." On her shoreline I said, "You used to go down there every evening and feed the ducks. Do you remember?" "Oh, yes," and she would smile like she was remembering. I talked about the loons and she said she remembered them. One picture was of a young Caroline out on the dock and Mother's black lab in the lake swimming. I said, "Oh, there's Caroline; and look, there's your dog, Cindy, do you remember how much your dog loved to swim?" She smiled and said yes. There was one of Mother standing in the yard and I said, "There's you!" She said yes. Usually she wouldn't even look at a picture of herself but I could see that she was really studying it.

Mother was pretty much holding the calendar and I was flipping the pages even though I had to slide each page from under her fingers. After going through the entire calendar I noticed that she had her fingers firmly between two pages. I waited a moment then she slowly flipped the pages to that spot. The picture she had turned to was of her log house; just a small section of it. Near the house was a long wooden planter on legs. In the winter she used this planter as a deer feeder. But now it was full of beautiful, colored blooming flowers. I stayed quiet as she looked at the picture. We sat there for so long that I thought she had fallen asleep. But she didn't; she was just looking down at the picture. I took this time to study her. She was wearing a pink sweatshirt that had some embroidery on the top front area. I was surprised because it was quite warm outside. She had on some light blue jeans. I hadn't seen them before so maybe they're new. They looked really big on her, especially in the hips and legs. She was also wearing dark socks, no shoes. She usually always has at least one little spot on her face that looks flaky. She had very few top eye lashes and no eye lashes on the bottom at all. Her eye brows were very sparse. While ears seem to get larger with age the inner part of Mother's ears looked smaller. The inner edges of skin around the ear opening actually looked heart shaped (I actually compared my own ears later in a mirror and I was right). Her hair was short, of course, and tucked behind her ears. I marveled once again at her long, tapered fingers. Her skin is so creamy looking. It used to be tan and weathered looking.

She seemed to be almost in a trance. I wondered what was going on in her mind. She finally roused a bit and said, "That was fun." I said, "Yes, we always had fun there," although I wasn't sure if that's what she meant. I think maybe a series of scenes were going through her mind, like a slideshow, and that's what was fun. I wished I could get her to tell me what she's seeing. She maneuvered her fingers between the pages and flipped to the next picture. I had explained this picture to her earlier but I did it again. "This is your garden." Pointing, I said, "This was your statue of St. Francis." The cement statue was quite large. I pointed out the different flowers in the garden. She looked at the picture for quite a while. I began looking at it again and then way off on the side, in the shade, I could see Mother. I was surprised because I hadn't seen her there before. I pointed and said, "Oh look, there's you sitting in the shade." She smiled and said yes. I wondered if she had already seen that. We sat there for a while, Mother still looking at the picture then I got up and looked in the drawer of her nightstand to see if I could find the other calendar.

Just then a nurse came in and said, "I have a root beer float for you and some pudding. Oh! A turtle!" Chelsey was sitting nice and neat right beside Mother. Mother looked up and smiled. The nurse handed Mother the small glass of root beer (medicine) and she started to drink it. "Oh, that's good." The nurse asked Mother what the turtle's name was and I told her. She then started talking real fast about wanting a turtle when she was a kid or something. That always happens; I always get turtle stories when someone sees Chelsey. The nurse was still holding her spoonful of pudding although it looked more like peanut butter. She held it out to Mother and she took a bite. Then she said, "Well, Sally, I didn't know you liked turtles." Mother looked up in surprise. She didn't remember that Chelsey was sitting next to her of course. I said, "Well, she's mostly a dog person." "Oh, you like dogs?" Very clearly Mother said, "Yes. I like dogs." Then the nurse asked Mother where she got the turtle; in a pet store? Mother just had a blank look on her face. You'd think that if Mother actually had a turtle the nurse would already know about it. I said, "It's a tortoise and she's mine. I got her in a pet shop…" "Here Sally. Finish your pudding and I'll let you get back to visiting." The nurse rushed back out of the room. I have to admit, Chelsey did look cute sitting there right next to Mother, like they were best of friends. I went back to looking in the drawer but couldn't find the other calendar, nor could I find her glasses. I asked Mother if she was done with that calendar and when she said she was I put it back on the wall.

I went and opened the closet and saw a large plastic bag containing all of the cards. I took it down but when I turned around I saw that Mother had discovered Chelsey. I couldn't tell what she was doing but it looked like she was pinching Chelsey's face. I hurried back over and said, "What are you doing, trying to figure out what she is?" She said yes, and she stopped. I sat back down wanting to make sure she wasn't going to do anything else. Mother sat quietly and closed her eyes. "Are you tired?" "Yes." "Would you like to lie down and take a nap?" "No." We sat quietly side by side, Mother with her eyes closed, swaying slightly. A couple of minutes later she put her left hand on the bed to steady herself. I said, "Would you like to lie down?" She just smiled and said no, eyes still closed. A few minutes later and her left arm shot out from under her, and she was barely able to keep from toppling over. I laughed and said, "Are you ready to lie down now and take a nap?" She smiled again and said yes. I put Chelsey back in her tote bag then helped Mother lie down; lifting her legs up on the bed, making sure her head was on the pillow. When she settled I leaned over and gave her a big hug and told her that I love her. She hugged me back then started to say something. I waited and she looked me straight in the eyes and very clearly and with determination said, "I love you." My heart fluttered. I smiled and said that I would be back soon. Promise. I think that I was probably floating on my way back outside but I also felt very sad that I was leaving her once again. It's so hard to leave her.

We had gassed up before going to the nursing home so we just headed south out of town. As we drove I filled Tom in on my visit, then we rode in silence. We didn't stop until we reached Owatonna and then we pulled into the huge Cabela sporting goods store. We were on the hunt for something to keep Chelsey warm at night while we're camping at the motorcycle races. Going all over the store we finally settled on some heat patches. They come from the same company that makes those small pocket heat packs. With the patch you just peel off the back and stick it on the outside of your clothing. It's supposed to stay warm for up to twelve hours. We'll try it. We'll stick one inside her bed somewhere where it won't touch her. We also had some fishing gear for the boys for Christmas and Tom found something he wanted. At the checkout I watched as the young man in front of me paid for his fishing rod. The woman clerk asked if he wanted to purchase a warranty and he said yes (it was cheap). Then she asked him if he had a Cabela card and he said no. He swiped his credit card and she asked if he wanted to round up his change for conservation (8 cents). He said sure and then he was on his way. Last time we were there the woman working in the restaurant gave us the paperwork for a Cabela card but it was actually a VISA, not a member's card.

My turn. The clerk started ringing up my stuff and asked if I had a Cabela card. "No." "Do you want one? You can get $15 off today's purchase and there's a 5% cash back." "No."

"Really? You can get $15 off today's purchase." "No." "Are you sure? You get 5% cash back." "No." She had everything rung up and it came to $25.11, which I pulled out of my purse. Then she turned to her computer, fingers poised, and said, "Can I have your phone number, starting with your area code." I said, "Why do you need that?" She got all flustered and said, "Well, they don't need it, they just want it, but they won't call you." I knew why they wanted it—for demographic reasons, but I don't give out any information that I don't have to, besides I thought that was illegal now. I said, "No." She said, "No?" "No." Then she said, "I don't suppose you have an email do you?" "No." "Would you like to round up your change for conservation? Your purchase is $25.11." "No." "No?" "No." Maybe I would have if she hadn't been giving me such a hard time about everything else. Handing her the money I said, "I'm giving you the change." She said, "Oh," and took my money. There was a young couple standing in line behind me and they were really watching all of this. I wondered if they thought I was being a bitch or if they knew they were going to get the same treatment. This took so long that Tom had walked over to the bathroom and was back in time to see the end of my ordeal. There was also a long line of people waiting behind the young couple. I know the woman probably gets a commission for each Cabela card she's able to procure but, first of all, they're not up front about it being a VISA. I'm not about to get another credit card, and I shouldn't be harassed about it. I doubt we'll go back there; there are plenty of other sporting good stores.

That put me in a foul mood and I was actually glad when we passed out of Minnesota. We stopped somewhere in Iowa, gassed up, and grabbed a sandwich and some cookies. Making sure we drove the speed limit we passed out of Iowa and into Missouri. Tom drove as far as Chillicothe then pulled into the EconoLodge. It was 9:45. Tom was too tired to even fight the price, plus the place was nearly full. After all the taxes it was almost exactly $70. Not a bad price really. The room is on the ground floor luckily and we quickly unloaded the truck. The room is nice, with two beds and new looking furniture. Tom left to get us some dinner and I put Chelsey in her bath and fixed her food. Tom came back with a big bag from Dairy Queen. Steak fingers with fries, Texas toast, and cream gravy, yum. That's what it said on the box anyway—steak fingers. However, the steak fingers turned out to be chicken strips! Oh well, they were still good. Tom said they were trying to close for the night so they probably just grabbed what they had left.

After Tom finished eating he climbed into bed and Chelsey cuddled right up to him. After a while I climbed in also to watch a little TV and Chelsey left Tom and came over and cuddled up to me. That was so sweet. I've been thinking about Mother of course. I feel bad about leaving her the way I did. I should have stayed with her until she fell asleep. The look on her face was so sad. I knew she didn't want me to leave, but I knew she couldn't stay awake any longer. Still, it was a good visit. I need to start stretching those visits out as long as I can. When she gets up and starts walking I can walk with her. And I'll try to keep some kind of conversation going that may keep her interest a little longer and maybe she'll stay awake a little longer. I already miss her, and I want another hug, and another 'I love you.'

May 24, 2011
Tom got up early this morning and went outside for his walk. He brought back coffee. We weren't in much of a hurry so we watched TV as we drank, and then started packing up. Tom went out and cleaned all the accumulated trash out of the truck then came back in. I was getting myself ready when there was a knock on the door and a Hispanic woman's voice said, "Housekeeping!" We were stunned and didn't say anything. She knocked again, louder, "House-keeping!" Tom didn't open the door but said, "Yes?" The woman said, "I'll come back later." Tom was mad and said, "That should be illegal." I said, "It's only 9:30 isn't it?" Needless to say we didn't rush our departure.

We were truckin' along Missouri and all of a sudden we were in Malta Bend. It caught me by surprise and I said, "Malta Bend!" Tom said, "So?" "We have to stop at the Waggin' Wheel for lunch." It was a little early for lunch but it's not usually open when we're driving through, and I love that place. We pulled in and found an empty table among a big group of men sitting at various tables. The lunch special was taco salad and we got to pick all of the items we wanted on it. I'm a picky eater so I didn't get anything fancy or spicy. Tom is just the opposite. It was really good and we pigged out then we were back on the road. We didn't stop again until we got to the Missouri/Arkansas border then we stopped at Wild Bill's and got gas and coffee. Then our usual stop at the Armory Ann's rest area outside of Russellville.

We got home about 6:00. We unloaded the truck but I'll unpack tomorrow. I'm tired, but I haven't been really sleepy; I missed my computer too much. Computer work is now done and just now I turned on the weather channel. I sure have been watching that a lot. Right now a tornado is crossing northern Arkansas, going through the small towns of Ozark and Denning. It'll take too long to get any details so I'm going to bed.

May 25, 2011

Oh my God! I turned on the weather channel and the line of storms that went through last night did some damage in northern Arkansas but it also hit Sedalia, Missouri hard. The video showed what looked like a roller skating rink with only the floor left standing. I can't believe how lucky we've been. All of these storms recently crossed our route to Minnesota. Our timing has been perfect. Sedalia is the only town hit that we actually drive through, and often spend the night. I have a huge desire to keep my butt at home.

May 29, 2011

We were up at Tommy and Trisha's today for her birthday. She prepared fix your own taco salads. It was really good and as everyone was eating the conversation turned to the recent tornados. Tom was working today, cleaning up some of the storm damage nearby, and just had the time to run over for the birthday celebration. All of a sudden everyone started talking about storm cellars and how everyone is planning on getting one. They began asking Tom about the different types, the prices, and what's involved in installing them. Tom answered their questions as best he could and said he would check into the different types and costs, etc. He explained that around here you really can't install the underground ones because the ground is too rocky and shifts easily. Then he said that the ones on top of the ground are better and explained how they are made of concrete and how they're installed then said, "That's the kind Janet and I are going to get because the water stands on top of the ground when it rains." I thought, "What? You never mentioned that to me." Then I thought, "Where are we going to get the money?"

In Minnesota nearly everyone has a basement and there's no trouble just running down there. One summer day Mother had yelled, "A tornado! Everyone get in the basement." I was down there in a flash, but no one else was. I ran back up and everyone was standing outside on the steps looking at the sky. I thought, well I have time. I ran to my bedroom and got my clarinet and a few other precious items and took them downstairs. I went back up, everyone was still outside looking up, I still have time, and so I started bringing my clothes downstairs. I made several trips and got all of my clothes down there. I went back up, everyone was still outside, looking up at the sky, and Mother said, "It's gone." Everyone came back in the house and I started bringing all of my stuff back upstairs, and no, no one would help me.

      June 3, 2011
I was reading a story in a magazine; I don't know if it was true or fiction but it doesn't matter. The man in the story was talking about how he had to put his mother in a nursing home because of dementia caused by a series of strokes. When he first brought her to the nursing home he brought photographs and knickknacks to make her feel more at home. Once she sank deeper into dementia and aphasia he added baby toys: a ring of plastic beads filled with water, a set of plastic keys—anything that she could press and move with her fingers, which remained active, "their constant dance both frenetic and graceful." Talking about visiting her he said sometimes tears would leak from her eyes as she

babbled, unable to express the feelings that rose up inside her.

That is so Mother! I felt that man's pain, that's for sure. Aphasia is the loss of the power to speak, through damage to the brain. So, there is a medical term for that. That was interesting about the baby toys. I didn't realize all the finger movement was connected with strokes. I need to try that, bring her some baby toys, and see what happens. But I wonder if it would be too distracting for her; would she just work the toy to the extent that she wouldn't do anything else? I don't know, but I'll bring her something on the next trip. Does that explain Mother's need to always have something in her hands, like the red plastic Christmas ball, or the little cups?

June 5, 2011
This weekend we were at the motorcycle race at Boston Mountain, near Pettigrew. As we were driving up there yesterday afternoon we went past a lot of the tornado damage in the forests on the mountains. In one spot all of the power lines next to the road were leaning over, supported here and there by tall poles. I guess with such widespread damage it will take awhile before everything is repaired. In other areas there were just numerous tress snapped off, even at a lot of the houses huge trees were down.

As we were driving somewhere between Ludwig and Ozone a large black animal started running across the road in front of us. I thought it was a dog but as we got closer I thought it looked strange for a dog. All of a sudden Tom yelled, "Bear!" He had already slowed way down and as we got to it the bear (which was huge!) was scrambling up a hill on our side of the road. As we watched the bear got near the top but started losing his footing in the soft dirt. He looked back at us and finally got some traction and disappeared over the top of the hill into the woods.

The thought of my camera flashed through my mind and I thought, "It's somewhere in the back seat." The back seat was loaded full of our camping equipment along with Kelley and Zakary's racing gear. As we continued on our way I said something about the camera and Tom said he had put it right where I could get it but I didn't because I was in shock. I said, "I wasn't in shock. I was in awe, and I just wanted to watch the bear." But I did place my camera where I could reach it easier—just in case. I said, "So, there really are bears in Arkansas." I was joking of course, they're all over. This was just the first time we'd seen one in the wild.

Mother really loved bears. One time she told me that she was driving down her road, going home, and she saw a bear nearby in the woods. She stopped her truck right on the road and grabbed her camera and started taking pictures. Then she got out of her truck to take more pictures. I was a little concerned about her safety if she would actually approach one (but they're so cute!), and yes, I'd probably be that stupid also. I remember seeing those pictures of the bear. I wonder if I can find them and show them to her. That would be fun.

June 12, 2011
Scott, Ruth, and the boys were here this weekend. They spent the night then early this morning Scott and Ruth headed out for a canoe trip down the Caddo River with friends. I love watching Ruth and Trevor together. Trevor is 14 now and they have such a close relationship. It's not unusual to see them cuddled up together on the couch. My generation didn't even want to be seen with our parents. I wish I'd had a better relationship with Mother; but I was a bad teenager, I gave her a lot of grief. Tommy is really close with his kids also. And those boys take their kids almost everywhere with them, even to rock concerts! Not the youngest ones (yet) but the other three attend concerts with their dads. I can't imagine attending a concert with my parents at that age. It's so funny to think about.

Tommy and Scott grew up with Rock music. I remember my first concert. It wasn't really a concert, more like a mini-concert, up at the high school. Emily and I were in junior high and we rode up with Nancy and one of her friends. The band was fresh out of Canada still trying to hit it big. They were awesome and I fell in love with Rock. I was already a Beatles fan but experiencing it in person was a totally different thing than watching it on TV.

At the end the band said they were going over to the community college and playing at their dance. They urged all of us to join them. Oh, I wanted to go so bad. Nancy wasn't going, of course, so I hunted down a pay phone and called Mother and asked if I could go. She said, "Do you have a ride?" I said yes. I didn't, but I figured I could get someone to take me over there. She said, "Do you have a ride home?" I said, "I'm sure I can find one." And she said, "If you don't have a ride you can't go." And that was the end of that. I would have walked home if I'd had to if she would have let me go. And I never got to go to another concert all through school. Bummer.

June 17, 2011

I was digging through the storage building today and found a picture of Mother that I had forgotten about. It was actually a professional portrait. I wonder who talked her into that; her church maybe. Didn't churches used to have all of their members photographed for a directory? Anyway, it's a good picture although there are some small holes where I guess insects got busy. It's still in the original paper holder instead of in a frame. I brought it in, cleaned it up, and put it on a shelf in the living room. She was wearing a long sleeve white blouse with pleats down the front, and a red ribbon tied in a bow under the collar. Her hair, showing some gray, was just below her ears, and looked like she had a fresh perm. She had a beautiful smile on her face. In the lower right corner of the photograph is the date 1992, which would put her at 66 years old. I'm trying to remember what was going on that year.

June 21, 2011

I got an email from Kippy last night. She said the house she used to live in just burned down in one of the big Texas wildfires. There are actually 29 wildfires burning in Texas right now; 173,000 acres have burned so far. She said that was one of the reasons they had left that area (the fire threat). The house had been really nice and sitting right in front of a large forested area. I remember her excited phone call when they had moved, "I own a forest!" They now live in Corpus Christi in a fancy apartment building, half a block from the beach. They don't have to worry about forest fires; just hurricanes (think iron sliding doors on their balcony).

When I was in junior high the house across the street from us burned down. The structure itself didn't burn down but the inside was totally burned out. We were in school at the time and when we got off the bus we didn't even notice it. But Mother was waiting for us and she told us about it. We didn't know the family very well but the lady was very nice and she graciously let us go inside and see the damage. It was so bad; just charred walls in the living room. And I'll never forget that smell. They had two or three kids. The youngest, Gary, was a year older than David. He was a bad kid, always getting in trouble. The family had to move into a rental home while their house was being rebuilt but they couldn't find one in our school district so they asked Mother and Daddy if Gary could stay with us until the end of the school year. My parents agreed. I was kind of surprised that Mother would agree to that and I was also a little scared; I didn't know what to expect. Gary moved into the basement with David. He had a tall metal barrel that held his rescued possessions. Everything smelled like smoke. It was a little strange at first. He was pretty much a stranger, with a reputation for getting into trouble, and he had just experienced a tragedy. Our dinners were definitely quiet the first few days. But Gary turned out to be quiet and very polite to my parents. By the time he left we were all kind of friends.

Last night they were predicting some extremely bad weather for today so this morning I turned on the weather channel. We were in the clear but some bad stuff was hitting Minneapolis and St. Paul. Our neighbor had a storm cellar installed yesterday. So, of course, tornados are on the top of our minds, especially what we should do if we're in danger. At least Mother is oblivious about any storms raging outside her walls.

July 5, 2011

I was reading through some old emails today and came across some from Emily. These particular emails started right after Mother fell and broke her hip. It was interesting to revisit these conversations, well Emily's anyway; I didn't save any of my emails to her.

> February 23, 2000: Hi Janet, very interesting reading about malnutrition. The symptoms seen to coincide, don't they? Make sure someone follows up on pursuing that. I was glad to hear that David was there and Jason, too. And I was very pleased that they had her up moving around already.

Mother had been diagnosed with malnutrition at the hospital. When my brother found her that day there was a potpie in the oven but the oven hadn't been turned on; it looked like she had been subsisting on bananas and candy bars.

> February 24, 2000: Hi Janet, I just talked to Mom, actually the nurse first. The nurse said she was going to move to a nursing home this afternoon. She said she has become more scattered while she's been there. When they ask her to stand up, she sits down. When they say sit down, she stands up. Nancy and David were there this morning but had already left (maybe went to the nursing home I'm guessing). Mom sounded very confused and didn't really know what was going on. She reminded me of Mark's dad when he got older. He moved into a nursing home after his last visit here. When we would talk to him, he really didn't quite know who he was talking to. It would seem like he knew, but as soon as we hung up, he would not know. He wouldn't retain it at all.

> February 25, 2000: Hi. Got your email. I guess you'll let me know what nursing home Mom goes to and hopefully more info from a doctor. I hope Mom doesn't have to stay in the nursing home too long. People just do so much better when they're in their

own homes. I talked to Mark about me going to visit when our house sells and of course there's no problem with that. It would be really nice if you and I could be with Mom at the house at the same time. And even nicer if Nancy and David could be there also. I'm assuming that you told Nancy about keeping me informed about everything. Thanks for that.

February 26, 2000: Hi Janet. Thanks for the update. Well, our Mom sure keeps everyone hopping doesn't she? You know, I guess I thought we'd have years to go before we would have to deal with these kinds of decisions and concerns. But, oh well. Life certainly slipped by. If you get an address for Whispering Pines (sounds like a soap opera place) please send it along to me. I'm glad the doctors didn't think it was Alzheimer's, either, and I'm sure that malnutrition was a factor in her condition. Maybe I'll call Nancy this weekend some time, just to touch base with her and maybe give her some moral support. I know what you mean about feeling helpless in not being able to do anything. But you're right that we can't feel guilty. We physically can't do anything about it. And David sure takes good care of her.

Mother stayed in the nursing home until her insurance ran out and that's when she came down here. It was actually the Pine River Nursing Home.

March 7, 2000: Hi Janet, thanks for the info. I'm soooo glad that Mom is doing better. I would hate it if she couldn't have gone home. I was wondering who has been taking care of her dog. Is someone staying at her house? And is Jason still going to live with her? That would be an answer. She could live at home and we would be sure she was alright.

We were still hoping at this point that Mother would be able to go home.

March 14, 2000: Hello! I'm glad Mom is doing better and getting around. I guess I'll call her and try to talk to her.

That was all of the email messages at that time. Emily and her family were in the process of moving from Oregon to California. When she first started writing she was very excited about having an email address for the first time. Plus, she had just become a new grandma, also for the first time. Then she got busy, very busy.

The emails brought back a lot of memories and that big question: "What were you doing when your Mother fell?" I actually had the flu. I remember Nancy calling and telling me what happened. My heart sank. I wanted to jump on a plane. One day near the beginning of my illness Ruth came over after picking little Trevor up from daycare. She started washing my dishes and cleaning the house. It was snowing. Trevor climbed up on my bed and watched out the window at the dazzling snow falling. He was so excited. It was his first time seeing snow. The next day the weather was beautiful. Tom set my lounge chair up in the backyard, snow still on the ground, and made me and the iguanas go out. He said we all needed fresh air and sun. I put my robe on over my pajamas and out we went. I was running a fever and that crisp, cool air felt really good. The iguanas, of course, soaked up the sun.

My flu went on and one. It lasted about a month. Eventually I ended up in the emergency room diagnosed with the flu and dehydration. Dehydration is a strange experience. I felt like my body was cooking from the inside out. They had to pump a bag or two of glucose into my veins. Which was not pleasant. They had sent a nursing student in to hook up the IV and because of the dehydration she couldn't find a vein in my arm. She had to call for help. The next nurse couldn't find a vein either and she had to call for help. Finally, the master vein finder arrived and saved the day. So, did the stress of Mother's condition exacerbate my condition? Probably. I was so worried about her and felt totally helpless. It was actually June of that year before I could go and see her although I was able to talk to her on the phone occasionally.

July 8, 2011

Dear Mother, the wildlife activity around here has really picked up. The indigo buntings started arriving a few weeks ago. Last week Tom saw a fawn walk out of the woods behind my office, cross the yard, then calmly walk down the driveway. It was about 6:00 pm. A couple of days ago a rabbit stepped out of the tall grass with her young one. They stood there until mama was sure we'd both seen them then they turned and disappeared back into the tall grass.

We've been seeing occasional hummingbirds but nothing like we're used to. In the last couple of days one finally came in and staked out his territory, running off all of the other hummingbirds wanting a drink. As I was watching the hummingbirds a large redheaded woodpecker landed on the tree next to them. I had just registered what it was when another one swooped in. The first one came off the tree and chased it off. That was such a thrill! We hardly ever see woodpeckers. A few minutes later a scrub jay landed on the same tree. We only see one of these each year. As I sat there I watched other birds staking out their territories. It's like spring is finally here; only three months late. Tom and I believe it's due to the tornado outbreak that swept through this part of the country the end of April. Maybe all of the birds were blown off course. I wish you were here, Mother, to experience all of this with me. I know you'd be as excited as I am. I love you Mother.

July 9, 2011

I just finished reading the novel *Turn of Mind*, by Alice LaPlante. It's just hitting the market. I had no idea what the book was about when I started it. I received it in the mail so I could write a review about it. I didn't read the book jacket or the back cover; I just started reading it. I was really surprised that the main character and narrator is a woman with Alzheimer's. There is also a murder mystery weaving throughout the story. The book is really good. Some of the things really touched me.

The woman was a doctor, a hand surgeon, so there is a lot of technical stuff she remembers. In the first part of the book the woman is living at home with a caretaker. In the second part her family moves her to assisted living. There are several things that really resonated with me and helped to clarify some of the things Mother is going through:

> She talks about the prosopagnosia, her inability
> to distinguish one face from another, was
> getting worse. She could not hold on to features,
> so when a person was in front of her, she
> studied them; trying to do what every
> six-month-old child is capable of doing: separate
> the known from the unknown.

> The only thing that helps is walking.
> What the people there call wandering.

> She was finishing up her lunch when someone
> pulled up a chair and sat down. It was a face she
> recognized, but she was in a stubborn frame
> of mind and would not ask.

> Her visitor says, "People think it's just
> forgetting your keys. Or the words for
> things. But there are personality changes. The
> mood swings. The hostility and even violence.
> Even from the gentlest person in the world. You
> lose the person you love. And you are left
> with the shell."

> Someone asks, do you know where you are? She
> does, but it is in pictures. No words. She doesn't
> see her present situation, but something from
> the past.

> She needs to walk. If she can't walk she will
> scream.

> Her mind was full of fantastic images, some in

lurid color, some in black-and-white. It was like watching a compilation of movie clips filmed by a lunatic.

The visions came and went. She would prefer them to come and stay, to linger. She enjoyed those visitations. The world would be a barren place without them.

The woman was dreaming. Not really present.

"Each day slower then the one before it. Each day more words disappear. The visions alone endure."

July 13, 2011

I was working in the storage building again and came across a small wooden plate Mother had painted for me. She had used the rosemaling technique on it. The background is a red brick color. There are blue flowers with gold stems. It's really pretty. On the back are her initials and the year 1981. She still had Ken's last name then. I wonder what was going on for her that year. I know she used to take a lot of different artistic classes.

July 18, 2011

There was an article in the newspaper today entitled, "Falls, eye test may give clues to Alzheimer's." The article, written by Marilynn Marchione for *The Associated Press*, states that scientists in Australia are reporting encouraging early results from a simple eye test they hope will give a noninvasive way to detect signs of Alzheimer's. Although it has been tried on just a small number of people and more research is needed, the experimental test has a solid basis: Alzheimer's is known to cause changes in the eyes, not just the brain. Other scientists in the US also are working on an eye test for detecting the disease.

A separate study found that falls might be an early warning sign of Alzheimer's. People who seemed to have healthy minds but who were discovered to have hidden plaques clogging their brains were five times more likely to fall during the study than those without these brain deposits, which are a hallmark of Alzheimer's.

Brain scans can find evidence of Alzheimer's a decade or more before it causes memory and thinking problems, but they're too expensive and impractical for routine use. A simple eye test and warning signs like falls could be a big help.

The eye study involved photographing blood vessels in the retina, the nerve layer lining the back of the eyes. Most eye doctors have the cameras used for this, but it takes a special computer program to measure blood vessels for the experimental test doctors are using in the Alzheimer's research. Researchers compared retinal photos of 110 healthy people, 13 people with Alzheimer's and 13 others with mild cognitive impairment, or "pre-Alzheimer's," who were taking part in a larger study on aging. The widths of certain blood vessels in those with Alzheimer's were different from vessels in the others and the amount of difference matched the amount of plaque seen on brain scans. Earlier work has shown that amyloid, the protein that makes up Alzheimer's brain plaque, can be measured in the lens of the eyes of some people with the disease, particularly Down's syndrome patients who are often prone to Alzheimer's. Eye doctors often are the first to see patients with signs of Alzheimer's, which can start with vision changes, not just the memory problems the disease is most known for. Other signs could be balance and gait problems, which may show up before mental changes do.

There was a study tying falls to a risk of developing Alzheimer's disease before mental changes show up. The study involved 125 people, average age 74, who had normal cognition and were taking part in a federally funded study of aging. They kept journals on how often they fell and had brain scans and spinal taps to look for various substances that can signal Alzheimer's disease. In six months, 48 fell at least once. The risk of falling was nearly three times greater for each unit of increase in the sticky plaque that scans revealed in their brains. The researchers say that falls are tricky because they can be medication-related or due to dizziness from high blood pressure, a blood vessel problem or other diseases like Parkinson's. Falls also can cause head injury or brain trauma that leads to cognitive problems. Older people who hit their heads and suffer a small tear or bleeding in the brain might seem fine but develop symptoms a month later. The bottom line is that if you see somebody who's having falls for no particular reason the person should be evaluated for dementia.

August 7, 2011

Man, it's hot around here. A few days ago it was an amazing 114 degrees. It doesn't even cool off at night. I told Tom today that I'm ready to go to Minnesota. Things are going good with the business. So, as soon as he can fit in four days off we'll go. I hope it's soon; I really want to see Mother. While shopping the other day I bought one of those infant water filled rings. I want to see what Mother will do with it.

August 8, 2011

Tom said he went to sleep last night watching the movie "Harold & Kumar go to White Castle." He said it made him want to eat some of those hamburgers. I said yuck. I ate at White Castle one time and thought it was so bad that I never went back. It was like eating mushy, unidentified meat. Mother and David loved that place. They would sometimes treat themselves and find one of the restaurants and pig out on those awful burgers. I wonder if she'd still like them. Probably, she seems to like everything these days. Maybe I'll take her one—and tell her it's a secret, that she has to sneak it.

August 9, 2011

Daddy would have been 85 today. During WWII he served in the Navy. He left right after graduating from high school, not even 18 years old yet. That was in June of 1944. After two years, in June of 1946, Daddy entered the Coast Guard, serving on the WWII ship the Barque Eagle. In the fall of 1947 Daddy was going to reup for another term but Mother said if he did she wouldn't be there, that she was "tired of waiting." He resigned and they were married that December.

They moved into a small cottage in his parent's backyard. The first item they bought was a television. Their friends would come over and they'd all have to sit on the floor to watch it. Nancy was born while they lived in the cottage. I think Grandma Ruth may have been a difficult mother-in-law to have. If Mother was at their house visiting and it was time to nurse the baby Grandma would try to convince her to just nurse right there in front of everyone. Mother always declined (politely I'm sure).

I remember the small cottage. While visiting Grandma and Grandpa I would sometimes go inside. It always stood empty and had a large screened-in porch. The main house was nice but had a tiny postage stamp size yard. There was hardly any space between the row of houses and everyone was enclosed behind fences. Grandma always hung her laundry out to dry and had a wire clothesline that ran the length of the backyard. Sometimes we brought our dog along and we'd hook the leash onto the wire and she'd run back and forth through the yard. There was a large wooden staircase leading down from the back door. Grandma would sit near the bottom and feed peanuts to a squirrel she had trained to take them right out of her fingers. At that time Grandma always wore housedresses.

Mother and Daddy bought our house in the suburbs when she was pregnant with me. I don't think she was as thrilled with my pregnancy as she was with the first two. I guess the funness was gone by then, plus she was having to go to work to help support the growing family. When she felt she had put in her nine months she went to her doctor and asked him to do something to speed up the process, to make that baby come out. He said no and sent her home. When the time finally came it was already night and everyone was in bed. Mrs. Knutson, from next door, was really watching Mother, waiting for the dash to the hospital. But Mother didn't want Mrs. Knutson to know what was happening, she knew she'd get on the phone and tell all of the neighbors. Mother wanted to make the announcement herself. So, she wouldn't let Daddy turn on any of the lights. In the darkness they hustled Nancy and David out of their beds and into the car. Daddy dropped Mother at the entrance to the hospital where she was placed in a wheelchair and whisked away. He then drove all the way to his parents' house in Minneapolis, dropped off Nancy and David then made a mad dash back to the hospital to welcome me into the world. I was born at 11:36 pm. Mother shouldn't have been surprised at what she got: a clingy little girl who didn't want to leave her side. And as it turned out, a night owl; someone who hates early mornings and prefers the dark of night, when the only sounds are nature.

August 13, 2011

Some believe that we decide our life path before we're born. We decide what life lessons we want to learn; what karma needs to be worked out. If this is so I have to wonder why Mother chose this particular journey. Why would she choose to spend her last years in a fog, unaware? But maybe it wasn't for herself that she chose this path, but for us, her family. Some also believe that we choose our families before we are born; that we enter the world as a group. So maybe we, the family, have life lessons to learn from this, karma to work out.

Not just Mother, but anyone in her position, anyone who is unable to care for themselves. How do we treat her (them)? With love, or indifference? Do we want to help her and be a comfort to her? Do we want her to feel our love and compassion? Do we visit her because we really want to be with her, or because it will look good to others? Do we visit at all, or just ignore her? Do we feel her pain? Do we try to make her feel good, or don't we care about that? Do we CARE? Do we <u>really</u> care about her, or is that just too much work?

Mother used to visit her friends in the Pine River nursing home and those who had moved into assisted living apartments, on their way to the nursing home. She had no ulterior motives; she just wanted to spend time with her friends. She never felt sorry for them. When she'd talk about them to me she'd just say something like, "so and so moved into…" When she ended up in the same nursing home she didn't seem to mind. She knew all of the staff and she knew all of the residents. They were already her friends.

But, it's not just the family that's being tested (are we being tested?); it's also the caregivers. Does the caregiver really care for her patients, or is it just a job? How do you treat your patients, and I mean really treat them? Do you treat them with love or indifference? Do you really try to help them, or just get the job done? Do you give comfort, or just do what has to be done? When you bathe your patients, do you do it with tender care or do you see it as just a nasty job that has to be done? Do you visit with your patients even if nothing needs to be done, just because? Do you try to make your patients feel good or do you ignore them if nothing is needed? Do you feel their pain? Do you CARE? Do you really care about them, or is that too much work?

So, how are we doing? How are we doing as a family? How are we doing as a society? How are we doing as a nation? How are we doing as a world? I don't believe that when we die God judges us. I believe that when we leave this world we judge ourselves.

August 17, 2011

Mother died last night. To say I was stunned would be an understatement. David called at 10:30 and told me. He said he had gotten a call from the nursing home in the afternoon saying she wasn't feeling well and was having trouble breathing. They had started her on antibiotics and sent her for chest X-rays (somewhere in the nursing home). The nurse told David that it would take quite awhile to get the results, that it could be 9:30 or 10:00, and that they would call him the next day. David said no; call me as soon as you get the results. He got the call around 8:15 and the nurse said Mother had pneumonia, that her lungs were full of fluid, that it wasn't good. She asked David if he was coming, he said yes he was coming, and she said, "I hope she'll still be here." She wasn't. She went that fast. The nurse said Mother had been walking around earlier, acting her normal self. Mother of course would never complain about anything. Even at the end the nurse was sitting there talking to Mother, then she had to leave the room for a moment and when she got back Mother was gone. That fast. It's a blessing really, that she went that quickly.

After watching Mother struggle for over 10 years, in the end she chose to not subject her family to the pain of watching her die (was her mind clear at the end?); instead slipping away while completely alone. I would have liked to have been with her when she passed; I would have liked to have been holding her in my arms. But it was her decision. Surely she was told that her son was on his way. Now my last memory of her won't be of her dying, but the last time I saw her alive. Her last words to me were "I love you," and that's the memory I'll carry with me. I love you Mother.

August 19, 2011

We're now on our last trip to see Mother. The final farewell. We left the house just after 4:30 and went and picked up Tommy. We're on our way to pick up Scott. Tommy was able to get three days off work so we'll leave back out Tuesday afternoon. Scott could only get one day off so he will be flying home Monday night. Emily and Annie are flying in tomorrow evening and out Tuesday evening. We'll pick them up at the airport on our way in and we'll drop them at the airport on our way out of town. I'm traveling with two of Mother's pallbearers. The other pallbearers will be Jamie, Jason, Rebecca, and Annie. I have been surprisingly calm, but I know that will change the closer we get. I'm already feeling the need to find some ginger ale.

Other than Tom I haven't told even one person that Mother has died. I had Tom call the boys and it went from there. I can't say it. I just can't say it. I'm afraid I'll break if I do.

August 20, 2011

We stopped finally last night in Marshall, Missouri. It was already 2:00 by then. We had wanted to stop in Sedalia but the state fair was going on and all of the motels were full, except for the Best Western. They had one room because the guy with a reservation didn't show up. But the room was $150 and Tom said no. That's about twice what it should have been. So we had gone on. Scott did most of the driving last night then Tom drove for a while. Tommy dozed a lot then was well rested for the last stretch. It was amazing how, except for Tommy's dozing, everyone stayed awake and the conversation rarely ended.

We were back on the road by 9:30. We stopped for gas and next to the station an Amish woman had a table set up and was selling baked goods. Her black carriage was standing behind her and the horse tied up to a nearby tree. The woman had a boy with her about 10 – 12 years old. Tom sent me over to get some bread. The woman had a lot of items to choose from. I bought a loaf of honey oatmeal bread, a bag of chocolate chip cookies, a bag of coconut oatmeal cookies, and a small jar of cherry jam. Life goes on. I guess.

After picking up Emily and Annie we stopped at the motel and checked in and unloaded our luggage, and then drove to David's and dropped off the girls' suitcases. We talked for a minute but it was already 9:00 and we were all starving. The six of us went down to Perkins and ate then we dropped the girls back at David's. Now we're back at the LaQuinta; the boys have their own room here. My head is swimming; I'm dead tired, but not really sleepy. I feel in a state of shock, almost numb. Tomorrow afternoon is the visitation and the funeral is Monday morning.

I wasn't ready for this. I need more time! There were things I wanted to tell her, stories to share. Gifts I wanted to give her. Places I wanted to take her. I wanted to walk with her and sit with her. I wanted to watch her and watch with her. I have cards I wanted to mail her. I wanted and needed to tell her again and again, that I love her. I needed to know that she understood that. And I wanted and needed her to tell me that she loves me, although I did understand, every time she told me. Did she get the same warm feeling in her heart? And there were so many more hugs I wanted to give her.

And I wanted more hugs from her. I'm really going to miss those hugs.

August 24, 2011

We're back home; got in tonight about 6:30. My head is still swimming, but the shock is wearing off, I'm quick to tears. Everything went well. I guess. Seeing Mother lying in her coffin was like a knife going through my heart. I burst into tears when I saw her. It's even hard writing about it. Judy and her family were the first to arrive at the visitation, and then Mike. A couple of Emily's friends were there. David's neighbors all came together. He's so lucky to have such a great support group. There were a few women from the old neighborhood. Shirley, who had seen the obituary and had started making phone calls. She's always been so nice. And Beverly was there with her husband, Bernie. I hadn't seen her since I was a teenager. She really had been Mother's best friend. Our two families had spent a lot of time together, including camping trips in Crosslake. Beverly brought us some old black-and-white photos of Mother on one of those camping trips smiling and wearing a bathing suit. She really looked good. Beverly moved out of the neighborhood before we did but she and Mother had always kept in touch with each other, until Mother no longer could I guess. It was nice seeing her.

David had gone to the nursing home to pick up Mother's things and the large plastic bag holding all of the cards and her jewelry was missing. I had wanted those cards. Waiting for me at David's house was the card I had mailed to Mother the day before she died. The nursing home had forwarded it to him. I was so afraid I'd receive it here stamped 'Deceased.' The day we left David handed me another card I had mailed. It was dated a week earlier than the last one. They had never given it to her.

Besides immediate family, only Mike and a couple of David's neighbors attended the funeral, although the entire neighborhood group was at the reception afterwards, which was at the American Legion Hall in Osseo. Mike rode with us to the cemetery and along the way he talked about when he first moved in with us when he had left the Air Force and how Ken had given him a job at the service station. We had fun with Mike in the house. He even did beer runs for me until Mother caught on and made him stop. Mother's resting now next to his dad.

Right before the funeral was to begin I went and talked to Mother, my final good-bye. As I stroked her hand I told her how much I loved her and that I'll really miss her. I talked about our last visit together. At the end I said, "Don't forget me Mother, and you'd better be there waiting for me when I pass over!" I wondered who had been there waiting when she passed. A couple of nights before she died I had done a meditation to help me go to sleep. In the meditation I was swimming in the ocean. I was by myself, just swimming and diving in the water. I was surprised and very happy when Mother suddenly joined me. We began swimming together, then I said, let's go down. We began swimming towards the bottom. Down, Down, Down. As we neared the bottom I saw that Mother was having some trouble. She seemed to be in distress a bit and looked a little frightened. I said, "Mother, in meditation you can breathe under water." I sat down on the bottom and Mother relaxed, joining me. Then two dolphins swam up to us. We got excited and began petting their snouts and stroking their sides. I said let's ride them. I helped Mother climb on one of the dolphin's back, having her lay forward and wrapping her arms around the head, and then I got on the other one. The dolphins took off swimming through the deep water giving us quite a ride. Then the dolphins surfaced and swam towards the shore. Mother and I dismounted and walked to a sandy beach. Mother sat down at the edge with her legs in the water, the waves washing over them. Just then Aunt Laurie stepped out from behind a huge rock next to Mother. It was so nice to see her and we were all smiling at each other. I was ready to continue on but Mother looked like she didn't want to leave. I said to Aunt Laurie, "Will you stay with her?" And she said, "Yes, I'll stay with her." That was it and I went to sleep. I know that Aunt Laurie was still with Mother when she passed and that brings me comfort.

Final Thoughts

I am totally amazed at the lack of compassion from people when an elderly person dies. It's like when someone becomes elderly they no longer matter—they're just nothing. And that's how they treat the death – like it's nothing. Even most of my own extended family has acted this way. There was no compassion, no reaching out, and not a word of sympathy; just complete silence. Complete silence makes you think no one cares about your feelings. Yes, Mother was elderly. Yes, she had dementia. Yes, she was in a nursing home. But! We still lost our Mother! And our pain is still just as strong as if she had been young and vibrant. To ignore her death, to not even mention it, is about as cold as you can get.

That's what our country has become. Cold. Uncaring. Uncompassionate. There was not even one caring word from the nursing home staff; the same people who took care of her every day. She lived there for four years; four long years. Was there not one person who felt a loss, or did they look at it as an empty bed soon to be filled by the next person (nonperson) on the waiting list. I really believe that a nursing home should at <u>least</u> send a sympathy card to the family so that they know that the loss life was valuable. Not just a phone call saying come and settle the bill. Don't any of the caregivers feel some kind of an emotional bond to the People they take care of?

How sad the people of this country has become that all life is not valued. I know that there are some compassionate caregivers out there. But from what I see the majority of nursing home employees are just that—paid employees, just doing their job to get that pay. How do we change it? I don't know. If family members aren't even compassionate (or even willing to visit) how can we expect total strangers to be compassionate? How can we get our family members to be more compassionate? We can start by more visits to family members in nursing homes. Let the grandkids get to know the elderly grandparent (or great-grandparent) even if they have dementia. Dementia doesn't change who they are.

Dementia doesn't change our love for that person. Entering a nursing home shouldn't be locking them out of the world. They still need to feel loved and want to return that love. If people would visualize themselves in that position maybe things would change. If visits aren't possible write letters, send cards, make your own cards. Have your children and grandchildren write letters, make cards, draw pictures – anything that the person can hold in their hands so that they know someone is thinking of them, that they are still loved and valued.

About Dementia

Dementia is a syndrome caused by cell death. Dementia mostly affects older people although it is not a normal part of aging. Dementia causes loss of cognitive abilities such as memory, attention, language, logical reasoning, and problem-solving. Light cognitive impairments, such as poorer short-term memory, can happen as a normal part of aging as we slowly start to lose brain cells as we age beyond our 20s. This is known as age-related cognitive decline, not dementia, because it does not cause the person or the people around them any problems.

All dementias are caused by brain cell death, and neurodegenerative disease (progressive brain cell death that happens over a course of time) is behind most dementias. There are different forms of dementia. One form, Alzheimer's dementia, is caused by "plaques" between the dying cells in the brain and "tangles" within the cells. Both are protein abnormalities: a build-up of "beta-amyloid" in plaques and the disintegration of "tau" protein in tangles. Vascular dementia is a second type, and it can be caused from brain cell death caused by conditions such as cerebrovascular disease, such as a stroke. This prevents normal blood flow, depriving brain cells of oxygen. Vascular dementia can also likely be affected by blood pressure; it's associated with multiple small strokes and other problems with the blood vessels. Mixed dementia refers to a diagnosis of two or three types occurring together. A person may show both Alzheimer's disease and vascular dementia at the same time.

Dementia can also be caused by certain diseases such as Parkinson's Disease, thyroid disease, drug toxicity, and others as well as brain injury, strokes, and multiple sclerosis. A brain tumor is another cause. Post-traumatic dementia is directly related to brain cell death caused by injury. Studies show that an overload of toxic heavy metals in the body such as mercury, lead, cadmium, and arsenic, can cause dementia. Aluminum exposure has long been suspected of being a cause (naturalnews.com).

Dementia is not temporary confusion or forgetfulness that could result from a limited infection, an underlying illness, or side effects from medications. Dementia typically worsens over time. There are over 5 million people in the Unites States with some form of dementia. It is reported that as many as 1% of adults over the age of 60 have dementia. It has been estimated that the frequency of dementia doubles every five years after the age of 60. Research shows that some methods, such as lifestyle changes, can be a benefit for those with dementia by lessening some cognitive problems. There is currently no cure for dementia although there are medications that can slow progression of cognitive changes; however, they cannot prevent the eventual worsening of the condition. Today's medications only temporarily ease some dementia symptoms.

Dementia doesn't kill people but it is often an underlying cause of death. Severe dementia can make it difficult for people to move around or swallow properly. That increases the risk of pneumonia. Pneumonia is one of the most common identified causes of death among dementia patients. Dementia patients may forget to take critical medications for other health conditions. They may not be able to explain that they are feeling symptoms of other ailments such as infections. There may be more falls, resulting in serious injuries.

Recent research has shown that memory loss may not always be the first warning sign of dementia. Changes in behavior may be an early clue. Researchers at the University of Calgary have outlined a syndrome they call "mild behavioral impairment" that may be a sign of approaching dementia. They proposed a checklist of symptoms to alert doctors. Usually these symptoms may not be the only early detection. Dementia creeps up slowly ravaging the brain a decade or two before the first symptoms appear. Early memory problems called "mild cognitive impairment" can raise the risk of developing dementia later. Worsening memory is often what triggers the person, or the person's family, to seek medical help.

What's new, say the researchers, is the concept of pre-dementia "mild behavioral impairment" that may signal degeneration is starting in brain regions not as crucial for memory. The symptoms that qualify for the new checklist are new problems that linger at least six months, not temporary symptoms or ones explained by a clear mental health issue or other issues such as bereavement. The symptoms include apathy, anxiety about routine events, loss of impulse control, flaunting social norms, and loss of interest in food. If the checklist is validated it could help doctors better identify people at risk (Lauran Neergaard, *The Associated Press*).

There is now questions regarding the beta-amyloid plaque theory of causing Alzheimer's. According to recent research (Isabelle Z. from naturalnews.com, August 15, 2018) the long-standing theory of beta amyloid's crucial role is being called into question as more than 100 drugs that attack the protein have failed to treat and prevent Alzheimer's. Beta amyloid therapies can clear amyloid plaque, yet patients do not see any significant improvement in cognition. Patients also continue to progress further into the disease. It's possible that the beta amyloid protein was never really the problem in the first place; that the plaques are not the target – they are biomarkers. Amyloid protein could still be a factor in the disease, but some experts believe that a different one, such as tau, or even the apolipoprotein E (ApoE) gene could play a more important role; it could even turn out that a complex interplay is taking place between various abnormal proteins and other factors.

Research continues.

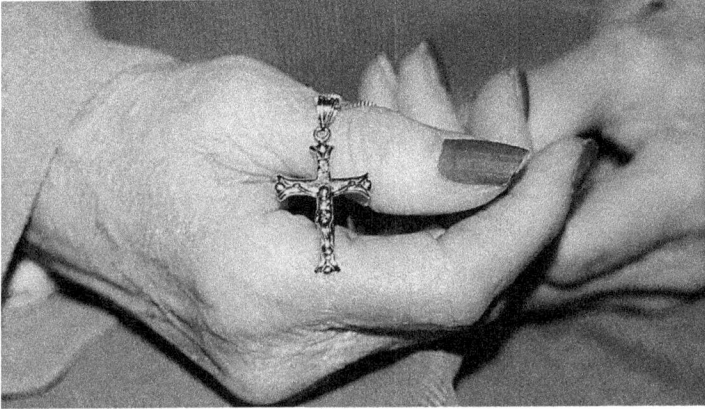

Janet S. Gould holds a Bachelor of Science Degree in Behavioral Science from Our Lady of Holy Cross College in New Orleans, Louisiana. She also holds an M. A. in Transpersonal Studies from Atlantic University in Virginia Beach, Virginia.

Other works include:

Catching the Dream: A Parent's Guide for Children's Dreams

Slumbertime: A Parent's Guide for Children's Sleep and Sleep Problems

www.ingramcontent.com/pod-product-compliance
Lightning Source LLC
Chambersburg PA
CBHW070901030426
42336CB00014BA/2284